A History of the Western General Hospital

To our spouses, Jenny and Peter.
To all those inmates, patients and staff, known and unknown who are the History of the Hospital.

A History of the Western General Hospital

Craigleith Poorhouse
Military Hospital
Modern Teaching Hospital

MARTIN EASTWOOD
ANNE JENKINSON

Foreword by John Connaghan

JOHN DONALD PUBLISHERS LTD
EDINBURGH

ISBN 0 85976 423 0 (Pbk)
ISBN 0 85976 430 3 (Hbk)

A catalogue record for this book is available from the British Library.

Typeset by WestKey Ltd., Falmouth, Cornwall
Printed and bound in Great Britain by J.W. Arrowsmith Ltd., Bristol

Foreword by John Connaghan, Chief Executive, Western General Hospitals NHS Trust

Writing the foreword to this book is both an honour and a pleasure and I am sure that turning its pages will also be a pleasure for many readers as they are carried on an enthralling journey through time.

In detailing the history of the Western General Hospital, this book also charts the eventful history of the community it serves and shows how the hospital has continually adapted to meet the changing needs of the community. Just as we may read this book and reflect on the Western General's past achievements with a sense of pride, so may we be proud of the hospital today. From its humble origins, the Western General has developed into a world-class centre of expertise, a major teaching hospital at the leading edge of developments in NHS care.

The best history books are the ones which bring the past to life and which show how the past has shaped our present, and I am delighted to say that this book falls comfortably into this category. Its chapters chart the many developments in medical care and administration witnessed by the Western and there are descriptions of exciting as well as traumatic times.

The latest adaptation in the evolution of the Western General Hospital came in April 1994 when the Western General and Royal Victoria Hospitals were established as the Western General Hospitals NHS Trust. I firmly believe that NHS Trust status is the right kind of management structure, as Hospitals should be managed locally with Clinicians playing a key role in the management decision-making process at the strategic as well as operational level. The new system of Clinical Directorates is now beginning to bear fruit with a real sense of commitment and innovation being experienced in the hospital.

Teamwork is essential to the provision of a quality service and one of the themes that emerges from this book is the evolution of teamwork within the Western General. Today, the Trust's multi-disciplinary approach to care encourages staff participation wherever possible in the continuing evolution of our services. Our team approach within the hospital is reinforced by our links with the community and the wider public. It is impossible to overstate the importance we attach to our links with the University of Edinburgh and the Medical Research Council. There are benefits to patients through our relations with Health Boards, GPs, Lothian Health Council, voluntary organisations and all other organisations that have an interest in seeing the best for the NHS and the public it serves.

The hospital has stood up well to the test of time and now it is ready to face a new century that will see it revitalised. We shall wish to build on the excellent work previously carried out under Lothian Health's Acute Services Strategy. Indeed at the time of writing our plans are well advanced to spend some £100 million over the course of the next 10 years in refurbishing the Western General and creating new ward, theatre and investigative facilities.

Of course, a hospital can only ever be as good as its staff and I am confident that the Western General has the calibre of staff to achieve our goal to end the millennium as a centre of excellence; to enter a new century and a new era of health care with the continuing recognition of being an organisation that sets the standards for others to match in terms of providing a caring, quality NHS service.

I offer my congratulations to Dr Martin Eastwood and Mrs Anne Jenkinson, and to everyone who played a role in the publication of this book. Not only is it fascinating to read, it is also a fitting testimony and tribute to the many thousands of people over the decades who have shaped the Western General's services and who are united through their shared commitment to improving people's health.

Edinburgh, 1995

Acknowledgements

We would like to acknowledge the unstinting help we have received from staff, both past and present. The people who have assisted are too numerous to mention by name, but we would particularly acknowledge the following for the many hours they have spent reading through the text and giving constructive advice:

Mr Clifford Burden, Communications Officer, Western General Hospital
Dr Nick Gordon, Consultant Anaesthetist, Western General Hospital
Dr Arthur Kitchen, retired Consultant Cardiologist, Western General Hospital
Dr Michael Matthews, retired Consultant Cardiologist, Western General Hospital
Mr Jack Newsam, retired Consultant Urologist, Western General Hospital
Dr John Scrimgeour, Medical Director, Western General Hospital
Professor Adam Smith, retired Consultant Surgeon, Western General Hospital

We have been given excellent cooperation from the following during research and in getting illustrations produced on time:

The City Archivist, Edinburgh City Chambers
The staff of the Edinburgh Room, George IV Bridge Public Library
The Medical Photographers, Western General Hospital
The Scottish National Dictionary Department, University of Edinburgh
An unknown member of the audience at a lecture who corrected a fallacious impression of the original site of the St Cuthberts Poorhouse.

Contributors

Dr Peter Abernethy
Dr J. L. Anderton
Dr Bryan Ashworth
Dr Jeanne Bell
Mr J. S. Boxall
Professor David J. H. Brock
Dr F. Buckley
Miss C. Cameron
Dr T. M. Chalmers
Mr U. Chetty
Dr F. R. Clark
Mr John Connaghan
Dr G. Crompton
Miss Isabel Duncan
Dr M. A. Eastwood
Professor John O Forfar
Dr Martin Fraser
Professor J. D. Gillingham
Dr Alex Gordon
Dr Nick Gordon
Dr Cameron Gould
Dr D. B. Horn
Mrs Christine Johnson
Dr Alex J. Keay
Dr Arthur H. Kitchin
Mr Ian Laing
Professor Allan Langlands
Dr John Law
Miss F. MacDonald
Dr Hugh MacDougal
Sister Catherine Macgregor
Mrs I. MacKenzie
Mr I. M. C. Macintyre
Dr M. Mackie
Miss Betty McLean
Dr John G. Macleod
Mr Tom McNair
Dr Michael B. Matthews
Dr M. V. Merrick
Professor J. Douglas Miller
Professor W. I. C. Morris
Mrs Isobel Nairn
Dr J. Newsam
Mr S. J. Nixon
Sister Christine Orr
Dr Paul L. Padfield
Dr W. H. Price
Professor Vaughan Ruckley
Rev Mr M. Schofield
Mr W. G. Scobie
Dr John Scrimgeour
Dr T. R. D. Shaw
Mr David Shirling
Mr W. Sircus
Dr Brian Slawson
Mr W. P. Small
Professor A. N. Smith
Dr R. G. Smith
Professor J. Smyth
Dr M. Steel
Professor John A. Strong
Dr W. Tomaszewski
Dr G. T. Vaughan
Professor Henry Walton
Professor Charles Warlow
Dr David J. Webb
Dr J. N. Webb
Mr Charles Wood
Professor Sir Michael Woodruff

Contents

Introduction

The history of the Western General Hospital is in many respects a history of the Public Health provision of medicinal care in Scotland and Great Britain. It is a different story to that of the great Voluntary Hospitals such as the Royal Infirmary. Both reflect the public conscience channelled through quite different pathways. The Voluntary Hospitals relied on individual generosity which was given in abundance. In contrast the Public Health Hospitals system depended very much upon the tax payer. This book describes the development of the Craigleith Poor Law Hospital which arose from the charity system in western Edinburgh. This system grew from concern for the people living in the slums in the Canongate, the Pleasance and the High Street. The Poor Law provision was for those who could no longer cope either physically or economically. It served the poor and particularly the poor wanting. For over forty years this massive building quietly got on with looking after the poor from 1868 until 1914. Everything about this Hospital was local, even the stone from which it was built — Craigleith stone from the quarry not half a mile away — emphasised its local roots. All of that changed quite abruptly with the events of the 1914–18 War. During this period as a Military Hospital, wounded soldiers were brought from France by train into Craiglockhart Station and brought to the Hospital. We have a better feel of life in the military hospital through a collection of magazines published at that time. After the War the Hospital to some extent continued as a Ministry of Pensions Hospital for the Army and also as a Poor Law Hospital. In the 1930's the Law changed again and the Hospital became a Municipal Hospital. Even the name changed from the Craigleith Poor House to the Western General Hospital, emphasising the new status of the Hospital as part of Municipal caring. New building began in the 1930's with the first development being the Nurses Home. However the Second World War came and such ambitious plans were shelved. The Hospital again became in part a Military Hospital, this time for Polish civilians who had been driven out of their own country and were cared for here in Scotland. Throughout all these periods there was care for the destitute young. A red brick satellite building for many years was for the care of the orphaned and neglected children. During the Second World War it was named Paderewski and became the focus of the Polish Medical School at the Western General Hospital. After the 1939–45 War an absolute change took place with the inception of the National Health Service. The Hospital owes a great deal to the innovation of Sir Stanley Davidson who felt that the Hospital would provide for a whole new approach to the care of the sick. Such care was by the introduction of Specialist Units. This was a controversial step in Edinburgh, no less controversial for introducing doctors who were not Edinburgh graduates, a concept which had had little support previously, despite Edinburgh being a very cosmopolitan city intellectually. There are a number of Hospitals and systems which have developed in this way, the Mayo Clinic in the United States and the Hammersmith Postgraduate Centre in London. The Western General Hospital has never aspired to such distinction but has been an extraordinary development in terms of specialties. Each specialty, oncology, haematology, renal disease, gastroenterology, urology, neurology and endocrinology have all been in the forefront of ideas. Interesting academic developments came along with these specialties, the largest of these was the MRC Cytogenetics Unit. This was started before the huge advances consequent upon the finding of the structure of DNA and the evolution of molecular biology. At the core of this Hospital has been a devoted group of general surgeons and general physicians who have provided a quality of care which has enabled the Specialist Units to function.

One of the gifts to the present time by the original developers of the Craigleith Poor Law Hospital was availability of land. This has enabled the Western General Hospital to have a freedom for building which has not been possibile for other Hospitals. Consequently, there has been the construction of the Oncology Building, Neurosciences, the Nurses Home, the Outpatient Building, the Alexander Donald Building, Laundry, Microbiology.

Now we come to the next stage of the development of this Hospital in its status as a Trust. Ambitious plans are in hand to completely redevelop the whole system. This comes at a time when other revolutions are sweeping through medicine — the development of laparoscopic surgery, endoscopic approach to gastroenterology and the development of molecular biology, new treatments for cancer and the care of patients with strokes and other neurological conditions. All of these are present on site in the Western General Hospital.

1

The Origins of Poor Law Hospitals in Edinburgh pre-1868

The Poor Laws in Scotland owed their origin not so much to a desire to help the poor as to the need for some means of repressing the growing menace of uncontrolled mendicancy. For years prior to 1390 Scotland had been a nation under arms, then came the truce with England, and the troops were disbanded. Some of the ex-soldiers attached themselves to the nobles and fought their private battles. Others went about the country in beggar bands taking where they were not given.

The Act of 1424, while directed chiefly against the strong and masterful beggar also gave consideration to the aged, the infirm and the impotent poor. This was the dawn of the Poor Law but beyond legalising begging it failed in its purpose. Subsequent statutes in 1425, 1449, 1455, 1477, 1503 and 1535 reiterated the need for punishing the masterful and fit beggar with the law providing for imprisonment, corporal punishment, torture and even death. In Edinburgh in the 15th century the market keepers were armed with iron staves 'to beat the pests away'.

In the 15th century the Trinity College Hospital and St Paul's Work were both founded in Edinburgh. It is interesting to note that while the number of residents in the hospital was never large, in times of prosperity a number of out pensioners were maintained. When the hospital was finally demolished this latter system of out pensioners was adopted. Many elderly people were helped through the fund.

The conditions of entry to St Paul's Work were very restrictive if adhered to. All the inhabitants 'must in their outward life and manner be not with blame or other portable vice, of good fame and conversation, no blasphemer, swearer, drunkard, carter [old Scots for card player], dysser [old Scots for gambling with dice] or thief, idle vagabond person nor sturdy beggar but must exercise themselves in some honest trade or shift'. They were to be admitted if they were sick, old or impotent. Early in the 17th century this institution became a Workhouse, the first of its kind in Scotland. It later became a House of Correction for idle vagabonds.

In 1579 Parliament passed a law stating basic principles. These included the preparation of a Poor Roll, power to assess and the power to return the poor to their own districts. The power to assess was not greatly used as in 1740 only eight out of 800 parishes had levied assessments while even in 1929 there were still four parishes which never levied a Poor Rate.

Between 1693 and 1699 it was estimated that out of a population of 1½ million in Scotland, 200,000 were begging from door to door.

An Orphan Hospital founded by a merchant in 1742, remained on the original site which was 'without the City wall on the northern side of Edinburgh near the western end of the Trinity Old College Church'[1], where Dingwall Castle stood, until the site was acquired by the railway company in 1854, presumably for the Waverley Station. This provided specialist treatment for orphan and poor children.

Efforts were made in the early 17th century to teach poor children spinning and weaving at the factory at St Paul's Work, and this continued until 1750. The Charity Workhouse was removed in 1743 to Greyfriars and was managed independent of the Town Council. The cost of keeping inmates in the Charity Workhouse, opened in 1743, was rather less than 2s (10p) per week each, but even this was considered wasteful by writers of the day. This was supported by church door collections and other funds for the poor. Charity plays and dances to help the funds were fashionable for a while and the institutions suffered when they ceased. Parochial boards were established in 1845 with responsibility for supporting the poor. They consisted of elected members and representatives of the Town Council and kirk sessions.

New Town Widens Poverty Gap

With the building of the New Town, the movement of the better-off citizens to live in this prestigious development was initially slow. By the turn of the century the trickle had become a flood and the social gulf between the two towns, the New Town and the Old Town rapidly widened. It was most marked between 1815 and 1830. The exodus of the wealthier led to the subdivision of the old tenements between the artisan and labouring classes. The subsequent congestion and overcrowding was greatly aggravated by the large influx of Irish labourers for the construction of the Union Canal, begun in 1818, and later for the railway construction. A great fire in 1824 may have reduced congestion in the High Street but made things worse elsewhere. Dwellings which had been insufficient for one family were often occupied by two or more families because accommodation was so short. In addition to this there was a shortage of water and lack of sanitary conveniences.

There were additional health problems with the butchers and fish vendors in Fishmarket Close which was described as 'a steep, narrow, foul smelling ravine'. Candlemakers added to the general smell and inconvenience of the centre of the town.

The water supply to the city prior to 1819, when the Water Company was set up, was reasonably satisfactory. Water was obtained from private and public wells. From time to time further sources were brought in to supplement the public wells from Comiston, Swanston and Crawley (an aqueduct from Tala Reservoir, near Broughton). Water was distributed by water caddies who came round with barrels on their back filling other people's barrels, selling water at 1d a barrel.

Water closets were introduced in the New Town from 1824 from new and existing sources of supply. The public wells were deprived of their second and third pipes and restricted to one only. Public supplies were thereby reduced and this caused serious inconvenience to the poorer people because of the inadequate amount of water available, particularly during dry periods.

In 1850 Edinburgh had a population of 170,000, with an average population of 40 to the acre. This compared with Birmingham 41, Dublin 66, Manchester 79, Glasgow 83, Liverpool 93. However, there were areas of Edinburgh with population densities well in excess of these figures. In the Grassmarket the density was 240 people per acre, and 314 per acre in the Tron. Throughout the New Town there were many areas with very poor sanitation.

In the mid nineteenth century the old town of Edinburgh contained many overcrowded, squalid and grossly unsanitary houses. The death rate for some of the wards in Edinburgh at this time was over 37/1,000. There were frequent epidemics of preventable infectious diseases.

Some conception of this misery and destitution is recorded in an anomymous letter printed in the *Scotsman* of 4 November 1843:

> In the West Port of Edinburgh, a portion of the town comprehending some 400 to 500 families of the poorest description, fever has for some time been raging with a virulence altogether unparalleled. The consequence is that, at the present moment, a very large number of the inhabitants are worse-fed, worse-clothed, worse-provided for than any beast of burden — had it not been for the assistance rendered by the Destitute Sick Society, very many would have died of starvation.... An example of the Society's work is a family living in a garret, husband, wife, daughter and a woman who was deaf and dumb. When first visited, the wife was ill of fever, lying in a corner on the bare floor without a single article of covering except an old coat. When visited the next day, she was lying in the same condition and the same place, stiff and dead. A week later the husband, daughter and the deaf and dumb woman were all lying ill of fever in different corners of the room, without a single rag to cover them or a particle of straw beneath them, shivering with cold. With the greatest of difficulty they were admitted into the Infirmary and their distressed condition was truly pitiable.

Other examples of such extreme poverties were quoted, graphically described by such writers as Drs Chalmers, Alison and Alexander Wood, the Surgeon George Bell and the lawyer Henry Johnston. In response to this, philanthropic associations were formed. They built model dwelling houses for the working classes including Chalmers buildings at Fountainbridge and Dr Begg's buildings at Abbeyhill. An association for improvement of lodging houses successfully operated three 'model houses' in the West Port, Cowgate and Merchant Street. An appeal was made by nine city clergy for the provision of a water supply to every flat in the old town tenements.

The Act of 1845, which remained the principal statute until 1934 failed to make provision for the able-bodied poor. In 1921 the position became so acute that the Parish Councils defied the law which had to be amended temporarily by annual acts until regularised in 1934. Relief paid to individuals in 1845 was 1s 6d (8p) to 2s 6d (13p) per week, the total cost in Scotland being over £157,000 in 1846.

In 1858 and 1861 a motion was placed before the Lord Provost's Committee to appoint an Officer of Health. The Committee found it difficult to define the duties of the Officer of Health and it was even suggested that such an appointment was premature.

Public opinion changed following the collapse of a High Street tenement. At 1 am on Sunday, 24 November 1861, the whole of 99–103 High Street collapsed. Thirty five people were killed and many severely injured. During the rescue operations a young man pinned down by the debris shouted to his rescuers 'Heave awa', one top one bottom lads, I'm no deid yet'. This fortitude was commemorated by the sculptured head of the lad in the archway in the High Street.

The unprecedented public outcry was followed by public meetings, sermons were preached, letters were written to the press, all were critical of the inertia of the Council. On 25 February 1862 at a packed public meeting a deputation was elected to urge the Council to appoint an Officer of Health. The Council continued to procrastinate until 30 September 1862 when the police surgeon, Henry Duncan Littlejohn, was appointed Medical Officer of Health. At that meeting the Town Council voted to appoint the first Medical Officer of Health by only one vote (17:16). Edinburgh thereby followed the example of Liverpool and London to make this appointment. Health affairs were initially the concern of the Lord Provost's Committee to whom Littlejohn was answerable. He persuaded the Council to support a general Vaccination Act for Scotland in 1863 against smallpox. It was a committee to whom he presented his Report on the sanitary state of the city in 1865 which led to Lord Provost William Chambers' *City Improvement Act* of 1867. Later that year the *Public Health (Scotland) Act* came into operation, after which it was decided to set up a special Public Health Committee at the Town Council for accomplishing the sanitary business of the city.

In 1867 the Lord Provost of Edinburgh, William Chambers of Glenmoriston, called a meeting to consider

1. The practicality and possiblity of simplifying, economising and amalgamating the public Charities of Edinburgh;
2. Improving the condition of the really deserving poor.

Two sub-Committees were created to examine these problems.

The conditions in the High Street were appalling. One stairway in a tenement, the Middle Meal Market stairs contained 59 rooms. Almost all of these were separate dwelling houses which were entered by a steep, dark stone common stair. 56 families lived here, 197 adults and 51 children under the age of five. In the old Meal Market stair there were 31 rooms housing 22 families, 14 children under five years and 96 adults. In the Berkley Buildings, Mid Common Close, Canongate, there was a 'modern tenement' erected especially for the poor. There were thirty five rooms which housed 33 families, 101 adults and 24 children under 5. None of the rooms had a sink, running water supply or water closet. 13,000 families (comprising 66,000 individuals, a third of the population of Edinburgh) lived in single rooms. 1,500 such single apartments were each occupied by 6 to 15 persons, 121 had no windows, 900 were cellars. The annual death rate in this area was 400–500. The recommended space for accommodation at that time was 500 cubic feet of air. Few of these dwellings met this recommendation and probably a quarter had no ventilation at all. Water was a somewhat scarce commodity in the city as a whole, especially in the districts where the poor lived. Of 450 houses visited by the Committee only 97 were supplied with water and inmates had to carry the water a considerable distance. Women living in the fifth and highest floor had to carry their water up the close stairs. The number of houses without water, sinks and soil pipes amounted to 14,000 where 70,000 people lived. The children reared in the dark cellars and dimly lit alleys were quite distinct from those brought up in the New Town and in the new houses on the south side of the city. A proposed improvement was the appointment of a Sanitary Committee of the Town Council.

Initiation of Public Health Committee[2]

On 19 November 1872 the Public Health Committee was initiated with 15 members including a Convenor. The Committee worked in close conjunction with the Lighting and Cleaning and the Streets and Buildings Committees whose officials, the Inspector of Cleaning and the Burgh Engineer, worked with Henry Littlejohn and the Chief Constable in relation to sanitation and public health. Much of the Public Health Committee's early work dealt with the control of epidemic disease, Fever Hospital administration, nuisances, smoke pollution and taking proceedings against owners of premises which were in need of repair when sanitary provision of a proper water supply was required.

Henry Duncan Littlejohn was born in 1826 and died in 1914, graduating in Edinburgh in Medicine in 1847. After graduation he worked in general practice, and later became a lecturer in Medical Jurisprudrudence, a department established by Sir Robert Christison. This department consisted of Forensic Medicine and Public Health or Medical Police as it was then called. Littlejohn's professional philosophy was modelled on the pioneering work of the English reformer, Chadwick, who was not a doctor but a lawyer and Secretary to the Poor Law Commissioners. Chadwick had shown that impure water, bad drains and overcrowding caused disease in the community. After his appointment Littlejohn took the opportunity to rectify these problems and to educate public opinion on the importance of cleanliness and sanitation.

One of his important achievements was to urge Edinburgh Council to request what was the first Act of Parliament requiring the notification of specific infectious diseases. This was obtained in 1879 in the face of much medical opposition, which felt that such notification interfered with patient/doctor confidentiality.

He cleared out many of the old buildings that had been incubating disease for

300 years and made new streets through the worst parts of the Town. Coincidental with this smallpox and typhus disappeared from Edinburgh. He was also involved, in part, with the construction of the new City Hospital in 1903.

The Origins of Craigleith Hospital

In the mid 19th century St Cuthbert's Parish Poorhouse, which had accommodation for about 500 inmates, was in St Cuthbert's Lane — a site which was eventually covered by part of Princes Street railway station (now integrated into the Caledonian Hotel).

In the early 1700's a tax of £100 was levied on the Parish to help reduce 'the menace of beggars and to maintain those who had grown accustomed to living on the charity of other members of society.' Parishes in general, and St Cuthbert's in particular, realised that the sick, aged and crippled were the responsibility of the Parish. In 1739 the Heritors of St Cuthbert's objected to this levy on the grounds that the Parish's poor funds were sufficient to maintain those living on the landward side of the parish and that those living in the Pleasance, Potter Row, and Bristo Street should be maintained by the Town in whose suburbs they were living. Consequently the levy was abandoned and the ancient practice revived of identifying the poor with metal badges. This entitled them to solicit alms within the Parish. In 1744, 58 individuals wore this badge but the number of enrolled poor was 220. This cost the Parish £200 each year. The Kirk Session of St Cuthbert's asked the City Magistrate to augment these funds for the support of the poor through a share of the duty levied on ale sales.

Building of St Cuthbert's Workhouse

The Parish of St Cuthbert's opened a subscription list to collect funds for a Workhouse. This Workhouse was built between 1759 and 1761. It was a tall and ugly building on a site just off Lothian Road which more recently housed the Caledonian Railway Goods Station. St Cuthbert's Poorhouse came into being through the benevolence of the Poor Law provisions of the Parish of St Cuthbert's. The Workhouse cost £1600 to build and an annual subscription of £198 was raised. In addition a levy was made on the owners of various properties within the Parish towards maintenance. The annual cost of maintenance for each inmate was £4.1s.6d (£4.8p). The Institution contained a hospital school, and there were facilities for weaving, spinning and knitting.

The sick wards in the Poorhouse Hospitals were visited twice weekly by a doctor and by two trained nurses who supervised the patients. The actual nursing of the patients was by other inmates of the Institution.

By 1834 considerable dissatisfaction was expressed for the conditions in the Poorhouse. A new and more compassionate committee was formed and looked into the affairs of the Workhouse. It is interesting to note that the Governor, who also acted as the Chaplain, received £105 a year and the visiting doctor

£40. The new committee looked into all grievances and abuses. Amongst their recommendations was to supply the old ladies with a bodice, or stays for warmth and comfort. They also provided a handkerchief for each inmate. The infirm were allowed to sit on padded chairs, pictures were hung and all the old bedding straw was sold as manure. Children old enough to behave in church were issued with caps.

Commission to review Poor Relief in Scotland

In 1843 a Commission was appointed by the Government to review the administration of Poor Relief in Scotland. They reported that while conditions varied widely from one part of the country to another, the general standard was low. The principal recommendations of the Commission were incorporated in an Act of Parliament passed in August 1845 for the amendment and better administration of the law for the relief of the poor in Scotland. This allowed for the creation in Edinburgh of a Central Board of Supervision responsible for the relief of the poor. There was also the creation of parochial Boards whose duty was to make Rolls of the Poor, to name an Inspector of Poor and to determine the methods of raising funds requisite for the relief of the poor.

Three modes of assessment were legalised and it was left to the parochial Boards to adopt one of them, the most widely adopted being the first. One half of the assessment should be imposed on the owners and the other half on the tenants or occupants of land and heritages according to their annual value. The salaries paid to the Inspectors of the poor were modest. The *Poor Law Amendment Act* of 1845 had laid down that nothing therein contained should be held to confer relief on able-bodied persons out of employment the right to demand relief. In 1848 the Lord Advocate and Dean of Faculty advised the Board of Supervision that able-bodied persons accidentally or unavoidably thrown out of employment and thereby reduced to immediate want may be regarded as Occasional Poor to whom temporary relief may lawfully be given out of the funds raised by assessment; but that such persons cannot be admitted to the Roll of Poor entitled to parochial relief.

Problems arose in St Cuthbert's Parish resulting in unnecessary delay in disposal of applications for relief. In addition, it became increasingly necessary to provide suitable accommodation for the casual poor. In 1848 the Board of Supervision issued a circular recommending parochial Boards to make such arrangements. The circular pointed out that there was concern about placing paupers, suffering from fevers, in lodging houses occupied by the healthy poor or by independent labourers, as they rarely met with the quiet and attention they required. The *Poor Law Amendment Act* of 1845 required parochial Boards to remove all insane and fatuous paupers to an asylum or establishment legally authorised to receive lunatic patients. The Act empowered the Board of Supervision under special circumstances, in particualar cases, to dispense with their removal. The parochial Board had to provide for them in such other manner and under such regulations as to inspection and otherwise as shall be sanctioned by the Board of Supervision. The Board of Supervision sent medical gentlemen to visit pauper lunatics living with their relatives to determine whether it was necessary to have them removed to institutions. Only five such individuals were so removed.

With the growth of Poor Houses it was found that many lunatic paupers came to be retained in premises not licensed for that purpose and often unsuitable for them. The Board of Supervision wrote in 1850 that for a large class of incurable and harmless pauper lunatics, especially such as have no near relation with whom they can reside, a well-regulated Poor House affords a place of refuge most conducive to their own happiness and welfare and most advantageous to the community. The cost of maintaining such persons in Poor Houses was less than half of that of an asylum. Following the Report of the Lunacy Commissioners in 1855 the Lunacy Board allowed lunatics to live in detached or separate portions of Poor Houses. The Act of 1845 declared it to be appropriate that Poor Houses should be erected in populace parishes for administering more effectively to the wants of aged and other friendless poor persons, such as were infirm or unable to take charge of their own affairs. It authorised the parochial Board of any parish or combination of parishes that contained more than 5,000 persons to erect a Poor House. The advantages of the Poor House system were to:

1. Secure comfortable living to the improvident, the weak in mind, the friendless and the impotent poor.
2. Make the Poor Houses a stimulus to industry and an efficient school for educating and training the poor.
3. Check begging.
4. Reduce over time, the poor rates.

In Glasgow, when a poor person was declared destitute and wholly disabled from contributing to his own support, no means test was required. If the pauper resided in the house of a relative or friend there might be a great cruelty in compelling him to exchange such a home for the Poor House. In cases of partial disability where the pauper was willing to contribute all he could towards his own support, there did not appear to be any reason why outdoor relief should not be denied. It was probable that the cost of maintaining him in the Poor Houses would considerably exceed the amount of outdoor relief that could adequately support him with the aid of his own earnings. The parochial authorities were required to provide in a Poor House for the various classes of helpless person. They also had to test whether individuals were poor and disabled or whose disability was doubtful or exaggerated.

In 1846 a petition was presented to the Board of Supervision on behalf of James Nicholson, a pauper in the Canongate Poor House, representing that House to be unhealthy because of its situation. Nicholson, a man of 78 years of age, was suffering from sickness and was neglected by the attendants. Dr Charles Bell was requested by the Board to visit Nicholson who was filthy and in a most miserable state of discomfort. All the beds were dirty and ill-adapted for such an institution. Canongate Poor House gave a bad impression, not only in its internal arrangements but also in its locality and seemed a very unfit habitation for the debilatated and aged. Other doctors felt it was no worse than many of the other Houses in the parish. It would be better if the children were boarded in the country provided they were adequately cared for. The building appeared in some respects in a dilapidated state with cracked windows and required careful inspection and repair. The Poor Houses in operation previous to 1845 had been regarded almost exclusively as Alms Houses which afforded a comfortable retreat for the more respectable of the aged and infirm poor. These had been conducted in a manner corresponding with the purposes being contemplated. Each parochial Board that administered a Poor House had to appoint a House Committee. The management of the Poor House was to be under the immediate control of a House Governor and a Matron subject to the Committee. At least once every year, and as often as necessary for cleanliness, the House Committee was to cause all rooms, wards, offices and privies belonging to the Poor House to be lime washed and the cesspools emptied. The Poor House was to be visited by the House Committee at least once a year and answers to the following questions were to be recorded:

1. Is the House clean and well ventilated?
2. Do inmates appear to be clean, decent and orderly?
3. Are the infirm properly attended to?
4. Are the children making due progress at school?
5. Are the Medical Officer and Chaplain regular in their attendance?
6. Do patients in the Sick Ward appear to be in as satisfactory a state as their ailments admit of?
7. Is there any infectious disease in the Wards?
8. Are any of the children not vaccinated?
9. Is the established diet and hours of meals adhered to?
10. Is separation of the sexes and the various classes of inmates strictly enforced?
11. Are there any complaints against individuals or against the quality of provisions?

A Porter was to be appointed. His duties were to examine all parcels and goods and to prevent the unlawful admissions of any 'spirituous or fermented liquids' or other prohibited articles and to take care that no inmate entering the Poor House should take into it any spirit or other prohibited articles and for this purpose to search their person if he should think fit. The inmates were classified into five groups:

1. Males between the age of two and 15.
2. Males over 15 years of age.
3. Females between two and 15 years of age.

4. Females over 15 years of age.
5. Children under two years.

The rules for the discipline of the inmates said that all inmates, except for the disabled, those of unsound mind and children, were to rise, be set to work, leave off work and go to bed with such intervals for meals as were notified by the ringing of a bell. For three or four of the working hours of every day boy and girl inmates were to be instructed in reading, writing, arithmetic and the principles of the Christian religion. No inmate of the Poor House was to be allowed to possess or read in the Poor House any book or printed paper of any improper tendency or to play at cards or any game of chance. No noise was to be made when silence was ordered to be kept. There was to be no insulting of any persons or any pretence of sickness. A disorderly inmate could be required, for a time not exceeding two days, to perform one or two hours of extra work or be deprived for a like time of all milk or buttermilk or to be deprived for a period not exceeding three days of any such other articles of diet. If the inmate was refractory and who, for example, reviled or insulted any Officer of the Poor House or who attempted to bring into the Poor House prohibited articles, became drunk or climbed over a wall, then this might be punished by solitary confinement for a period not exceeding 24 hours. In 1862 there were attempts to regulate the freedom of Poor House inmates. Poor House inmates were required to ask for permission to leave the House for the purpose of attending divine worship or any other purpose. Religious instruction must be provided in Poor Houses. In 1860 the average weekly cost for maintaining Poor House inmates was 4s 5½d per person per week (23p). Of this sum food, fuel, clothing, light and all other necessities account for 2s 8¼d (19p) per week per person. Salaries of the officials, feu duties, insurance, repairs etc. come to 10d (5p)/ per week per person. Estimated rent of Poor House 8d (4p) per week per person. Medicine and medical attendants 2d (1p) per week per person. The Scotsman criticised the Poor Law system in a leader on 7 May, 1863. Poor Houses had two objects: to enable Local Authorities more effectively to administer the wants of the aged and infirm and to furnish a test of poverty. The system was unsatisfactory. The guiding impulse had been to test poverty. The average number of poor placed in Poor Houses in Scotland during the year ended 1862 was 7,843, and there were 1,812 (23%) deaths. Nine of every 100 paupers who entered a Poor House, whether intended for a long stay or short stay, died within the year. The inmates were deprived of their liberty, exercised in narrow yards enclosed by high walls subject to the will of others. The furniture was simple, the hours stated, the sexes completely separated. The diet was calculated to sustain life and no more. The leader doubted whether aged, sick and broken-down paupers could be sufficiently fed on 3½d (2p) per day.

Old Age Pension Act

In 1864, and the years immediately following, poverty was prevalent in Scotland and the incidence of pauperism high. The number of persons on the Poor Roll, together with their dependents, numbered 39 per 1,000 of the population and the proportion continued to rise until 1868 with 42 per 1,000. By 1875 it had fallen to 30 per 1,000, by 1884 to 24 per 1,000. There was little change between 1884 and 1910. By 1914, following the removal of the pauper disqualification under the *Old Age Pensions Act*, the figure fell to 21 per 1,000.

The recurring theme throughout the discussions was that inappropriate persons received charity. The fit paupers were to be excluded, unless they were very hungry and in dire straits.

The reduction in the number of registered poor was in part due to improvements in the general standard of living, the introduction of the Old Age Pension, and a more stringent administration of the Poor Law. Mr McNeil, one of the Board's Senior Officers worked to reduce the number of paupers in Scotland by ensuring that:

1. No outdoor relief whatsoever should be given to mothers of illegitimate children whose sole cause of disability arises from the fact of having such children.
2. Deserted wives should invariably be tested by an offer of a place in the Poor House.
3. When applicants are known to have families able to support them and offer of indoor relief should invariably precede any correspondence with the children.
4. A large number of persons in Scotland receive relief as paupers whose collateral relatives are well able to support them. He was persuaded that a judicious use of the Poor House in such cases could induce the relatives to perform the clear moral duty which devolves on them.
5. In addition, wives of persons sentenced to terms of imprisonment or penal servitude should be recommended admission to the Poor House.

Mr Andrew Wallace, the Inspector of Poor in Glasgow, identified those entitled to relief as widows with or without dependents, men disabled for work from sickness or infirmity, deserted wives with dependents, orphans and deserted children, single women with illegitimate children, and lunatics. In his parish widows accounted for 50% of the total, but there were various kinds of widows — some had grown-up families who ought to support them. In 1867 a Committee was appointed to prepare a report on the condition of the poorer classes of the city. The Committee was concerned to secure reform of existing measures of relief for the poor believing that almost any change must be for the better. The Report listed 15 causes which had operated to produce the lapsed classes that contributed so much to pauperism. These were:

1. Crowding together of the lapsed classes without association with the better class.
2. Their neglect by the legislature and by their employers.
3. Their outgrowal of Christian influences.

4. Their lack of education.
5. Intemperance.
6. Drinking customs and other causes leading to intemperance.
7. The licensing system.
8. Pawn broking.
9. The operation of the Poor Law.
10. Indiscriminate private charity.
11. Want of method amongst charitable societies.
12. Overcrowding of districts and of dwellings.
13. Want of water.
14. Want of light.
15. Want of proper arrangements for removing offensive matter.

The earnings of the industrious supported the idle and the dissolute, making no distinction between that poverty which had resulted from misfortune and that which originated in vice. It tended to diminish industry by giving to every pauper a right to maintenance whenever he sank to a certain level. It diminished frugality and providence. It destroyed the tie of relationships. It lessened the sympathy of the wealthy for the poorer classes by giving the latter a legal claim on the former. The Committee divided remedial measures calculated to restore the lapsed classes into three groups: Those which could only be applied by law and authority; those which could be applied only by a person superior to the sufferers in a social scale and those which could be applied by the labouring classes themselves, either by their unaided efforts or with the encouragement or assistance of others.

Individuals who might be sent to the Poor House were patients in the Infirmary alleging themselves to be destitute and who it might be considered expedient to discharge from the Infirmary on whatever grounds. A problem arose with the admission into the Poor House Hospitals of previous inmates of the Poor House who were suffering from fevers. The problem was highlighted by the need to care for individuals who had tuberculosis. The Inspector of Poor was an agent of the Parochial Board in whom rested legal responsibility for seeing that all applicants entitled to parochial relief did in fact receive such relief. During the period of the Craigleith Poor House there was an increasing tendency to offer indoor relief rather than outdoor to an increasing proportion of applicants. There was a widely held feeling that many of the less deserving poor were having things made too easy for them. The Convener of the Employment Committee, the Edinburgh Association for improving the conditions of the poor, wrote in 1868 that too many poor were being kept in relative comfort and idleness. There were in the Edinburgh City Poor House system 4,135 souls, the daily average being 604. During the course of that year the gross return from the productive labour of these inmates amounted to £498, equal to 15s 2d (76p) from the year's work of each inmate. The arrangements in Poor Houses for nursing sick and bedridden inmates was not ideal. Mostly untrained pauper nurses were employed.

There were great problems with personal cleanliness and purification of clothes. Many of the children admitted to Poor Houses had vermin and in the eyes of some the presence of vermin on children was regarded as a capital sign of the health of those who possessed them. The beds were placed barrack fashion in a dormitory. A urine tub was placed there for night use. The elderly couples were separated. Sir John McNeill in 1869 argued before the Select Committee on the Scottish Poor Law that the separation of husband and wife was not improper — if you want to establish a colony put them together, if you want to diminish pauperism keep them separate. In 1894 the General Superintendent of the poor remarked that if a respectable married couple could look after themselves or had anyone to look after them they were invariably granted relief at home. It was only dissolute or helpless couples who were sent to the House. It was therefore only the aged, helpless and respectable for whom separate accommodation was required. Children were apprenticed to local tradesmen. It was also agreed that if Poor Houses were to be retained as part of the administrative machinery they should be classified, one class being for the purpose of correction and the other for industrious poor — people who had been reduced to poverty not by any fault of their own.

For many years the emphasis in Scottish Poor Houses was very heavily on their 'test function'. When paupers were admitted to Poor Houses their money was taken from them. In 1889 the Board of Supervision came to the conclusion that this practice of removing money found on paupers admitted to a Poor House and applying it towards their keep was of very doubtful legality. When a considerable sum was found in the possession of an applicant the proper course was to withdraw relief on the grounds that he was not a proper object for it. The test became the prime object of the Scottish Poor House. There were the following three classes of persons for whom the Poor House was advocated as a test:

1. Persons suspected of concealing or misrepresenting the extent of their means and resources;
2. Persons regarding whom there was a doubt as to whether a disability rendered them incapable of maintaining themselves and their dependents without parish relief;
3. Persons of idle, immoral or dissipated habits.

Discussions Leading to New Poorhouse

This was the situation in 1865 which presented to Sir Henry Littlejohn. He concluded that two of the three Poorhouses in the City, the Canongate and the one providing for the largest Parish, St Cuthbert's, were in a derelict state.

The number of deaths during 1857 in St Cuthbert's Poorhouse was 97 and of these 21 were infants and children under the age of 5 years and 43 individuals over the age of 60. The young died of marasmus (wasting away of the body), diarrhoea and infection and the elderly of tumours, old age and debility.

One view was that the two parishes should combine resources for one poorhouse. The City, however, had recently acquired Craiglockhart Estate with a view to development. If 1500 inmates were all housed in Craiglockhart, the cost would have been just over £3 per head per annum, whereas if St Cuthbert's acted alone, the cost was estimated to be £5 per annum for each inmate.

Sir Henry Littlejohn suggested that the existing workhouses in neighbouring Parishes in the City should be replaced by a single new and larger building in a 'a freer and healthier exposure in a rural district' as a well organised and properly managed house to hold 600–900 inmates. In a house this size the responsible officers, namely the Governor, Medical Officer and Matron could at all times have personal communication with every inmate. There was also a concern that parishes would be combined as well as poorhouses. Hence there was an argument.

This suggestion in 1867 gave rise to a flood of the most bitter controversy. The head of a plan for the separate St Cuthbert's Poorhouse was Sir James Gardener Baird, Chairman of St Cuthbert's Parochial Board. His main protagonist was Dr Alexander Wood, a Heritor of St Cuthbert's and a Fellow of the Royal College of Physicians. Sir James supported the concept of a separate poorhouse for St Cuthbert's, whilst Dr Wood supported Sir Henry Littlejohn's plea for a combined poorhouse. A public meeting was held in January 1867, where there was a fierce argument. The Scotsman supported the combined idea. Despite this at a further noisy, difficult meeting on February 16, 1867, Sir James won the day and the amendment calling for a new poorhouse for St Cuthbert's was approved.

On 19 January 1866 an acting Committee of the St Cuthbert's Parochial Board, chaired by Sir James Gardiner Baird, met with their Architects (Peddie & Kinnear). The Committee were of the opinion that the Board ought to keep in view:

1. The 'singular suitableness' of the present site (i.e. Lothian Road) of the Poorhouse
2. The potential difficulties of obtaining a site for a new Poorhouse for a Parish which has a population of more than 95,000 people.

The original Poorhouse in Lothian Road was not designed as a Poorhouse but as a Charity Workhouse, whose function was to give overnight accommodation, supper and breakfast. In return a certain amount of work was expected. The lodgers foraged for themselves for the remainder of the day. New buildings had been erected for the 'fatuous' inmates. The managers had given some ground to the City of Edinburgh to make a street which crossed the ground. They later gave further ground for the erection of a Church. This meant that the Lothian Road accommodation for the Poorhouse was limited. The problem of space was compounded by the buildings being separated by the new street, so in effect there were two Poorhouses.

At this time (1866), the Caledonian Railway Company was looking for

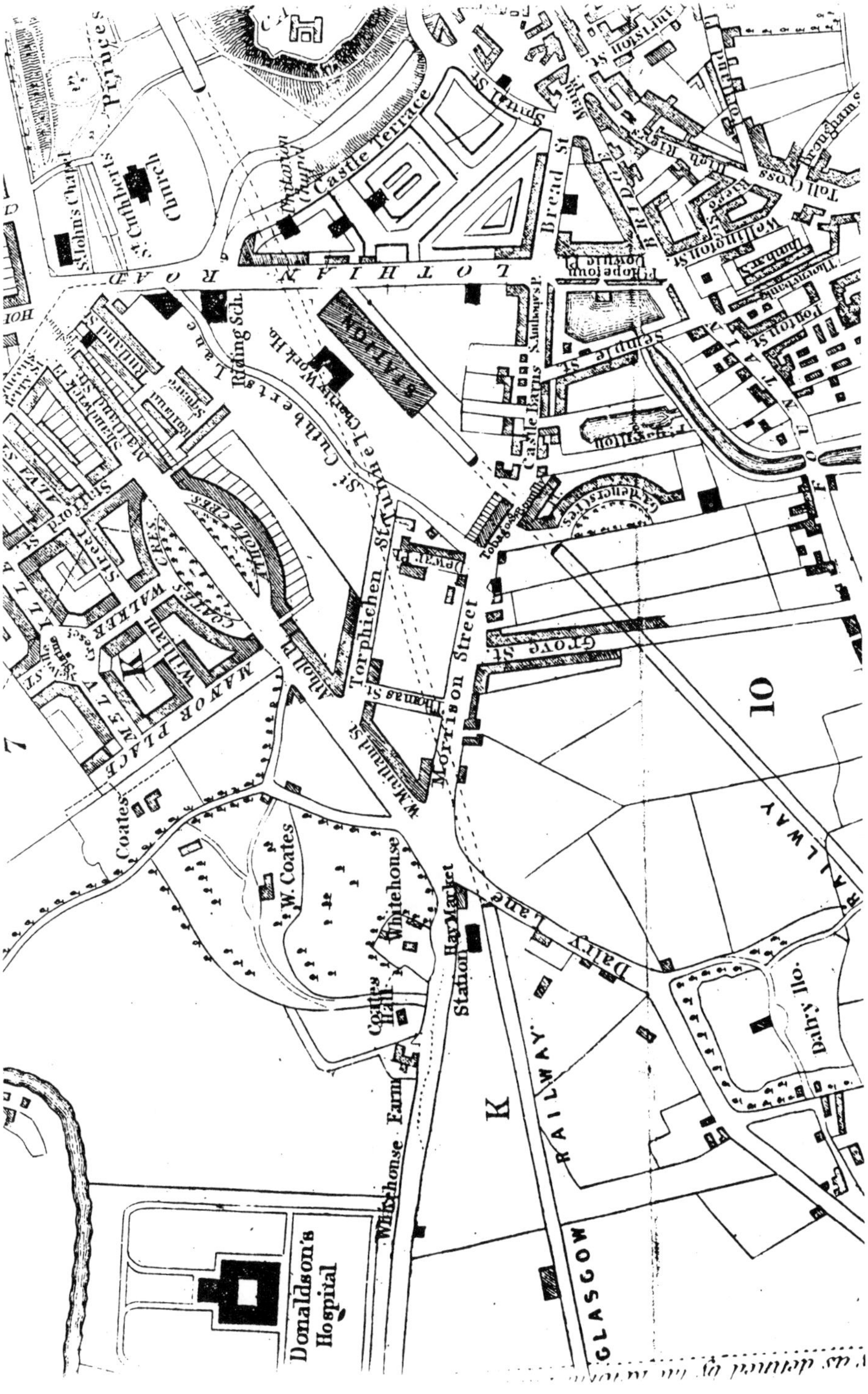

Charity Workhouse, off Lothian Road, 1858

ground to build a Railway Station on the Western side of the City. The chosen site was on the ground occupied by the poorhouse. The Lands Clauses Act meant that the Railway Company could requistion the Poor Law Hospital site. This would have resulted in the closure of the Poor Law Hospital and the evacuation of the Poorhouse inmates.

The St Cuthbert's Parish meeting agreed that a sub-Committee be set up to negotiate with the Caledonian Railway Company to petition against the Bill in the House of Lords and Parliament. They also agreed to select a site for the new Poorhouse and elected Sir James G Baird, Bart. as Chairman of the Board.

The Special Committee of St Cuthbert's Parochial Board negotiating with the Caledonian Railway Company eventually recommended that the Parochial Board:

1. Find a suitable site for a new Poorhouse to the satisfaction of the Parochial Board and the Board of Supervision;
2. That a new building be erected which was capable of accommodating the same number of inmates as the present Lothian Road Building but with statutory modern improvements and conveniences;
3. That the new site and buildings be ready for occupation before the Railway Company could move into the Lothian Road premises.

The architects estimated a sum of £54,635 as compensation. The Railway Company responded with a suggested sum of £25,000 compensation and valued the Poorhouse and its land, in 1867, at £115,000.

In April 1868 the agents of the Railway Company stated that 'the Railway Company are not prepared to concede the sweeping clause and demands made by the Parochial Board'. A compromise was to be decided in Parliament and was discussed before the Committee of the House of Commons.

The Parliamentary Committee met on the 29 May, counsel were heard and witnesses were examined at considerable length, on behalf both of the Railway Company and the Parochial Board. After two days the Chairman said that in the opinion of the Parliamentary Committee the Railway Company ought not to be liable for the whole expense of a new and improved Poorhouse and that if it were decidedly better than the old one, a certain proportion of the expense should be paid by each party.

The Railway Company had been held bound to find a suitable site for a new Poorhouse within the Parish to the satisfaction of the Board. All of this, including the building of the New Poorhouse had to be completed within two years.

The Railway Company informed the Committee of the House of Commons that they had obtained very suitable grounds on the Dalry estate.

These generous terms contrasted with the poor financial provisions of the Canongate Poorhouse. This was the background and hidden agenda to the quarrel as to whether two Poorhouses or one combined Poorhouse should be built, one Parish had money and the other did not.

2

Craigleith Poorhouse 1868–1914

A meeting of the Parochial Board of St Cuthbert's took place on the 25 June 1867. The Committee, Chaired by James Gardiner Baird, authorised the Board of Supervision to erect a Poorhouse for the Parish on the ground acquired from the Fettes Trustees at £16 per acre. The site consisted of ten acres of farmland at Porterfield, Craigleith, within their own parish, but in those days truly in the country.

The Architects for the project were Messrs Peddie & Kinnear who drew up plans for the building of the Poorhouse. The estimates for the work were:

	£ s d
Mason Work — W& A Beattie	£21,004
Joiner Work — Bell Scott	£7,371
Painting — C & F Moxon	£71
Plaster Work — John Webster	£1,324
Slater Work — Wm. Anderson	£747.18.0
Iron Work — James Tod & Son	£648. 9.6
Glazier Work — Davidson & Chisholm	£265.15.0
Plumber Work — Robert Kemp	£3,100. 0.0
	£34,534. 2.6

In order to pay for this it was necessary to borrow £8,000 in the first year. The expectation was that the new Poorhouse would be completed before the Lothian Road Poorhouse was handed over to the Railway Company.

The stone for the new building came from the now disused quarry at Craigleith. This quarry lay between Groathill Road South, Craigleith Road and Craigleith Hill Crescent. Stone from this quarry was used for building much of the New Town of Edinburgh, Nelson's Column and Buckingham Palace. The quarry was filled in during the 1960's and 1970's and for a long period was an unofficial nature reserve. This site is now occupied by a Sainsbury's Supermarket.

Opening of St Cuthbert's Poorhouse

The Scotsman of December 22, 1868, described the opening of the buildings:

> The opening ceremony of the new Poorhouse for the Parish of St Cuthbert's at Porterfield, near Craigleith, took place by the appointment of the Parochial Board on the 21 December, 1868. The Poorhouse was opened by Sir James Gardiner Baird, Bart, accompanied by a large number of the Acting Committee and others interested

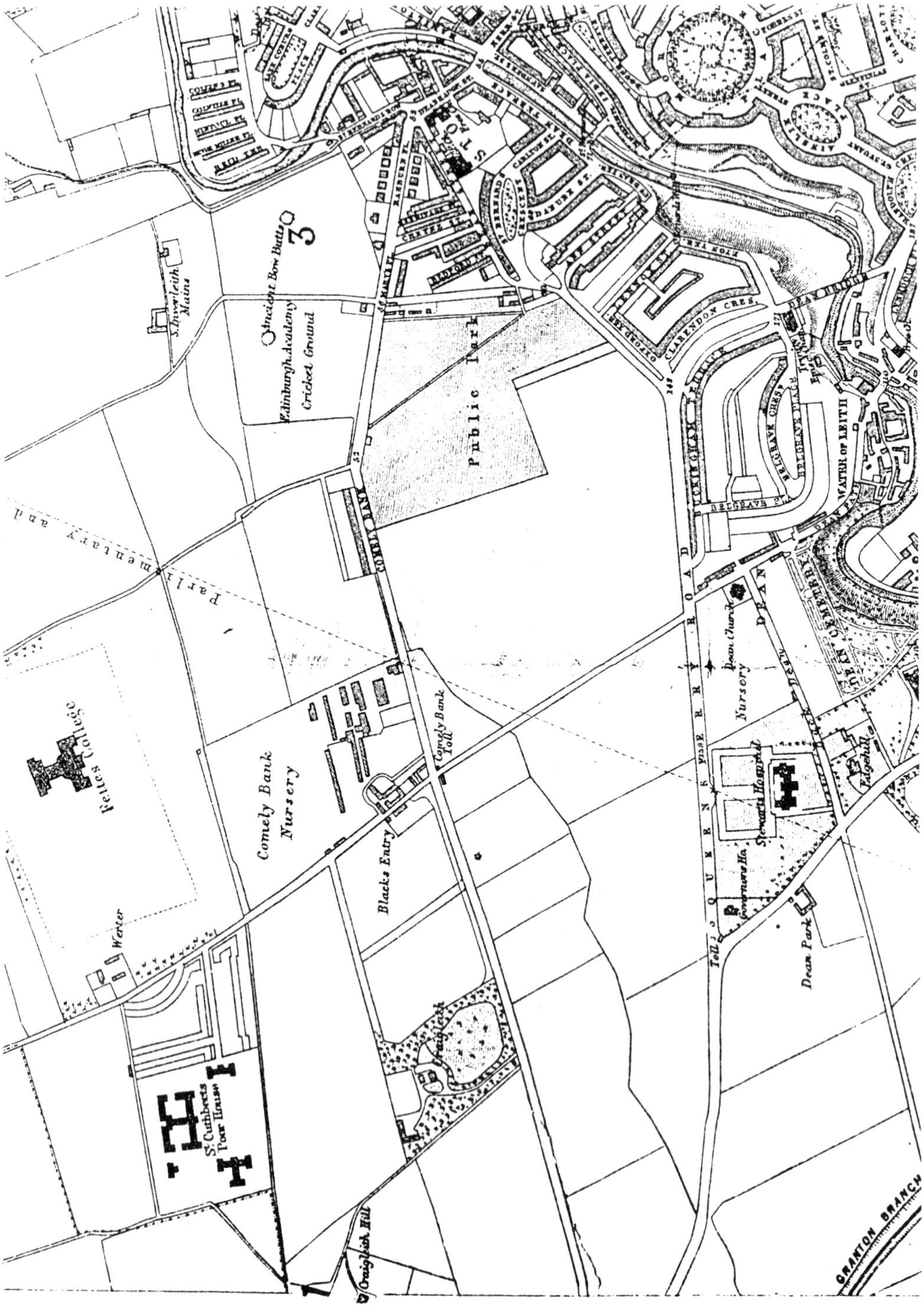

St Cuthbert's Poorhouse, Craigleith, 1878

in the Poorhouse and from the Parish for which it had been provided. The day was unpleasant, rain falling heavily and the consequence was that the newly formed grounds could not be visited. The transfer of a large number of paupers from the old house, many of then aged and infirm was accomplished under the supervision of the Governor, Mr Cowan. The total number removed was 410. The able bodied adults walked, the hospital patients, infirm and the aged were driven in cabs and vans and the children were also transported in vans. The removal of the inmates occupied three days, twelve days were occupied in shifting the goods and chattels. For the first month after the removal — from the 14 November to the 14 December — only six deaths occurred in the house, the number being considerably under the average for the season of the year. The total number of inmates at present residing in the house is 433, 132 men, 208 women and 93 children and infants.

The house was described by Sir James Gardiner Baird 'as handsome and commodious an erection as they would be justified in building for such a purpose. It had been erected on a site in their own parish as elegible a site as would have been impossible to find anywhere in the county of Mid-Lothian.' The accommodation was well ventilated, commodious and cheerful with beautiful views throughout the property.

Sir James continued his description 'To promote the happiness and comfort of the inhabitants they had adopted a thorough system of classification which would prevent the respectable poor from being annoyed or having their time infringed upon by those who were reckless or bad tempered, or who were inclined to make manifest the vicious cause which had brought them to poverty'. A hospital had also been built which appeared to him to be very handsome and commodious. He trusted that those who suffered from sickness and required to go to the hospital would find it a means of restoring them to health and strength. They also had ground to cultivate and workshops in which artisans coming into the hospital could be employed. Every article of wearing apparel, male and female, and every article of clothing distributed to the necessitous poor out of doors, was made by the paupers themselves within the house, with the exception of the boots and shoes. The inmates were employed to reduce the expense incurred in looking after such an establishment. It was also stated that a firm discipline would be necessary to repress the violent, to protect and respect the quiet, the weak and the infirm that they might live together in harmony and happiness.

The description in *The Scotsman* continued:

The inmates will have an allowance of plum pudding at dinner in addition to their normal supplies. They also will have an additional allowance of bread and cheese and ale, the children getting currant bread.

The site consists of 10 acres in addition to the large portion appropriated for the buildings, large spaces for airing yards and plots for shrubs and cultivation. The entrance lodge at the east side of the ground faces the Granton Road from which a new drive of about 150 yards in length has been constructed to the entrance gates. The whole ground is enclosed by a wall 10 feet high with the exception of the front of the Lodge where a large space at the entrance is covered with gravel and left open for vehicles.

There is a lodge in the main drive, a two story building on the southern side of the hospital which has an open archway. This gives house accommodation for the gate keeper and also the fumigator for filthy patients and their clothes. On either side of the lodge are the single storey probationary wards each 70 feet long, giving the lodge a total frontage of 175 feet. A small plot of ground is enclosed in front of each of the probationary wards and is covered with shrubs. South of this block is a hollow with a small stable and a shed for vehicles. The wash-house is supplied from a large rain tank and all the boiling and heating is done by steam. Along the drive at the west end there is the Infirmary (D Block) and the main building is to the right (North). A broad straight walk runs between the lodge and the infirmary and on either side, there are neatly planted strips of ground with grass borders. From the middle of this, another walk, similarly planted, passes to the main building. The space in the enclosure formed by three blocks is crossed by two walks which contain airing yards. There are terraces in front of the main building. In front of these are two large square grass plots, with gravel walks flanked by palisading between which is the airing ground for the decent and infirm inmates. Beyond these plots at each end are the airing yards for the boys and girls. The main building consists of four storeys with wings of equal lengths on each side. The tower, with a clock, rises from the centre block 120 feet in height to the top of the vane and 18 feet square.

The system of classification adopted in the house meant that each division be kept entirely distinct and separate from the others. The only area for general meeting is the dining room; leading into which are four doors, one in each corner through which different grades are admitted. Each division stair has its own accommodation and day room. The main building is in three storeys to the front with a fourth storey in the centre for the governor's house and one storey behind where the dining hall and chapel, kitchen, stores, washing-houses and workshops are placed, to which there is a back entrance. The principal entrance is in the centre of the south front through a covered porch. This is laid with Staffordshire tiles. Here is to be found the governor's office, clerk's room, waiting room, committee room to the front; and governor's and matron's stores to the back. The corridor down the centre east and west of the hospital is six feet wide giving access to the various parts of the building. Pauper inmates are entirely excluded from this area, except when being brought to the chapel and dining hall. On each side of the corridor are the day rooms and dormitories of the different classes; 18 feet wide and 11 feet 6 inches high, giving 500 cubic feet of space per inmate which was the suggested requirement. Each of these groups are accommodated in an area complete within itself and contained a lavatory, bath and water closets, and a separate stair with access to its own airing ground. The day rooms are all provided with fires.

Over the front of the main building a tablet stated: 'Erected by the Parochial Board of the Parish of St Cuthberts, Sir James Gardiner Baird, Bart, of Saughton Hall, chairman, 1867. Peddie & Kinnear, architects.'

The following is a description in *The Scotsman* of 22 December 1868

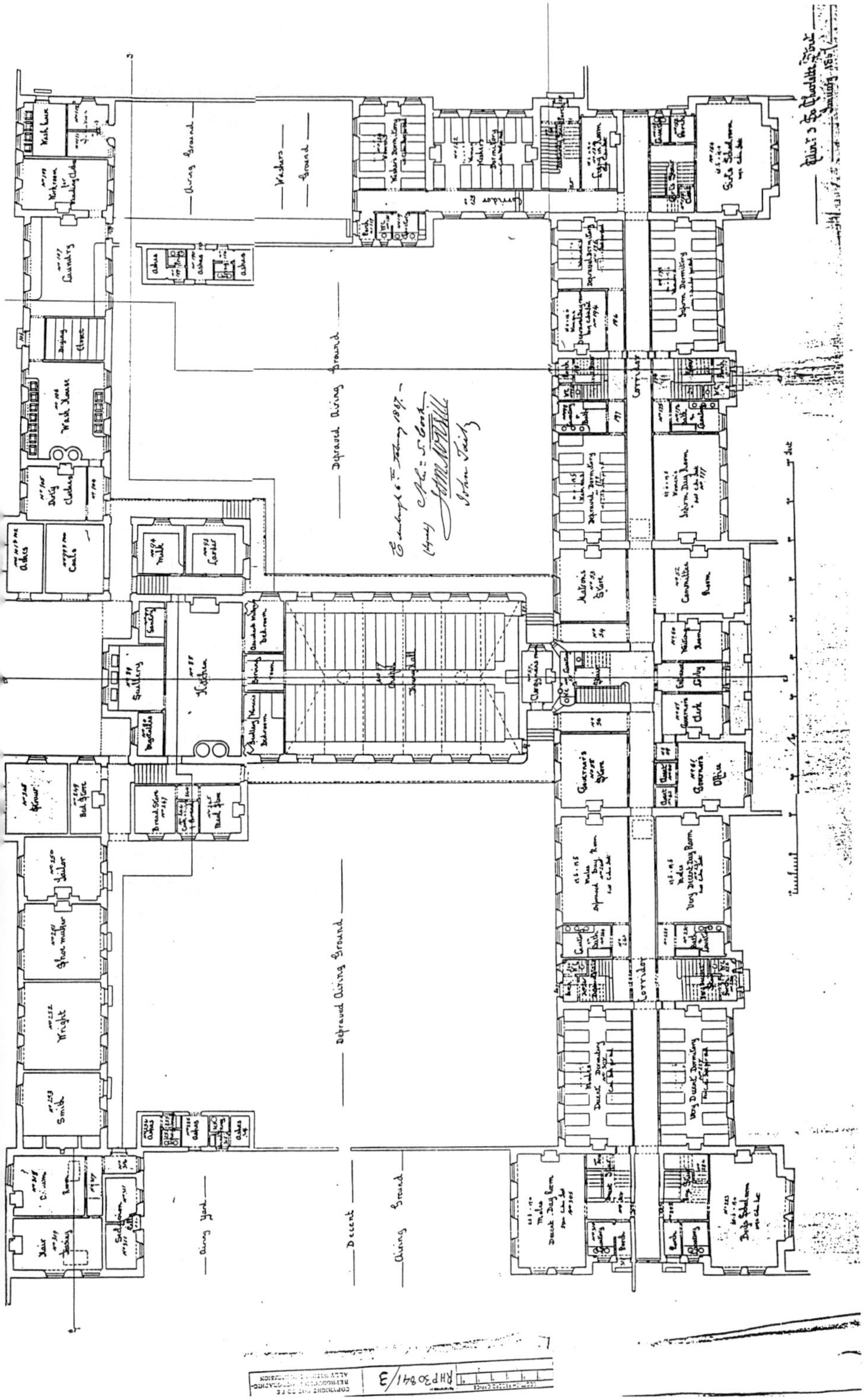

Original Plans, 1867

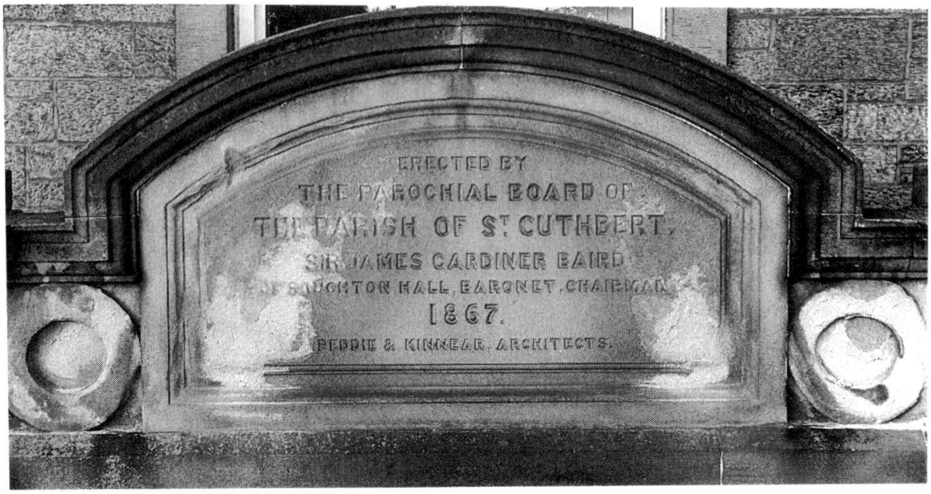

Foundation stone of 1867 – taken in 1995

> There is one day room, for the decent aged women. Here sat 20 or 30 clean and chatty old people, one aged 90 years. They wore warm tartan shawls and red woollen hoods over their white caps. Each sat in soft comfortable chairs or sofas. Several framed prints hung on the walls. The accommodation for the male inmates, which was on the west side of the building is sub-divided into four classes; very decent, decent, depraved and boys. There were more female inmates than males so that an additional wing was built northwards from the east end and divided into the following classes — sewers (decent), infirm, depraved, washers, bastardy, and girls.

This extension is the Frenchy (architectural term) forecourt which was designed by D & J Bryce, 1880; the father being the architect who designed the Royal Infirmary of Edinburgh. The style of this extension is somewhat different from the remainder of the building. For example the original building has simple stone spheres on the roof, whereas the added wing has spheres with carved garlands. In the centre of the main building, on the third floor, was the governor's house. Accommodation was also provided in the main building for Miss Ross, the matron, and a wing mistress. There was a school room both in the girls and boys department supervised by a master who came in the morning. The dining room was at the opposite side of the corridor from the kitchen and the food was delivered through service hatches and carried into the hall. The kitchen had a range of boilers, a large one at each end with smaller ones in the centre. Two side doors, centre door and passage were used for collecting and removing the empty dishes. A reading desk stood on a dais at the south end of the room with a platform extending from it on either side for the officials. Approximately 300 inmates could be fed in this hall. The chaplain's room was just off the hall. The large wash-house had a Morton's patent water lifter which pumped water from the rain tank in the adjoining yard. There were also two large boilers for steam which was taken to every portion of the premises by a ramification of underground pipes. There was a constant supply of hot water throughout the whole building. The heat for the washing, drying, cooking and heating, was provided by the steam pipes led from the general boiler house. The wooden washing machine lasted 35 years, being replaced in 1903 by earthenware tubs. The Infirmary (D block) is in the shape of the letter T and consists of a centre block with three storeys, three two-storeyed wings on the north, south and east side. The north and south were for ordinary cases and contained

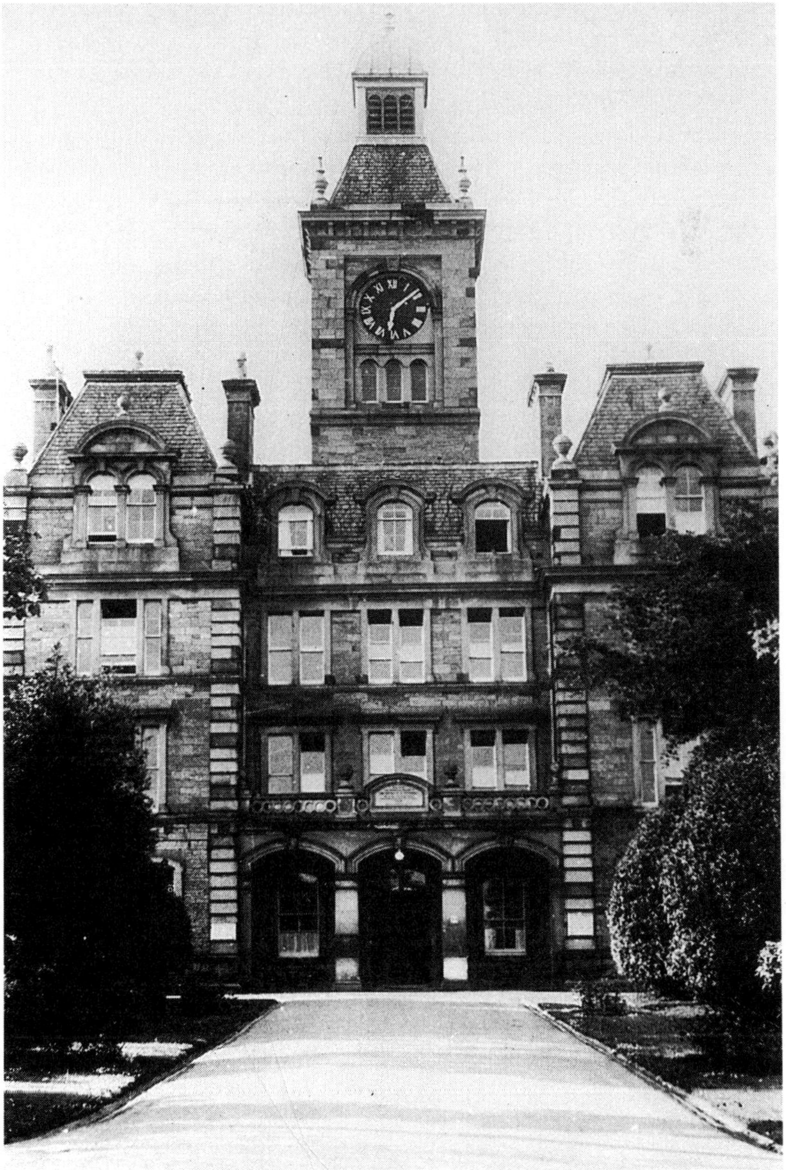

The clock tower, Western General Hospital

two wards, 76 by 23 feet, and giving a 1000 cubic feet per bed. At the extreme ends of each are the lavatories, baths and water closets. On the third leg of the T were the male and female fever wards, accommodating 40 patients, with 1200 cubic feet for each patient. In the centre block to the right of the entrance was the doctor's room. Close by were the children's wards and a whooping cough ward on the second floor. The kitchen was on a partly sunk level in the south wing. The whole building was surrounded by its own airing and pleasure ground in which there was separate means of access from the various wards for the different classes of patients. To the north of the Infirmary was the washing-house and laundry solely for the infirmary. There was a separate washing green separate for the the main building.

The total cost of the undertaking, including the laying out of the ground, but not the furnishing, was under £40,000. The whole was completed in little more than eighteen months. Dr Paul explained that the new building would not be a heavy burden upon the rate payers because of the sum obtained from the Caledonian Railway Company for the old premises. Furthermore the remarkable increase in house building in the parish over the previous fifteen years had resulted in more rate payers to share the financial burden.

Life in the Poorhouse

The life of the Poorhouse thereafter went on at an even pace and there are very few records of what actually happened. The main source of information was the Annual Report to the Board. Tables 1–7 give an indication of numbers and food.

Table 1. St Cuthberts Parish Poor Law Hospital, Lothian Road

Overall Poor Registered with the Board in 1866	
Adult poor in the community	1185
Children in the community	303
Lunatics	141
In licenced wards at the Poorhouse	42
In private homes	9
Ordinary inmates of the Poor House	427
	2107

Expenditure on feeding and clothing the adult poor was £9,059 consisting of

Oatmeal	£248
Barley	£58
Split and Barley Peas	£306
Tea and sugar	£241
Bread	£772
Milk	£280
Beef	£299
Vegetables	£14
Ales and Wines	£125
Beef, Steak and Egg	£177

Clothing, soap, tobacco and snuff were provided.

Table 2. Craigleith Poorhouse, 1870

Total number		1870
Adult poor		1167
Children at Board		291
Lunatics –	Public asylum	168
	Private Asylum	11
	Private house	10
Inmates in the Poorhouse		380
Admitted to the Poorhouse in the year		1574
Expenditure for feeding and clothing		£10,142

This was a self-contained community, segregated according to previous social background, adult and children, fit and unwell. Many of the support services, e.g. tailors, shoemakers, knitting and sewing, joiners and smiths (Table 4) were provided by the inmates.

It is difficult to obtain an idea of life in the Poorhouse. The average individual who entered or even worked in such an institution was not given to writing memoirs. Some idea of life and the reasons for admission are given in the Report of the Royal Commission on the Poor Law in 1909. The commissioners appear to have visited the Craigleith Poor Law Hospital.

The Royal Commission on the Poor Laws and Relief of Distress 1909 came to the conclusion in their far-reaching report for the whole of Britain that:

> it was very unpleasant to record that notwithstanding our assumed moral and material progress and notwithstanding the enormous annual expenditure amounting to nearly £60 million per year upon poor relief, education and public health, we still have a vast army of persons quartered upon us unable to support themselves and an army which in number has recently shown signs of increase rather than decrease. To what is this retrogression due? It cannot be attributed to lack of expenditure. Is this costly

Table 3. Craigleith Poorhouse, 1880

Total number on Roll		1985
Aged and infirm		71
Widows with Children		73
Deserted wives		53
Mothers with illegitimate children		24
Relieved on account of need of sustenance		849
Husband in jail		11
Parents in jail		3
Orphans		10
Deserted children		11
Out-of-door poor		975
Children at Board		224
Lunatics Public		284
	Private	22
	No. in Poorhouse	480
Admitted during the year		2536
Average number of inmates		651
Cost 3s. (15p) per week		

and elaborate machine we have established effective and, if so, where does it fail to establish its ends?

There was a distinction between methods of relief practiced by Boards of Guardians by 'indoor relief' and 'outdoor relief', between maintenance supplied in an institution and maintenance or part-maintenance by means of an allowance. The significance of the distinction lay in the principle that when the guardians granted relief in an institution, whether workhouse, infirmary or school, they made themselves entirely responsible for the lives of the recipients. The children were to be properly fed, clothed and educated; the patients in the infirmary were to be treated appropriately and made to carry out their doctor's instructions and the inmates were to lead a sober, clean and orderly life:

> The loss of liberty may be keenly felt and greatly resented, more especially in the workhouse; the loss of family life is hardly less serious for the children though they may not know what they miss.

The intention was that the workhouse was to be a miscellaneous institution, being a place where able-bodied might be set to work under conditions which should be the least harmful both to themselves and to the independent labourer. The inmates reflected the mixed character of the town population from which they were drawn. A thousand or more inmates of all types were gathered together in one of these large town workhouses. The problem of organisation and discipline required great skill and strength of character on the part of the master. In the

Table 4. Edinburgh Parish Council 1890

No. of Registered Poor		3670
Out-of-Door Poor in the community		1641
Children at Board in the community		542
Orphans		271
Adult Registered — Poorhouse		827
Lunatics Public		472
Wards		152
Private		307
Patients in Poorhouse	men	235
	women	227
	boys	42
	girls	32

The inmates worked as Tailors, Shoemakers, at Knitting and Sewing, and as Joiners and Smiths.

Causes of death in the Poorhouse during 1890 were —

Tuberculosis		1
Exhaustion		2
Disease of the nervous system		15
Cardiovascular and valvular disease		22
Respiratory disease	Phthisis	22
	Pneumonia	15
Alimentary		6

absence of these qualities institutions presented many painful features. The able-bodied were not occupied and spent their day in sullen idleness and the old people suffered from the general atmosphere of repression and gloom.

The chaplain of one workhouse said to the Commission:

> There is no doubt in my mind that life in the workhouse deteriorates mentally, morally and physically the habitual inmate. The life of these people is better described as more or less a miserable existence than a life. It must be admitted that the mental capacity of the average person who drifts into the workhouse is of a low order but in countless instances there is a gradual deterioration of intellect owing to the lack of almost all incentive to use the brain. The inmate finds the necessities of life provided for him with scarcely any thought or effort on his part. In the majority of cases, the sole idea is to fill the mind or to get as much to eat and as much sleep and get as large an amount of immunity from even the lightest task as possible. The young may arrive full of spirit, but rapidly deteriorate to lazy and unwilling to do anything, though physically able

Table 5. Craigleith Poorhouse 1890

Quantity of Food used in a Year	
Bread	103,675 loaves (1½lb each)
Sweet milk	16,388 gallons
Churn milk	10,029 gallons
Beef and Mutton	2,896 stones
Cheese	4,031lb
Oatmeal	413 cwt
Barley	125 cwt
Pease	82 cwt
Peasemeal	37 cwt
Rice	40 cwt
Potatoes	4ton 17 cwt
Fish	8,880 lb
Butter	3,973 lb
Eggs	18,200
Tea	2,449 lb
Sugar	80 cwt
Salt	68 cwt
The costs were:	
Coals	£53.12s.3d. (£53.62p)
Oatmeal	£39.3s.11d. (£39.20p)
Churned milk	£9.12s.6d. (£9.63p)
Butter and eggs	£3.1s.1d. (£3.06p)
Eggs	£15.11s.2d. (£15.56p)
Groceries	£3.9s.1d. (£3.46p)
Beef	£77.12s.0d. (£77.60p)
Tea	£33.17s.4d. (£33.87p)

3 bottles of port wine and whiskey were bought as stimulants.

NB 20 cwt = 1 ton
1 cwt = 112 lbs
2.2lb = 1 Kg
1 gallon = 8 pints : 1 pint = 473 ml

to work. Physically and mentally inmates degenerate. Varied employment helps to keep them interested in life but is not an absolute success. Married mothers will sometimes remain in the house for the good of their children and after some years lose all desire to leave the workhouse or they become mentally unfit to take up the duties of life again.

Table 6. Distribution of Occupancy in Craigleith Poorhouse in 1910

Males	
Ground Floor	33
First floor	46
Second Floor (Wing)	28
Third Floor	82
Attic floor	22
Boys	
First floor and top floor	25
Classified Wards	33
Females	
Ground floor	10
First floor	31
Centre back	3
Second Floor	30
Attic floor	19
Classified wards — ground floor	26
First floor	28
Second floor	18
Nursery – first floor	14
Children – first floor	15
– second floor	24
Hospital – Males	
Main building	21
Ground floor	31
First floor	14
– Females	
Ground floor	20
First floor	74
Second floor	9
The following Wards being Isolation and Probationary Wards were not included in the Main House or Hospital	
At Gate –	
Probationary – Beds	
Males Nos.15 and 17	16
Females, No. 51	9
Females, No. 51, with cribs for children	4
Venereal Ward	–
Males No. 26	7
Females Nos.2 and 61	4
Eruption Wards	–
Males No. 30	7
Females No. 55	7

Emigration

Emigration was a method of giving a new future to certain classes of children who were dependent upon the parish guardians. Boards of Guardians were empowered to procure or assist in procuring the emigration of orphans or deserted children under the age of 16 years. No emigration could take place until the child had consented before the Justices. The mode of emigration was through various charitable agencies, the Roman Catholic Emigration Agency, The Waifs and Strays Society, Dr Barnardos Homes, Miss MacPherson's Homes or one of the various well-known Emigration Agencies. The home in which the child was placed was chosen by the Agency through which the child emigrated. No payment other than the cost of travelling was made by the guardian. The child was practically adopted under contract.

Table 7. Provisions

	Year 1909	*Year 1910*
Bread	53,840/8oz loaf	41,265/8oz loaf
	378,529/6oz loaf	366,036/6oz loaf
	3,856/2lb loaf	4,428/2lb loaf
Sweet milk	20,932 gals	20,028 gals
Skim milk	11,746 gals	10,564 gals
Churn milk	4,510 gals	4,230 gals
Sugar	3,947 st	3,667 st
Oatmeal	554cwt 95lbs	499cwt 105lbs
Barley	131cwt 65lbs	119cwt 38lbs
Peas	93cwt	85cwt 81lbs
Peasemeal	45cwt 39lbs	42cwt 10lbs
Rice	59cwt 23lbs	59cwt 91lbs
Butter	5,348lbs 4oz	5,387lbs 4oz
Cheese	182lbs	234lbs
Potatoes	6 ton 70lbs	6 ton 477lbs
Fish	10,306lbs	10,151 lbs
Eggs	13,251	10,786
Tea	2,586 lbs	2,476 lbs
Sugar	88cwt 40lbs	87cwt 62lbs
Salt	90cwt 26lbs	85cwt 51lbs
Gin	–	–
Wine	–	16 glasses
Whiskey	8 6/12 bottles	18 5/12 bottles
Brandy	1 bottle	5 glasses
Soap (hard)	29cwt	23cwt 65lbs
Soap (soft)	90cwt 23lbs	81cwt 80 lbs
Tobacco	331lbs	294lbs
Snuff	23lbs	14lbs
Coals	867tons 9cwt	1017tons 16¼cwts
Dross	487tons 11cwt	1043tons 8cwt
Flour	34cwt 101lbs	33cwt 102lbs
Soda	51cwt	47cwt 106lbs
Cornflour	60lbs	90lbs
Lentils	27cwt 62lbs	22cwt 17lbs

Able-bodied men and women in the poorhouses were encouraged to emigrate to the white colonies, such Canada, Australia and New Zealand. During the period 1835–36 5,241 persons were sent out to the above countries at a cost of £28,000 from Britain.

In Scotland a pauper was admitted to a Poorhouse on an order signed for by the Inspector of the Poor. This Order was given only after a medical man had certified that the applicant was not in good health. There was a constant appraisal of the inmates of the poorhouse and they were discharged when the medical officer certified them to be healthy and able-bodied. These patients who were regarded as fit were called the turnouts or tests. The workhouse also sheltered a number of men whose mental capacities were below the average. These men constantly took their discharge from the workhouse and then returned, picking up a precarious liveliood outside for a few days, working at odd jobs. Some of these alternated between prison and workhouse with short intervals at liberty. A considerable number of those frequenting institutions were confirmed drunkards and persons leading an immoral life who came to the poorhouse to be cured of the diseases they had brought upon themselves and returned as often as they left.

Malnutrition and Diet

There were many poor in the city during this time. During the late nineteenth century ten per cent of the population were too poor to buy sufficient food for themselves. Such malnutrition, in addition to bad sanitation, inadequate overcrowded housing, insufficient land for farming, and a host of acute and chronic infectious diseases, led to rickets, poor stature, and high maternal and infant mortality. Adulteration of food and beverages by the unscrupulous, was widespread: flour with chalk, and tea with dried oak leaves.

In 1903 Patton, Dunlop and Inglis published a study of the diet of the labouring classes in Edinburgh, amongst whom a large proportion of poorly developed and undersized children and adults were found. They studied two groups; families with assured and adequate incomes, and the poor, who were unable to buy the necessities of life, either because of inadequate income or because of employment that was only casual. Some families living in poor housing on small irregular wages refused to take part in the study. The range of expenditure on food varied from 2.5 to 9.5 pence per man per day. The daily nutrient intake per man varied from 1,100 to 4,800 kilocalories. The wife and children of the poor families lived on tea, bread and potatoes, the tradition being that the man ate butcher meat daily. The larder was replenished with small quantities of food bought each day. Alcohol was a great problem, affecting work record and hence income. In contrast, the families of workmen receiving regular wages ate meals consisting of bread, potatoes, oatmeal, eggs, beef, mutton, ham, butter, herrings, cod and sugar. Fresh vegetables were confined to potatoes, cabbage, peas, rice and barley.

A further detrimental feature of the diet in Edinburgh before the First World

War was that over 12 per cent of samples of milk contained tubercle bacilli. The consequence was that the bovine, milk-borne form of tuberculosis occurred in 32.4 per cent of tuberculosis patients aged under 5 years, 29 per cent aged 5 to 16, and 2.9 per cent of adults.

The general mixed workhouse was regarded by many of the established working population as a way of obtaining ample food, sleep, unlimited idleness and low gossip to suit the inclination of the dirty, dissolute and vicious old man or woman who, as an alternative to a life of petty pilfering and assiduous begging, asked for the aid of the guardians of the Poor Houses to make out a not disagreeable life.

The practice in Scotland was that women having the care of children should, so long as such care is required from them, be wholly excluded from the category and stigmata of the able-bodied inmate of the Poor House. This enabled women who were widowed or destitute to be cared for in homes. Under the Law of Scotland from at least 1579, as definitely interpreted in 1864 by the Court of Appeal, it was illegal for the destitution authority to give relief in any form to the able-bodied or even to admit them to the poorhouse. This prohibition applied not only to residents but also to vagrants. Every applicant for relief, whether local resident or a wayfarer had, according to the regulations, to be examined by the parish doctor and certified on soul and conscience whether or not he was able-bodied. Only those men and those single women unencumbered with children and certified to be suffering from some ailment were admitted to the poorhouse. However, in reality the occupants of the Scottish poorhouses in the large towns in no way differed from those of the English general mixed workhouse. In practice it was difficult to prevent intolerable hardship to able-bodied men who were absolutely destitute and to their wives and children. In this way it was possible to obviate the dangers attendant on leaving the hungry at large without relief.

The Central Authorities officially advised the Parish Councils in 1878 that in the case of a really destitute person the Inspector of the Poor should not carry the letter of the law to an extreme. It was obvious that if a person was really destitute, they would rapidly become disabled from want of food. The Assistant Inspector sent cases to the Medical Officer who, in practice, usually accepted a very slight ailment as sufficient to justify a Certificate of Disablement. The Medical Officer certified the cases sent to him by the Assistant Inspector. The Medical Officer sat in an empty room into which came a succession of applicants all of whom had been already identified as destitute, i.e. without the means of subsistance. It was the duty of the doctor to reject them from every kind of relief if he was able to demonstrate that they were free of any complaint or infirmity that made them unsuitable for the Work House. His examination consisted, in practice, of asking questions. If the applicant presented some complaint such as sciatica, neuralgia or rheumatism that could not be tested by the stethoscope or similar instrument the doctor certified him at once. If the complaint was of a sore foot, then following an examination the doctor decided whether it was sore enough. Only the unfortunate novice who said that he would willingly work

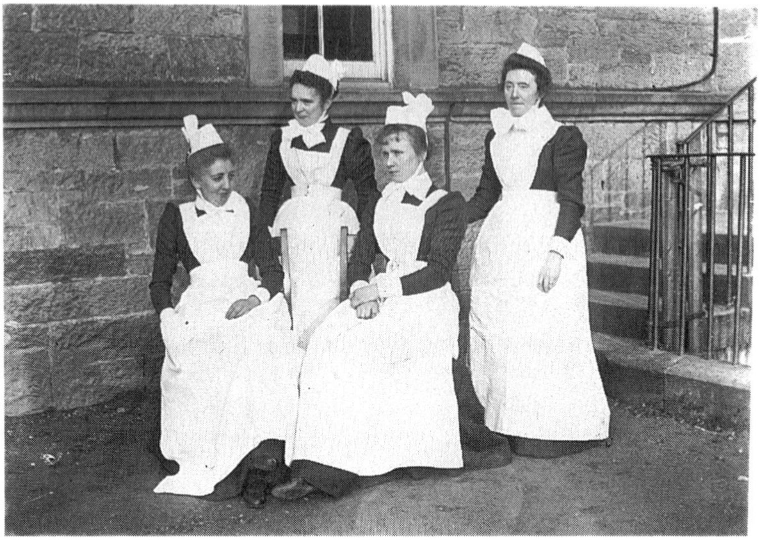

Four of the nursing staff of Craigleith Poorhouse Hospital, approximately between June 1899 and October 1901. Figures seated from left E. Crowe (Matron until approx. 1913–14); Helen E Hill (later MacMaster) Figures standing from left Maiden name unknown but married Guy Dick and went to live in Carluke; last nurse unknown.

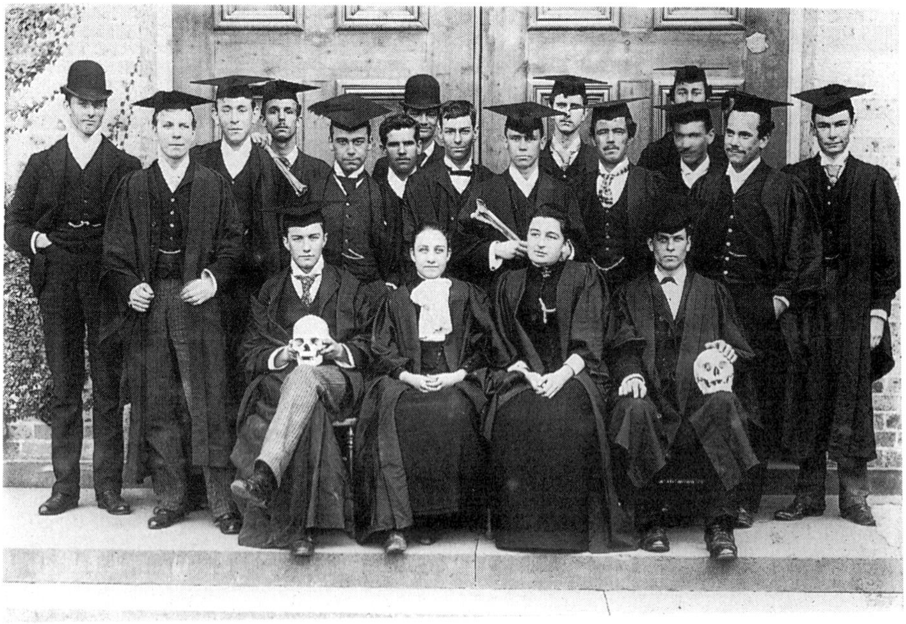

Group of students at Edinburgh University. Fourth from right of middle row and wearing a patterned tie, Hugh MacMaster from Sydney, Australia (married Helen Hill), and who visited Craigleith Poorhouse Hospital wards, presumably on University/ Royal Infirmary Perpetual Pass ticket. Taken between 1894 and 1901

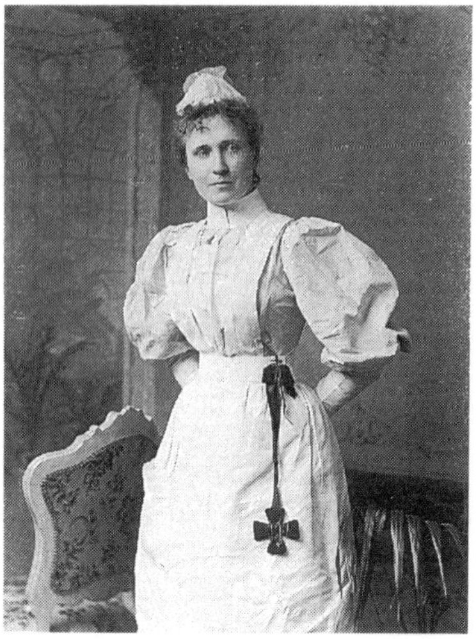

Helen Emily Hill (born 18.10.1875); nurse at Craigleith Poorhouse Hospital, married Hugh MacMaster. Taken July 1899

if he could get employment was rejected and turned into the street. Overall, 49% of the population of the inmates of the poorhouse were over 60 years of age. After visiting one of the Scottish poorhouses, almost certainly Craigleith Poorhouse, a sub-committee of the Royal Commission reported to the Royal Commission. The numbers admitted to the workhouse increased by 25% to 30% in the winter. The vast workhouse had only a single resident Medical Officer, a young woman. Aided only by a consultant visiting three times a week, her duties were to examine thoroughly every inmate on entrance in order to discover their exact state of health and the nature of any disease or infirmity; to certify which of the adults — all presumably non able-bodied — were fit for the test (work); to settle the diet and treatment of all persons actually sick; and to supervise the arrangements for the children and infants. In each of the workhouses the 'hospital cases' alone numbered between 200 and 300. In one of them at any rate there was a phthisical (tuberculosis) ward, a surgical ward, an ophthalmic ward, a lying-in ward and a male venereal ward all under the charge of the same young lady doctor who had the medical supervision of the rest of the establishment.

The nursing staff was not very good, extensive use being made of pauper inmates. In many of the large wards there were no trained nursing attendants, even in the day time. In one of these institutions there were only three night nurses for all the hundreds of patients. The operations, including some abdominal sections and others of apparent difficulty, were performed by the same young lady doctor with the help of the consultant who was a physician. No records of the patients' care or operations were kept. This young lady doctor also had to extract the teeth of patients when required. She was one of the earliest female graduates in medicine from Edinburgh (1896). There was still

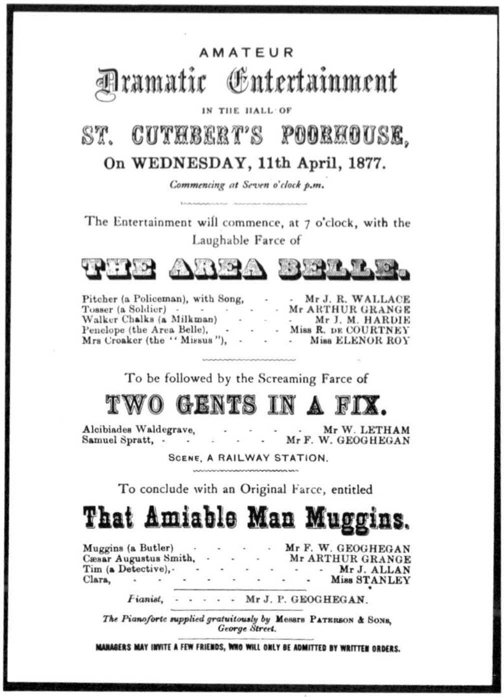
AMATEUR

Dramatic Entertainment

IN THE HALL OF

ST. CUTHBERT'S POORHOUSE,

On WEDNESDAY, 11th April, 1877.

Commencing at Seven o'clock p.m.

The Entertainment will commence, at 7 o'clock, with the Laughable Farce of

THE AREA BELLE.

Pitcher (a Policeman), with Song, - - Mr J. R. WALLACE
Tosser (a Soldier) - - - - - Mr ARTHUR GRANGE
Walker Chalks (a Milkman) - - - Mr J. M. HARDIE
Penelope (the Area Belle), - - - Miss R. DE COURTNEY
Mrs Croaker (the "Missus"), - - - Miss ELENOR ROY

To be followed by the Screaming Farce of

TWO GENTS IN A FIX.

Alcibiades Waldegrave, - - - - Mr W. LETHAM
Samuel Spratt, - - - - - Mr F. W. GEOGHEGAN

SCENE, A RAILWAY STATION.

To conclude with an Original Farce, entitled

That Amiable Man Muggins.

Muggins (a Butler) - - - - Mr F. W. GEOGHEGAN
Cæsar Augustus Smith, - - - Mr ARTHUR GRANGE
Tim (a Detective), - - - - - - - Mr J. ALLAN
Clara, - - - - - - - - Miss STANLEY

Pianist, - - - - - Mr J. P. GEOGHEGAN.

The Pianoforte supplied gratuitously by Messrs PATERSON & SONS, *George Street.*

MANAGERS MAY INVITE A FEW FRIENDS, WHO WILL ONLY BE ADMITTED BY WRITTEN ORDERS.

Concert programme – St Cuthbert's Poorhouse

so much prejudice that women had difficulty finding jobs and a few new posts were created specially for them, including the job at the Craigleith Poorhouse. Her son was Sir John Brotherstone, Professor of Public Health in Edinburgh University, who subsequently became Chief Medical Officer for Scotland. His daughter, Dr Helen Zealley, is the Chief Administrative Medical Officer for Lothian.

During 1890 Craigleith Poorhouse looked after 724 patients who were cured, relieved or died. This meant that two patients were admitted and two discharged each day. The individuals cared for were essentially the chronic sick. The hospital was overcrowded from time to time, hence there was a need to put less urgent cases on a waiting list. The needs of the Hospital were developing with more ill patients being admitted. A need for an operating (surgical) ward and small single room accommodation was identified.

In 1900, a Resident Medical Officer was appointed at an annual salary of £100. A Chaplain was appointed, the Rev. William Macdonald, with a salary of £150 a year. An assistant nurse was appointed at an annual cost of £20 and a trained children's nurse for £30 a year. The head nurse, Miss Robertson, was paid £60 per annum. A cook cost £25 per annum and this was increased to £27.10s (£27.50p). The salary of the Matron was raised from an initial salary of £50 to £70 per year in 1910. When Miss Ross, the Matron, resigned in 1910, her successor was Miss Robertson, aged 45 years.

The care of children was an important aspect of the work of the Craigleith Poorhouse. The children were subsequently either fostered or placed in apprenticeship. It is of interest that in an exhibition of the work of the pioneer photographer William Henry Fox Talbot there was a photograph of children gathered outside the Palace of Holyrood. Following the publication of this photograph in the *Edinburgh Evening News*, a letter was received from an elderly gentleman who said the photograph was of children from the Craigleith Poorhouse. This elderly man, Mr David Stewart, said his parents had died in 1904 and that David Stewart, his brother James and his sister Jane were taken to the Poorhouse, the brother being aged 10 and his sister 8. Foster parents were eventually found for them as was the case with other children. It is possible that the children's section of Craigleith Poorhouse was temporary rather than children being taken there for the whole of their upbringing.

Children aged 14 were sent to service or to apprenticeship and tools were purchased for them. There were 90 children in Craigleith at that time — 53 boys and 37 girls. They are remembered as grey-clad and smelling of carbolic.

From the opening until about 1885 the building was known as St Cuthbert's & Canongate Poor House. Thereafter until 1895 it was just 'St Cuthbert's'; then from 1895 it was known as Craigleith Poor House until the start of World War I in 1914 when it was renamed 2nd Scottish General Hospital, Craigleith.

3

Military Hospital 1914–18

From 1914 to 1918 the Hospital was requisitioned by the 2nd Scottish General Hospital, a Territorial Unit. The Poor Law inmates were transferred to Craiglockhart Hospital.

The hospital was to be committed to the care of sick and wounded British service men. The Unit was staffed by Edinburgh doctors and commanded by Lieutenant Colonel Sir Joseph Fayrer, who was at that time Medical Superintendent of the Royal Infirmary. The first military patient was admitted on August 14, 1914. These military patients were transported by rail to Craigleith Station which was located below the site of the present Holiday Inn Hotel.

As befitted a Military Hospital, the provisions were sparse, spotless and the whole enterprise was conducted as a military operation.

The hospital section (D Block) of the Craigleith Poorhouse was provided with a surgical theatre suitable for the needs of the Poorhouse, but quite inadequate for a Military Hospital. An entirely new operating theatre with space for several surgeons was built, close to the main building and within easy reach of steam, water and electrical supplies. The main room measured 30ft × 20ft, constructed of wood and galvanised iron and covered with roof-felt under corrugated iron. The supply of sterilised water for the theatre was a problem, so ordinary domestic tanks were used. Captain Guy fitted a dental room at his own expense. Most of the surgical operations enabled recruits and territorial soldiers to return to active service abroad. Sister Macaulay was the theatre sister. The operating theatre was still being used in the 1950's before conversion to a Central Sterile Store Department, which is still housed in that building.

A recreation hut was built on the northern side of the Hospital which opened to patients on 1 August 1916. It consisted of an entrance hall, recreation hall (48ft × 28ft), reading and writing room (26ft × 20ft), billiard room (26ft × 20ft), attendant's room with cloakroom and store room for books etc.

At the mobilisation of No. 2 Scottish Hospital no special provision was made for pathological work in Craigleith Hospital. Materials for diagnosis were sent to the Laboratories of the Royal Infirmary and the Royal College of Physicians. Later, a laboratory was equipped, under the supervision of Major Boyd, in a small room in the hospital. Among the Unit personnel, skilled laboratory assistants were identified. Sergeant Pettigrew, formerly of the University Surgical Laboratory, assisted by Private Buchanan, and later Private Leeper, looked after the microscopic work of the laboratory which was situated in a small room opposite Lieutenant Baker's room.

There was an orderly room which provided an accurate record of daily,

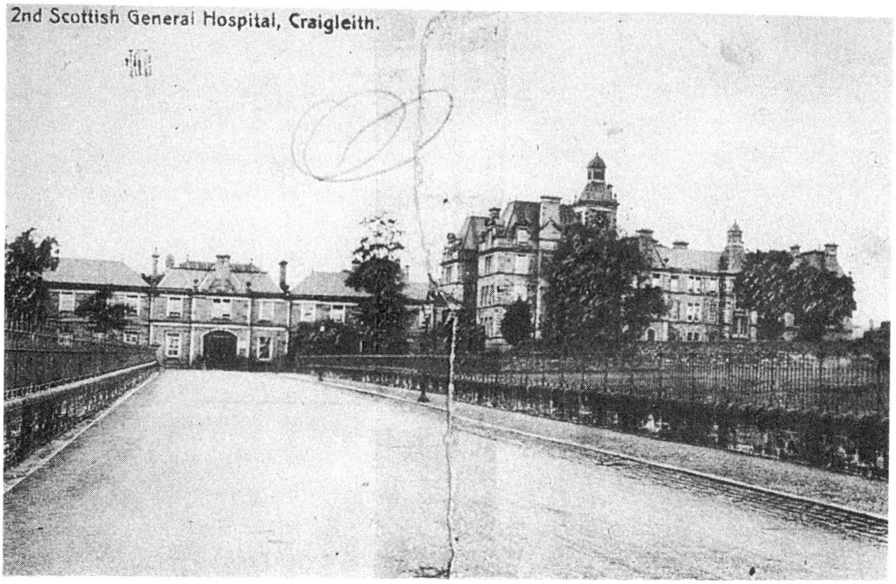

2nd Scottish General Hospital, Craigleith, showing gatehouse, flanked by admission wards and gardens used to feed the inmates.

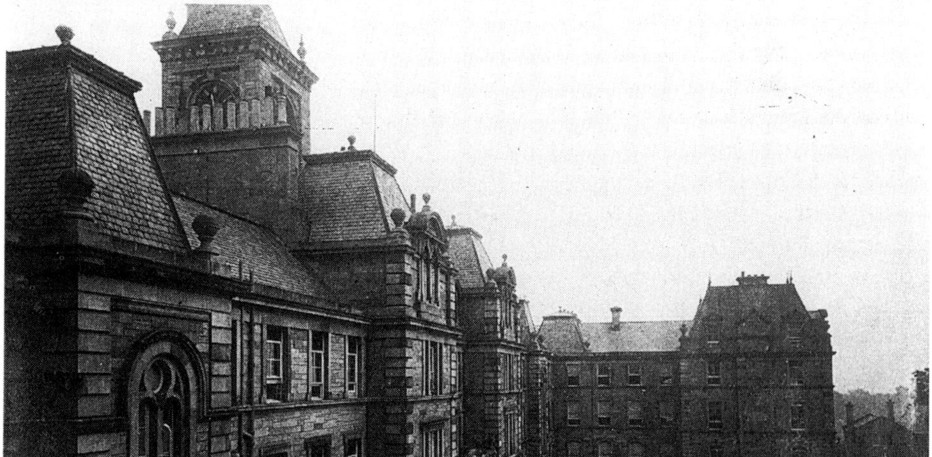

Craigleith Poorhouse – taken about 1914.

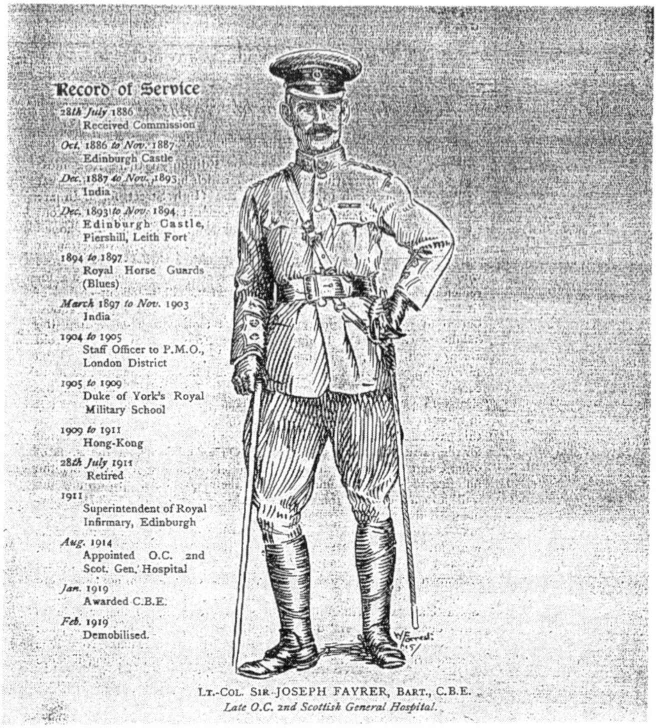

Cartoon in *Craigleith Chronicle*, with Record of Service of Lt.-Col. Sir Joseph Fayrer, Bart., C.B.E., Officer Commanding 2nd Scottish General Hospital, 1914–1918

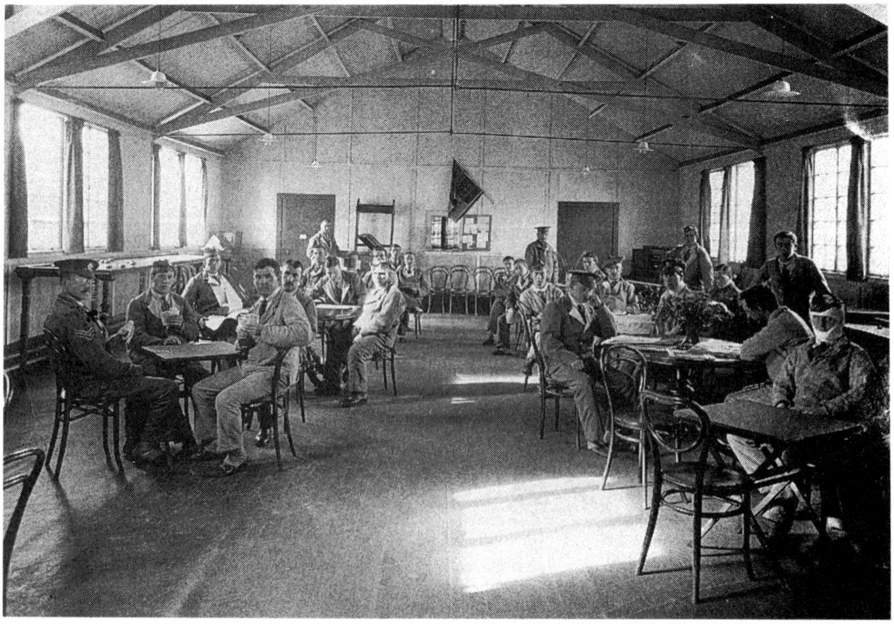

Recreation hall 1914–1918

weekly, monthly, quarterly and annual reports; the paying of patients' bounties; issuing railway travel warrants, and communicating with the Command Paymaster, the officer in charge of records and the patients' commanding officer.

The Hospital was very busy. From the day of mobilisation to June 1915, 5,464 home service patients and 941 Expeditionary patients were admitted, including Belgian soldiers. 60,560 hot meals were cooked, 1360 major operations performed, 1050 dental cases were seen, and 2823 teeth were extracted. During this time the Radiographic Department of the Hospital was established with a floor area of 150 square-feet — about half of which was assigned to the scullery. A ten-inch spark coil, with accessory equipment, transformed the current from the lighting mains to serve the X-ray tubes. 783 X-rays were taken over this period.

During the six months from 1 January to 30 June 1915, the Eye Department saw 1342 patients, Ear Nose and Throat Department 618, and 436 men were supplied with spectacles.

Some of the soldiers who died in the hospital are buried in the cemetery at Comely Bank.

A number of patients were moved to other hospitals: 359 to the Royal Infirmary, 70 to Leith, 256 to the Deaconess Hospital and 401 to Dalmeny. On Saturday 25 July 1915 the Flora Stevenson School was taken over and 103 patients transferred from the main building. For the duration of the war this facility was used for medical cases only. Some patients were moved into convalescent homes. A voluntary worker, Mr J. R. Wilson, W.S., devoted himself to the supervision of work connected with the convalescent homes.

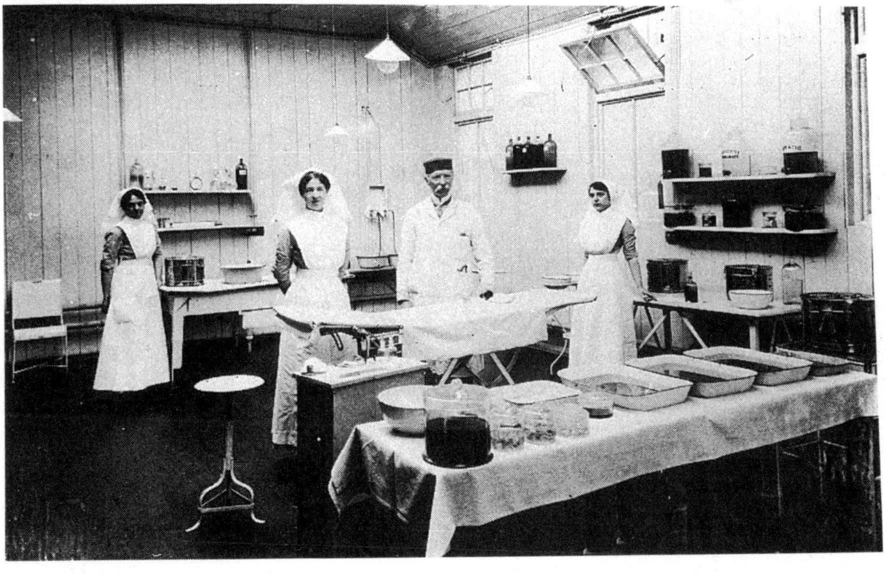

Operating theatre, Craigleith Hospital 1914–1918

One of the convalescent homes was Craigforth Convalescent Red Cross Hospital at Elie, accommodating 20 patients. Dr A. L. Pentland-Smith of Elie was the Medical Officer and the owner, Mrs Outhwaite, was the Matron. Facilities for playing clock golf, tennis and quoits were available.

One of the patients in Craigleith Hospital later received the VC; he was Lance-corporal Joseph Tombs who was decorated for 'conspicuous gallantry near Rue de Bois on the 16 June 1915'.

In June 1915 the staff included: Captain E. Bramwell, Captain G. L. Chiene, Captain J. Easton, Captain R. A. Fleming, Captain H. G. Langwil, Captain J. Millar, Captain H. Rainey, Captain A. Scott Skirving, Captain W. J. Stewart, Captain J. W. Simpson, Lieut. E. Allan, Lieut. D. Charteris Graham, Lieut. J. Donald Gunn, Lieut. R. L. Ritchie, Lieut. A. Watson Simpson, Col. The Rev. H. M. Davidson, Col. The Rev. J. A. McClymont, Lieut. Col. The Rev. Marshall Lang, Lieut. Col. The Rev. J. Mackintosh, Capt. The Rev. A. W. Ferguson, Capt. The Rev. A. E. Wallace.

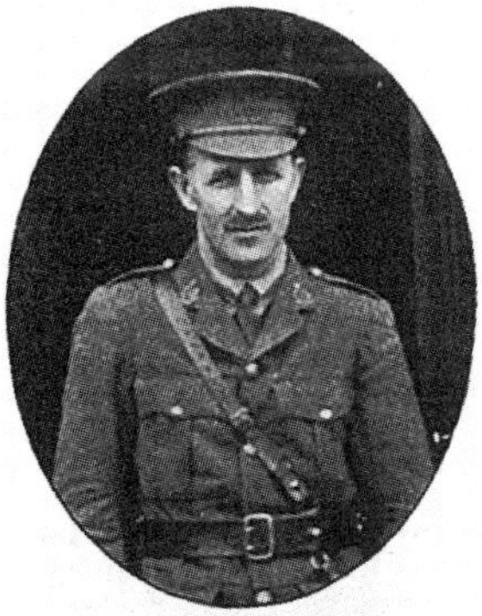

CAPT. J. W. SIMPSON.

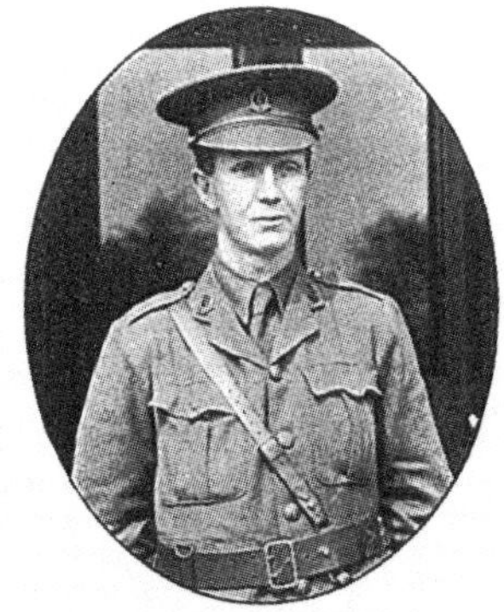

CAPT. W. J. STUART.

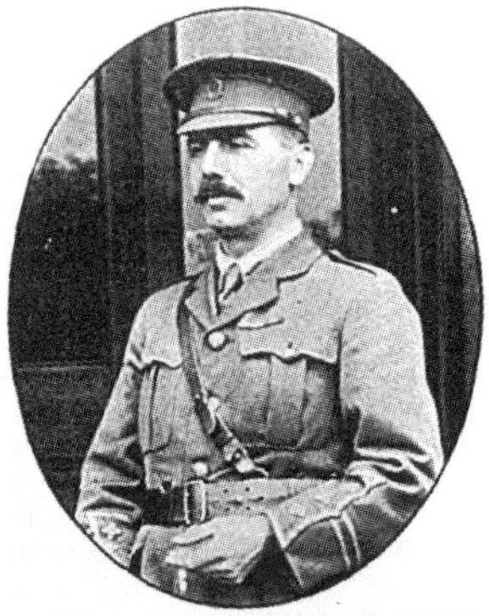

CAPT. A. A. SCOT SKIRVING, C.M.G.

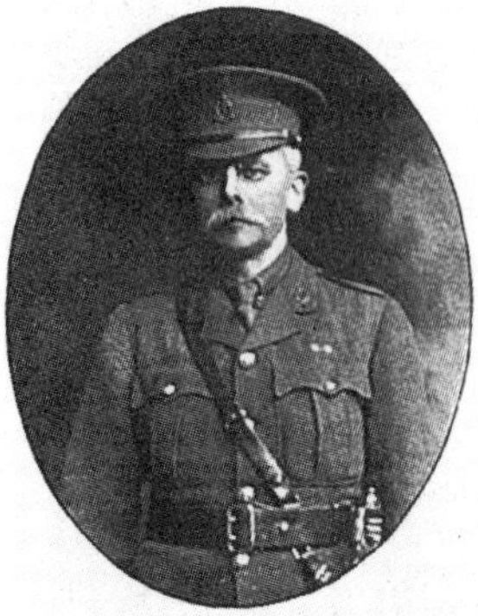

CAPT. R. A. FLEMING.

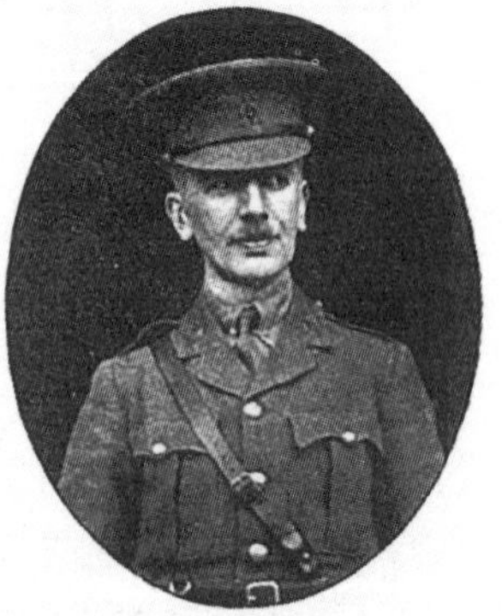

CAPT. E. BRAMWELL.

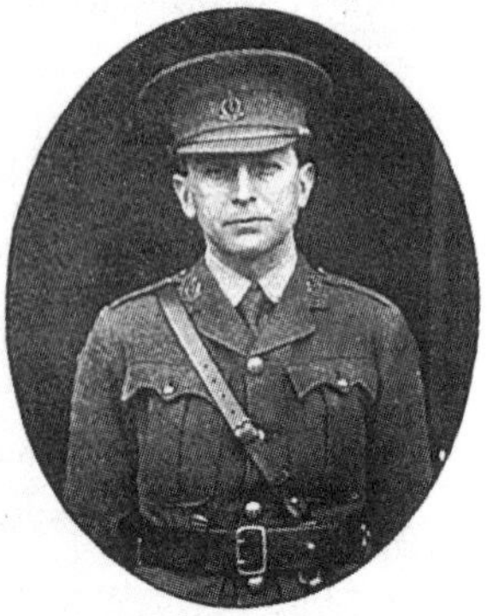

CAPT. J. EASON.

Six Captains on medical staff of military hospital

Nursing Staff

Few of the nursing staff were trained. The Matron was Miss Milligan and Assistant Matron Miss Humphries. Miss Milligan was sent overseas to the East in 1916. She was succeeded by Miss CW Millar who trained in the Royal Infirmary. Most of the nurses were local ladies who were volunteers. A photograph taken in 1918 of the entire staff showed many of the volunteer nurses. Voluntary work was very important; for example the Quartermaster was assisted by Mr Sutherland, C. A, during his spare time. The work included catering, clothing, storing of linen, washing and disinfecting of clothing, transport, the supply of provisions and equipment including furniture, linen, and instruments, and the care of arms and accoutrements etc.

When the war broke out massage treatment (known now as Physiotherapy) in the hospital was undertaken. by Mr and Mrs Almeric Paget. Miss French, daughter of Field Marshall Sir John French, who had just finished her training in Medical Gymnastics and Massage became Honorary Secretary of the scheme. Monsieur Soirrons of Belgium acted as a masseur during this time.

Concerts were given by the Kings Theatre Orchestra and other musicians. A gramophone with records was presented by Col. McClymont.

The Library Committee was given a monthly sum of £2 to supplement the fund for the supply of daily papers to the wards. The Library Committee was

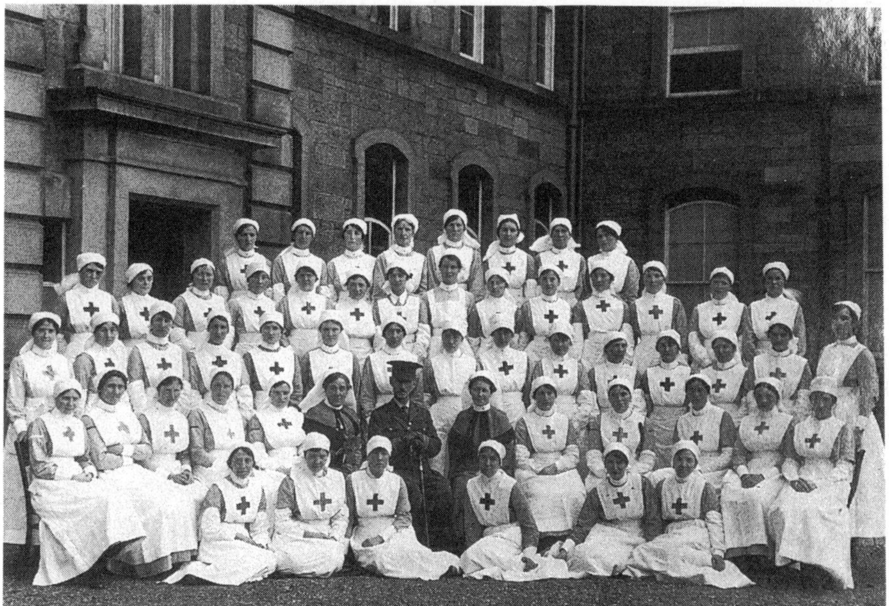

Lieut. Col. Sir Joseph Fayrer, Officer in Charge, with nursing staff at 2nd Scottish General Hospital (later Craigleith Hospital) 1914–1918

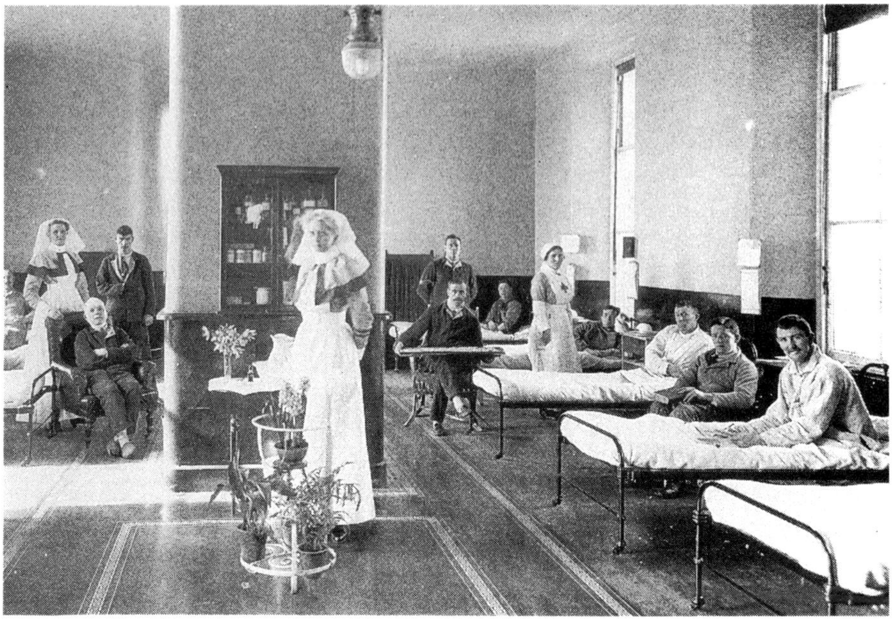

One of the Nightingale wards (possibly D1 or D2) 1914–1918

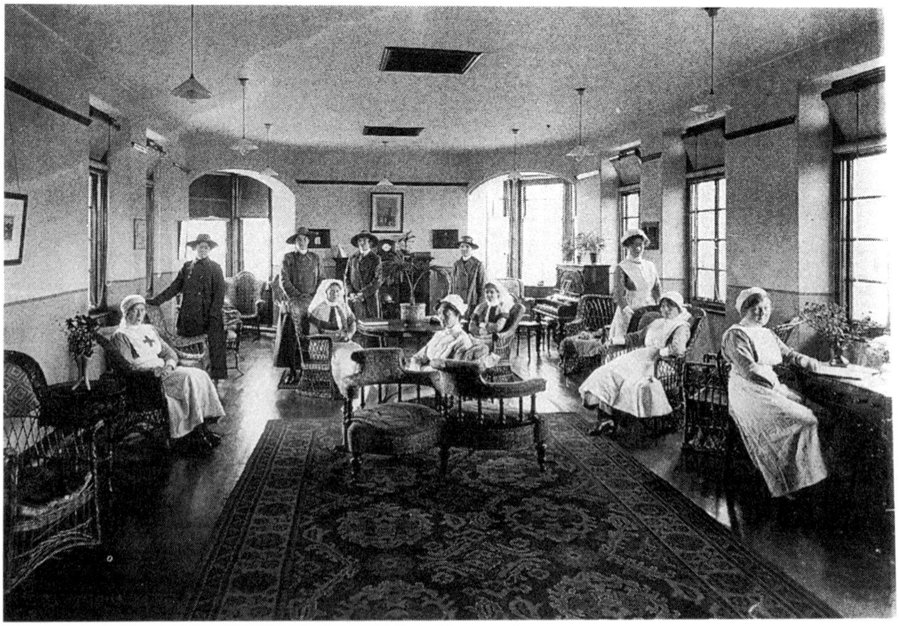

Nurse recreation sitting room, Craigleith Hospital

also ‘indebted to Mrs Anderson of 52 Palmerston Place for her constant kindness in making and mending picture puzzles’. The Committee was also grateful to Mr James T Stewart of Eglinton Crescent who provided the library with electric light.

There was a Sergeant’s mess with a billiard room. Cigarettes were provided by His Grace the Lord High Commissioner and ‘The Soldiers and Sailors of London Fund’.

Communion cups were provided by the Minister and Kirk Session of the Dean Parish Church, whilst Captains Fleming, Rainey and Miller acted as elders together with two elders from the Dean Parish Church.

A special service was held at the Second Scottish General Hospital on Wednesday 14 August 1915 to mark the first year of the war. Miss E Wemyss officiated at the harmonium (as she had done almost since the Hospital was opened). After the Benediction the orchestra played the national anthems of Belgium, France, Russia and Japan, followed by ‘God Save the King’.

On Christmas Day 1915, the wards were decorated both in Craigleith and the Flora Stevenson School. Carol singers made their round of the Hospital. From an early hour of the morning until late at night trolleys delivered loads of parcels.

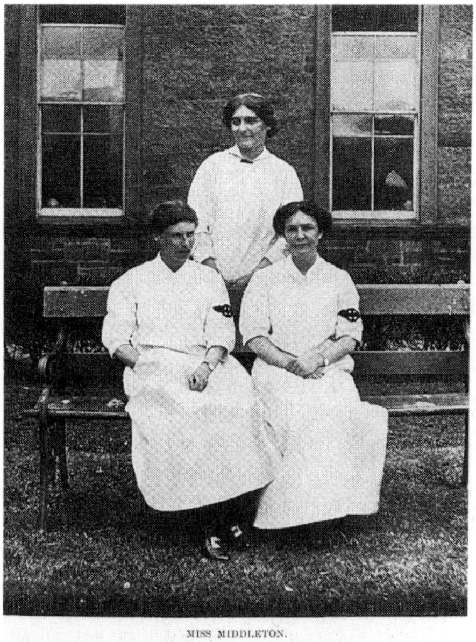

MISS MIDDLETON.
MISS LEITH ROSS. MISS M'CUAIG.

Volunteer nuses, Craigleith Hospital 1914–1918

The Craigleith Hospital Chronicle

One of the features of hospital life was the *Craigleith Hospital Chronicle* and the first editor was Nurse Annie Paulin. She was associated with the Hospital from 1914. She had come forward as a volunteer and had also persuaded many ladies among her friends to volunteer their services to the Hospital. She gathered a band of willing Red Cross ladies who assisted in the Ward, Master's Office and other Departments. When the idea of a hospital magazine was conceived, Miss Paulin was approached and asked to undertake the post of Editor. She accepted. She died in 1915, a young woman who clearly was deeply missed. The *Chronicle* cost 7/6d for an annual subscription and was printed and published by Messrs Oliver and Boyd. It was beautifully presented, complete with lovely end pieces and drawings. The names of men who had been through Craigleith and then subsequently killed in action were recorded. Their numbers gradually increased as the *Chronicle* developed. Advertisements were included for the All British His Majesty's Voice, Adams Non-rustable Sheffield steel knives from 63–65 Shandwick Place, John Croall Taxi Cars for Hire and Officers' Kits ready for service at Mauls (Now Frasers at the West End) costing £33.

In 1915 the Lord Provost of Edinburgh wrote in the *Chronicle*

> No class has excelled the zeal, devotion, self sacrifice and willingness to spend and be spent in the service of the Country than the medical profession. When speaking of the medical profession I, of course, include the noble army of nurses. The great merit of the Chronicle is the catholicity and variety of subjects treated. There is nothing of the sick chamber about it. There is much to make appeal to the conscience of the reader and make him ask the question 'Am I doing my duty in this great crisis?' Sandwiched between, there are appeals to the historic and patriotic sense, while the saving grace of humour is not wanting.

The *Craigleith Chronicle* described some of the staff in doggerel verse —

Anonymous Nonsense

I hear that when really annoyed,
Our distinguished friend Major F Boyd
  Makes his underlings quail,
  But most likely this tale
Of veracity's wholly devoid.

Captain Thomson has now gone away;
Why was it that he wouldn't stay?
  I've a kind of notion
  He's keen for promotion,
And is off to the thick of the fray.

Captain Stuart will certainly climb
To the top of the ladder in time;
  He's so thoroughly good,
  Without being a prude
(That last is a shocking bad rhyme).

Captain Dowden makes gloomy folks laugh,
With his cheery and good-natured chaff;
  Sure, he's Irish by birth,
  Which accounts for his mirth;
It's a pity he's leaving the staff.

Captain Fleming is rather a treat
To look at, he's always so neat.
  He goes up and down
  From his house in the town
In his motor, or else on his feet.

The *Chronicle* had repeated acknowledgement of patients being taken for outings by local volunteers. There were descriptions of the Massage Department, how to distinguish ranks in the Army and Navy, a bugler from a trumpeter etc. There was an account of how Newfoundland felt about the war. There were histories of Scottish Regiments: The Second Dragoons, The Royal Scots Guards, The Lothians Regiment, The Highland Light Infantry, The King's Own Scottish Borderers, The Cameronians, The Seaforth Highlanders, The Royal Scots Fusiliers, The Gordon Highlanders, The Queen's Own Cameron Highlanders (the 79).

There was an account of the Dardanelles, describing the scenery rather than the battles that took place. Thirty-four soldiers from Craigleith went on the Mediterranean Expeditionary Force.

In the May 1916 issue there was an account of the tragedy at Gretna in which a train full of Guards soldiers caught fire. The doors were locked and many of the soldiers on the train were burned to death.

As the *Chronicles* went on there were increasing descriptions of the reality of life both in Gallipoli and on the Western Front, the trenches, the bombing, the fear, the near misses and the wounded — they were the lucky ones. There was an article on 'Sphagnum Moss: Its use in Surgery'. Cavalry men also wrote of their experiences.

Interspersed with this magazine chit-chat there were rather stark accounts of awful experiences in the trenches at Mons:

> Picture yourself in a trench about 5 feet deep, fill this trench with muddy, evil smelling water to a depth of 4 feet; remember that 100 yards from you is an enemy who, you can assure yourself when you straighten your aching back, will send you per express messenger, ticket for another land.

There is an account of the gassing at Hill 60 in Ypres. Typical of the stories in the magazine was 'The Fortunes of War, or, A Week-end at the Front', ending with a shell landing in the trenches. The squad was bombarded, then gassed, losing a great deal of men from shell-fire, with shells landing all around and eventually a high explosive landed on the parapet above the man's head. The wounds he sustained sent him home. One wounded officer earned the Military Cross during the 12 hours he was with his regiment at the front.

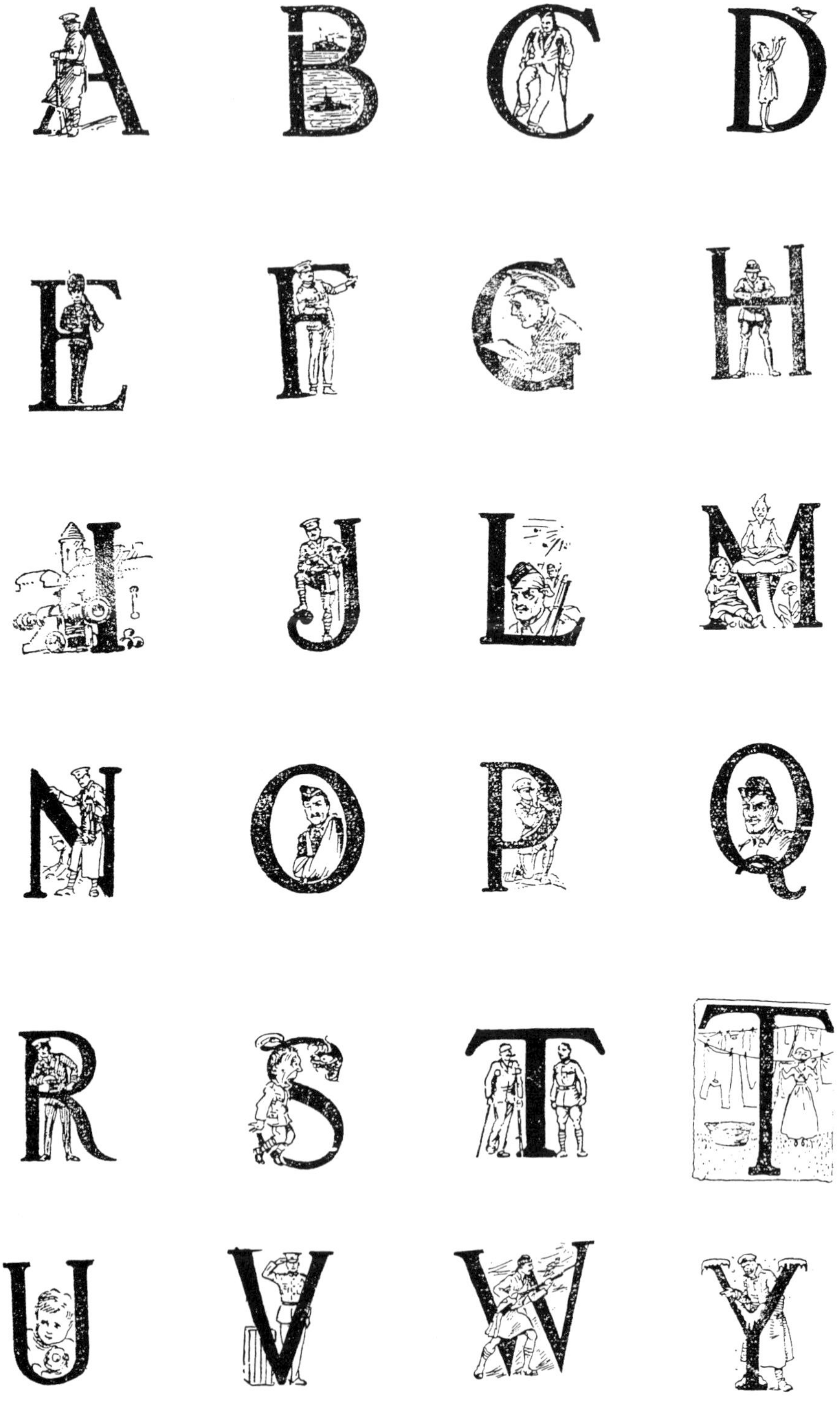

Capital letter cartoons used in the *Craigleith Chronicle*

There was another article by 1st Gordon Highlander, J. C. Macpherson, who returned from the front and who was killed in action in France during the severe fighting of the last week. The arrival of the first tank in September 1916 was described by Private William Paton, Scottish Rifles, a patient in G Ward.

Articles included 'Social Service among the Indian Troops in France'; 'Notes on the army' 'Use of water and land', 'Labour trouble in the time of war': 'We have it from the Bishop of London that every man who refuses to do his best in the production of armaments at home is guilty of the murder of his brothers in the trench'. These are strong words addressed to labour and labourers.

As the war continued a shortage of paper and rationing caused difficulties in producing the *Chronicle*. The frequency of its publication dropped from monthly to quarterly, reducing the paper by two thirds.

Craigleith Hospital Chronicle

Reckless Rhymes in Warlike Times

By VIVIAN PHILLIPPS.

WILHELM, War Lord, Chiefest Hun,
Is revered by every one.
Nothing quite so wise and good
Ever yet in trousers stood.
If you doubt this, ask his Bosches—
They will tell you this no "tosh" is;
Only ribald British laughers
Dare to mock this Prince of Strafers.

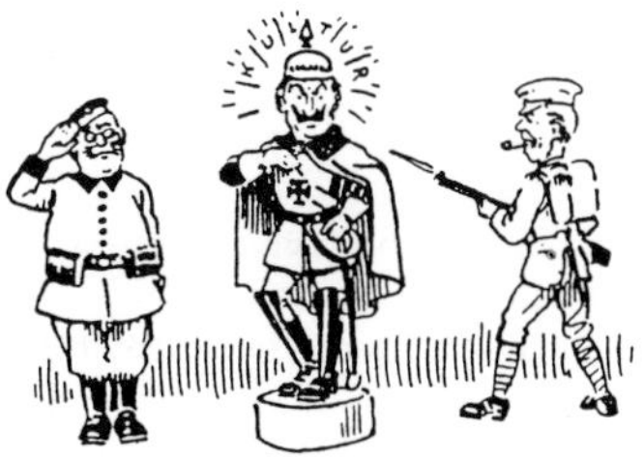

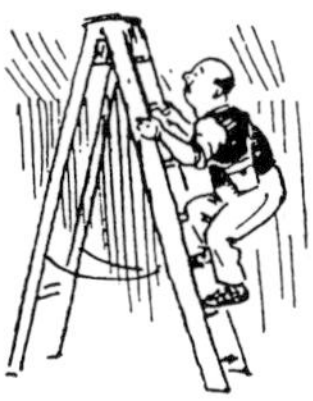

Uncle seized the kitchen steps,
Clambered up to see the Zepps;
Presently a bomb fell "plumb"
On poor uncle's cranium.
We, his nephews and his nieces,
Found him all in little pieces.
Still, what is the use of whining,
Every cloud has a silver lining;
Though we wish him with us still,
He has made a first-class will.

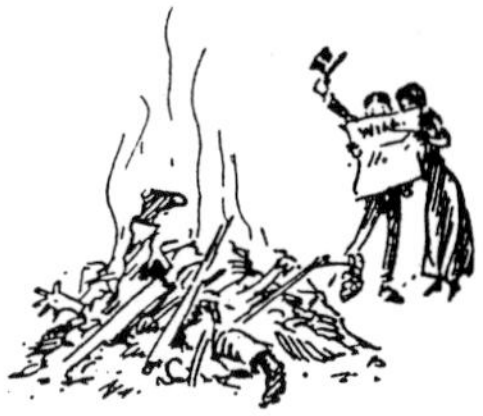

24

'Reckless Rhyme . . .' from *Craigleith Chronicle*

In the penultimate copy of the *Craigleith Hospital Chronicle* there was a poem by Sgt. Bevington of the Lancers.

Beds

At Craigleith there stands a big Hospital
Where the nurses are angels, 'tis said;
They are gentle and kind, but shine best of all
In the way that they make up a bed.

Three nurses in snowy white aprons,
Embroidered with crosses in red,
Are busy all day with their duties,
And, my word! they can make up a bed.

When I'm lying in bed with a fever
And awful bad pains in my head,
As soon as I drop into slumber
Once more they will make up the bed.

One trips in the ward with the porridge,
One slices and 'maggies' the bread,
One carefully dusts the piano
(Not forgetting to make up the bed).

One straightens my locker untidy,
One sees that I'm properly fed,
One washes my features with soapsuds,
Then they all have a go at the bed.

Should I die, and perchance go to Heaven
(Or some place where 'tis warmer instead),
I wonder if three little nurses
Will follow and make up my bed.

So when I return to my unit,
And the last fond good-bye has been said,
I'll always remember those nurses
And the way that they made up my bed.

The final volume devoted to Demobilisation appeared in Spring 1919 *Craigleith Hospital Chronicle*, Volume VI, Number 36. One of the main objects of the *Chronicle* was to provide funds for extra comforts for patients and over £350 of surplus profits were contributed. A special achievement was the extension of the billiard room in the Red Cross Hut at a cost of £70 and grants given to the library and tobacco funds.

A feature of the final copy of *Hospital Notes* was the announcement of marriages. Christmas 1918 was celebrated by repatriated prisoners of war, some of whom had spent four years in captivity. The returned prisoners included French, Italians, Portugese and Indian soldiers. The final pages were devoted to news items, the last article being 'Hun Hypocrisy' and the last poem was 'Farewell, Craigleith'.

End of the War

Craigleith underwent many changes in the months prior to Spring 1919. On the 1 December it became a Clearing Station for repatriated prisoners of war, following which the hospital became a Central Dispersal Hospital. This was a busy time for the clerical staff but less so for the medical and nursing staff. The Commanding Officer, Lt. Col. Sir Joseph Fayrer who commanded the Hospital throughout the War was demobilised in February 1919. He was succeeded by Lt. Col. D. J. Graham.

Major Webster was the Officer in Command and handed the hospital back to the Parish Council. On receipt from the Army, temporary buildings on the airing yards were removed. In February 1920 the Council received compensation in respect of fair wear and tear. The Red Cross Recreation Hall which had been such a great success, behind the main building, was retained.

The minutes of the Parish Council in 1919 recorded that the Rt.Hon. Winston S Churchill, Secretary of War, wished to make a permanent record of thanks for the use of Craigleith Hospital for valuable and patriotic assistance. This certificate was framed and placed in the Poor House.

Table 8. To November 1915 the number of patients treated in Craigleith and Auxiliary Hospitals

Craigleith		*Deaconess Hospital*	
Expeditionary	2,056	Expeditionary	286
Mediterranean	106	Mediterranean	58
Home service	8,310	Total	344
Canadian	19		
Australian	5	*Leith*	
Belgian	67	Expeditionary	95
South African	1	Mediterranean	14
Total	10,564	Total	109
Royal Infirmary		*Dalmeny*	
Expeditionary	609	Expeditionary	592
Mediterranean	91	Canadian	1
Canadian	37	Mediterranean	101
Total	754	Total	694

4

The Origins of the Western General Hospital 1919–39

Legislation & Council

The Craigleith Hospital reverted to its former role as a Poor Law Hospital in 1919 and also continued under the aegis of the Ministry of Pensions.

The problem of the support of the unemployed, poor, sick and elderly continued to be a topic for debate throughout this period until the second World War. The *Evening News* of May 1935 reported that Sir Godfrey Collins was

> of the view that in Britain the general public , although they were suffering, nevertheless received greater assistance in housing, old age pensions, unemployment relief, health insurance and other social services than the people in any other country in the world. Edinburgh is contributing annually £400,000 for public assistance. This is equal to the cost of public lighting, cleansing, the fire brigade, public libraries and public parks combined.

Sir James Leishman drew attention to the enormous cost of the Poor Law in Scotland and pointed out that:

> There are limits to the cost and burdens resting upon our country and industry. While it is true that vast sums have been spent on social services the rate payers of the city can hardly feel satisfied that they have to pay five times more for public assistance than they do for housing.

In 1936 the Children's Home in Craigleith cost £4,300 and in 1938 the cost of the Craigleith Children's Home was £4,000.

In 1938 the scales of relief available to the recipients of outdoor assistance were such that where a recipient was not living as a member of a household of two or more persons, the rate for a male or female was 15s (75p) a week. If the recipient was living as a member of a household of two or more persons the householder and wife received 24s (£1.20p). Members of a household received different rates according to age: if over 21, 10s (50p); over 16, 8s (40p); over 14, 6s (30p). A boarded out apprentice had his wages made up to 15s (75p). A lunatic received 12s 6d (63p); a mental defective with relatives, 10s (50p). Clothing was issued in special circumstances and the medical officer had power to grant medicines and nutritious diets. There was also assistance and care for blind persons. The work of looking after the poor of the city was under the control of the Corporation.

Following the amalgamation of Leith with Edinburgh in November 1920 the Public Health Committee was reconstituted with 16 members including Convenor. Five standing sub-committees dealt with a variety of issues including general public health, port health, infectious disease control and hospital affairs, and special schemes including maternity and child welfare.

In 1928 the Edinburgh Parish Council converted the Hospital for general hospital purposes.

The long-standing function of a Public Health Authority was primarily preventive medicine, including a duty to prevent the spread of disease. The Hospital functions of the City Corporation were the provision of isolation or fever hospitals, and hospitals for the care of sick poor. This changed with the passing of the *Local Government of Scotland Act 1929* which removed the distinction between preventative and curative medicine. A local health authority was established to maintain general hospitals for the treatment of the sick, thereby removing the stigma of being a Poor Law patient. The former Poor Law Hospitals at Craigleith (Western General Hospital, Pilton (Northern General Hospital) and Seafield (Eastern General Hospital), formerly administered by the Parish Council, came under the aegis of the City Public Health Committee.

As a consequence of the Local Government (Scotland) Act 1929 the Parish Councils were abolished. The county became the administrative area except in burghs with a population over 20,000. Edinburgh, which had extended its boundaries in 1920, assumed the duty of looking after the poor through the Town Council.

Craigleith was taken over by the Public Health Committee on 16 May 1930.

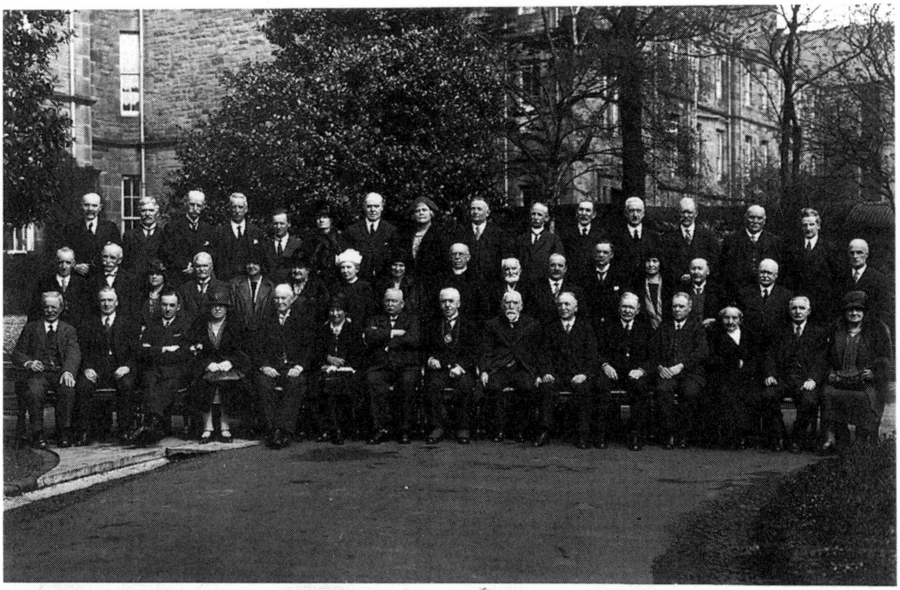

Back Row—(Reading left to right)—D. G. Cormack J. R. Forsyth, J.P. J. R Milne J. Gardner W. Smith Mrs E. MacIntyre J. Cunningham Miss M. C. Geddes
A. White Scott C. M'Guire C. C. Plain, J.P. H. Duncan (Depute Inspector and Clerk) J. Campbell, J.P. J. G. Veitch J. S. L. Kerr

Middle Row—(Reading left to right)—W. Brogan J. Nicoll Miss C. R. Sinclair (Inspector's Secretary) J. Nairn, J.P. Mrs I. Deas Mrs F. Johnston, J.P. Miss M. Lawson (Matron, Craiglockhart)
Miss M. R. J. Cornwall Rev. G. Dodds, B.D. G. Balfour, J.P. G. C. Easton, J.P. G. Mackie, M.B.E. Miss E. B. Campbell (Matron, Children's Home)
W. Galloway J. Pringle (Governor, Seafield) W. Young (Governor, Craiglockhart)

Front Row—(Reading left to right)—J. Puttinger A. Thomson Dr R. Bailey (Medical Superintendent, Gogarburn) Miss S. L. Munro, J.P. J. Slater, J.P. Mrs H. Melville
Col. A. Young, C.B.E., D.L., J.P. (Chairman, District Board of Control) J. Duncan, J.P. (Chairman, Parish Council) C. Waldie, S.S.C., J.P. J. D. Robertson, J.P.
H. Maclean W. M. Mowat (Inspector and Clerk) Mrs M. J. Boémé W. Waterston Mrs S. Purves

Edinburgh Parish Council and District Board of Control April 1930

At this time 271 beds were made available at the Hospital. Arrangements were made to admit general medical and surgical patients, with wards for gynaecology and children. In 1932 Craigleith, Pilton and Seafield Hospitals were renamed the Western General, Northern General and Eastern General Hospitals under the generic title of Municipal General Hospitals.

As the activities of the Hospital increased, the new Management completely renewed the drainage and heating systems, and re- equipped the operating theatre and X-ray departments. New departments of dentistry, massage, electro-therapy, ophthalmology, ear, nose and throat, and urology were introduced during 1932–1933. The statistics for the cases cared for during the 1930's are shown in the tables. The average number of patients present in the Hospital in 1936 was 558 and the cost per inmate 16s 5d (83p).

Following the Local Government reorganisation in 1934, further services were added to the administrative responsibility of the Public Health Department of the City of Edinburgh. The Municipal General Hospital scheme included indoor medical care of the poor and sick poor under the immediate supervision of the Medical Superintendent of the Municipal General Hospital, Dr J. W. Keay, uncle of Dr Alex Keay, Department of Paediatrics, Western General Hospital.

The Corporation decided that patients who could do so were expected to contribute to the cost of their stay in hospital. The maximum charge being

Statistics for the Year 1932 — Western General Hospital

		Admitted	Discharged	Died
Adults:	Males	329	252	55
	Females	294	279	31
Children:	Males	408	402	15
	Females	411	396	13

Table to show results of treatment or termination of illness in 1932

Number of cases treated		1,689	
Cured	422	Not improved	624
Improved	283	Died	114
Remaining under treatment		246	

Causes of Death

	Adults	Children
Diseases of Heart and Blood Vessels	23	0
Cancer or other Tumour	28	0
Diseases of Brain and Nerves	13	1
Diseases of Lungs	8	14
Diseases of Digestive Organs	7	6
Diseases of Kidneys	6	0

In addition, surgical conditions resulted in nine deaths, senility two deaths, and among children, congenital disabilities seven deaths.

Total beds	280
Average number of occupied beds	233
Average length of stay, in days, per patient	28

twenty one shillings per week (£1.05p). The Hospital could then be viewed in quitc a different light from that of the former Poor Law Hospital. Anyone could be admitted and receive first-class treatment. Patients who disliked the idea of going into a free hospital, yet found nursing home charges beyond their means, took advantage of the facilities offered them in the 'Western General'.

A serious problem had arisen because of the long waiting-lists of the Royal Infirmary and it was felt that the Western General Hospital had a contribution to offer to its solution. It was expected that as the various plans of the city matured that ' "Craigleith" like "Laurison", will yet be synonymous with the great art of healing that is Edinburgh's pride.' There was testing for Edinburgh citizens according to means £2.12.6d (£2.62p) for patients belonging to other Local Authorities and £3.3s.0d.(£3.15p) for private patients.

The voluntary side of the hospital was developed by voluntary organisations. Friends of the Hospital produced concerts, arraged outings for convalescent patients in motor cars or wheel chairs, airings for babies and gifts.

Description of the Hospital in 1933

An article in the *Edinburgh Evening News* in June 1933, commented that the general public were not aware of how efficiently the hospitals under the control of Edinburgh Public Health Department were run. The author of this article had a tour of the Hospital accompanied by Dr Guy, Medical Officer of Health, Dr Keay, Medical Officer of the Western General Hospital and Professor Wilkie.

> There were 300 patients being treated in medical, surgical, maternity and children's wards. There were nearly 100 children in the hospital, not all sick and some 'tinies' being kept there because they were too young for admittance elsewhere. In one ward full of babies there were twin girls who looked about four months old but were actually one year old and they were suffering from malnutrition. In the case of some children their mothers were in hospital elsewhere, and others in institutions of various kinds. There were 21 maternity beds and the equipment provided was up-to-date. All the wards were beautifully kept and walls painted in pastel colours and everywhere lightness.

At the time of this article the staff at the Western General Hospital comprised three resident doctors, two 'clinical students', ten sisters, eight staff nurses and 50 probationers. Medical students, including women students, were given the opportunity of residing in the hospital for periods of three months.

Nonetheless in 1933 it was obvious that the hospital did not meet teaching hospital standards and that mere alterations were insufficient.

Rebuilding Plans

Plans were drawn by the City Architect for the complete but phased rebuilding of a 700-bed hospital on the site of the existing hospital. The estimated cost for rebuilding the hospital was £500,000. This development ran in a north-south direction, in contrast to the east-west direction of the original building. The first phase, the building of a new Nurses Home for 160 nurses and 50 domestics, started in 1936. A mortuary, chapel and kitchens, started in 1937. All were completed by 1938.

In 1935 the gatehouse was modified to allow ambulances to enter. In December 1937 it was agreed to build a Recreation Hall with the same coloured bricks used on the south front of the Nurses Home, and that a covered way should be provided between the recreation hall and the nurses' home.

Plans for a new one-storey mortuary — adaptable to two storeys if required — for pathological work were submitted.

In 1938 a new boiler house was built — designed by Sir Basil Spence.

On 1 February 1938 a familiar story began. The Medical Officer of Health submitted a report on the present policy authorised by the Corporation of reconstructing the Western General Hospital. He 'echoed long-expressed views' that the reconstruction at the Western General Hospital should be deferred and that a completely new hospital be built in the south side of the City. The next phase scheduled for 1939 was permanently cancelled by the outbreak of war. The old hospital had to continue almost without alteration in its role as part of the Department of Health's Emergency Scheme.

Sir Stanley Davidson described the changes which occurred in the Western, Eastern and Northern General Municipal Hospitals in the *Royal College of Physicians of Edinburgh Chronicle*, July, 1975. In October 1938 he had returned to Edinburgh to take up the position of Professor of Medicine, having been in Aberdeen University as Professor for the previous eight years. He was also appointed Director of the Medical Wards of the three Municipal General Hospitals — the Western, Eastern and Northern. This was at the insistence of the Lord Provost who was an important member of the University Court who had heard derogatory remarks about the catering, nursing and medical services in these hospitals. Sir Stanley was asked to investigate these problems and write a report for him and the Medical Officer of Health in regard to the correctness and potential for improvement of these views . The report was never made but it was felt that the sad state of affairs was not the fault of the medical and nursing staff but that of the system under which they had to work.

Development: Medical/Surgical Units

In 1932 Dr Keay, the Medical Superintendent, saw advantages for the Corporation and the patients in these hospitals if some association was forged between the Corporation and the University Medical School. The concept of a joint venture was accepted provided the hospitals were not administered under any provisions of the Poor Law. It was agreed that Professors of the Medical School were appointed directors in the Hospital in their speciality. University staff were appointed to clinical and teaching functions in the hospitals and students were allowed to be taught in the hospitals. The University paid the salaries of the Consultant staff, the Corporation contributed a sum to cover expenses.

Towards the end of that year, four main units were created: medical, surgical, obstetrics and gynaecology and children's wards, each unit having a Consultant with two or more assistants, both for the treatment of patients and for teaching. The directors of these units were: Medicine — Professor W. T. Ritchie; Surgery — Professor David Wilkie; Obstetrics and Gynaecology — Professor R. W. Johnstone; Child Life and Health — Professor Charles MacNeil.

Col. Keay was succeeded by Dr R. B. McMillan who was in charge of Eastern, Western and Northern. He then went south during the 39/45 war. Dr A. J. Slessor, his successor, died in office. The last Medical Superintendent was Dr Sandy Donald who had been the Assistant Superintendent at the City Hospital.

Some of the assistants to the Professors at that time became famous: *Surgery* — Charles Illingworth, who became Regius Professor of Surgery in Glasgow, Bruce Dick and David Band: *on the medical side*; Dr J. G. McCrie, for many years Dean of the Faculty of Medicine in Sheffield; Dr Ranald Murray Lyon, Physician, Royal Infirmary, Edinburgh; Dr Melville Arnot, Professor of Medicine in Birmingham; Dr George Percival, Professor of Dermatology, University of Edinburgh; Dr John Henderson; Professor W. T. Ritchie, Cardiologist.

Included in the senior staff in Medicine were Dr B. O. Campbell and Dr Norrie Robson who subsequently became Vice Chancellor of Edinburgh University; Dr T. Y. Finlay and Dr W. S. N. Craig in Paediatrics and Dr Traquair

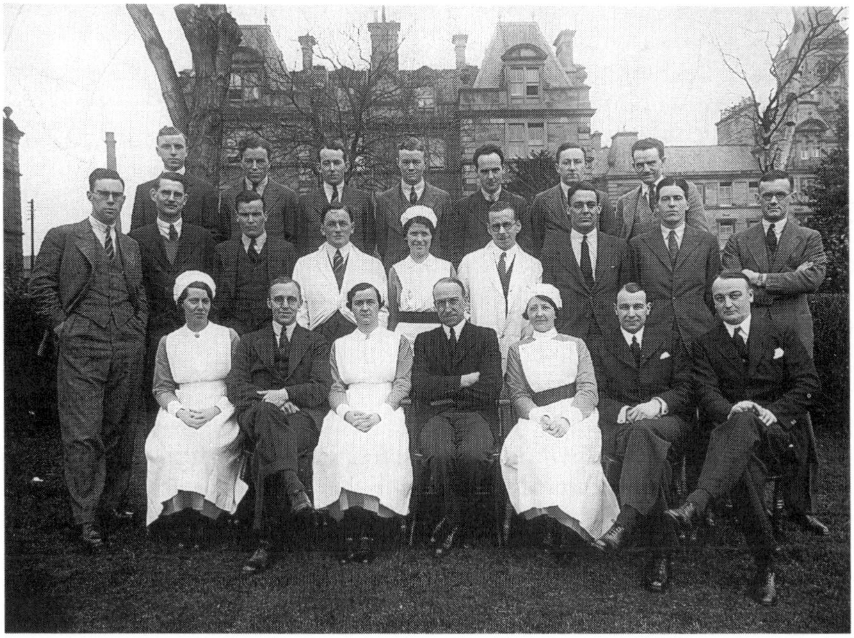

Group which includes, in front row, Dr CFW Illingworth, Professor David Wilkie, Mr David Band, Mr Bruce Dick; 1936

Thin in Obstetrics. Mr Andrew Logan started a thoracic clinic here at the WGH. Dr Archie Duncan moved to Cardiff from his post as head of Obstetrics and Gynaecology to become Professor of Obstetrics. He returned to Edinburgh to be executive Dean of the Faculty of medicine. Mr Mason Brown was the Senior Surgeon in Paediatrics; Dr Charlie Scott became an ENT surgeon. Dr W. I. C. Morris, another obstetrician, moved to the chair of obstetrics in Manchester.

It was agreed that acute medical, surgical, paediatrics and maternity cases were to be treated at the Western General Hospital; sub-acute cases at the Northern General Hospital and chronic cases at the Eastern General Hospital. In all there were 900 beds: Western General Hospital 280; Northern General Hospital 260; Eastern General Hospital 360.

During 1930-1931 a sub-committee of the Public Health Committee met Professors Wilkie and Ritchie to discuss increasing the Hospital establishment. This included the introduction of a biochemistry laboratory, stenographer, pathology and bacteriology services, medical equipment and outpatient facilities and increasing the number of resident doctors. A sum of £3,500 was recommended to meet the increased running costs of the improved services.

Additional assistant physicians were appointed and the nursing staff numbers were strengthened by the addition of a sister tutor, a theatre sister, X-ray sister, night sister, three staff nurses and 19 probationary nurses.

All physicians undertook obstetrics and gynaecology. Four residents ran the hospital with 12 students. The living-in cost was 25/- (£1.25p) per week. Residents lived in the gatehouse. This gatehouse was also the out patients department and had a tin roof.

In 1932, on the surgical side, the greatest number of patients were operated on for diseases or conditions of the abdominal organs, followed by affections of bones and joints. Medical cases were chiefly diseases of the respiratory, circulatory and nervous system.

By 1934 the number of cases treated was 2673 compared with 1689 in 1932. Of the patients treated, 35 per cent were children. The surgical operations had increased from 87 in 1932 to 887 in 1934. By 1935 the number of cases treated in the Western General Hospital was 3080, 34 per cent of whom were children. Most of the children were admitted suffering from diseases of the skin, respiratory disorders or malnutrition.

In 1934 the total number of X-ray examinations was 1167 compared to approximately 480 in 1932.

Clinical research was also important. Mr Charles Illingworth wrote on carcinoma of the colon and rectum. His other interest was in obstructive jaundice and he was able to confirm recent work that attributed the risk of haemorrhage in these cases to a lack of prothrombin. Vitamin K was used to rectify the prothrombin deficiency in a number of cases, and this proved a valuable method of pre-operative medication to overcome the risk of haemorrhage.

Mr Bruce Dick investigated pulmonary tuberculosis, and was also able to divide pleural adhesions by means of the thoracoscope. One of the problems with tuberculosis was that the lung stuck to the pleura surrounding the lungs which made for problems with breathing. This could be separated out by a tube inserted between the ribs. Mr Dick worked on the surgery of the thorax with successes in the treatment of certain types of pulmonary tuberculosis, in which therapy by artificial pneumothorax had failed.

Mr David Band was interested in diseases of the urinary tract including the treatment of certain types of prostatic disease by transurethral operative procedures. He looked at the pathology and treatment of prostatic enlargement and transurethral operations, and the treatment of early cases with hormones.

A maternity unit was established at the Western General Hospital in 1932, under the direction of the Professor of Midwifery. In the first year there were 59 deliveries in the Unit.

The maternity department looked after 89 cases in 1932 which included 59 deliveries (42 normal, 17 abnormal), post-partum puerperal admissions 7, deaths — mothers 1, infants 2. One mother who died had delivered a premature child before admission to hospital. There were no cases of puerperal sepsis (infection after childbirth) during the year. In 1934 the maternity department treated 241 patients. In 1935 there were 29 antenatal beds in maternity hospitals in Edinburgh, 9 of which were in the Western General Hospital.

In 1938 the maternity department abortion cases totalled 63 and there were 26 other complicated pregnancies. There were nine deaths of toxaemia of pregnancy, one death from cardiac failure under anaesthesia and one death from pulmonary embolism.

There was a continuous appraisal of needs. In April of 1938 tenders for the supply of X-ray apparatus at the Western General were submitted and the tender was awarded to Watson & Sons, Edinburgh and London, for an apparatus made by themselves at a cost of £1,468.9s.

The operating theatre was re-equipped during 1938 and 87 operations were performed. 53 of these operations were major operations and 34 minor operations. A general anaesthetic was administered in 79 operations, three operations were carried out with a spinal anaesthetic and five operations were under local anaesthesis.

The dental department treated 59 patients, 48 children and 11 adults.

Teaching: Students

Teaching of undergraduate medical students began in 1933. Residential accommodation for twelve students was provided at the Western General Hospital for students undergoing the newly introduced three months 'hospital experience'.

The hostel was a great success. This scheme entailed living at the Hostel for three months and to be involved in hospital clinic work. The success was such that the directors of the hospital units suggested that accommodation for forty students should be provided. The scheme for the training of students from the University was extended in 1937. Medical students attended daily practical tuition at the Western General Hospital as part of their University curriculum.

Developments: Nursing

After 1925 the poorhouse hospitals provided a training school for probationer nurses. This was recognised by the General Nursing Council for Scotland, but the lack of surgical nursing experience did not allow for full nurse registration. In 1927 arrangements were made with the Royal Samaritan Hospital for Women, in Glasgow, and the Dunfermline and West Fife Hospital for surgical nursing experience to be gained by nurses requiring State Registration.

In 1923, following the issue of the Scottish Board of Health conditions for certificate and registration of Health Visitors, the Scottish Branch of the Institute sent a quarter of their nurses each year to the Scottish School of Social Study and Training for the probation health visitors certificate. These facilities were greatly extended in 1930 when the Corporation provided two weeks of extensive training in infant hygiene at the Western General Hospital Childrens Wards; one week on school medical work, one week at the tuberculosis dispensary, one week at the ante natal clinic and three weeks district visitation with health visitors. These continued until the outbreak of the Second World War when considerable modifications were required.

In 1933 the Western General Hospital was recognised by the General Nursing Council for Scotland as a full training school for nurses for the general part of the Register. In 1937 the first group of nurses sat their examination and 19 out of 21 candidates passed their Final State Examination.

In September/October 1938 there was a shortage of nurses at the Eastern General Hospital despite repeated advertising campaigns. The Medical Officer of Health considered the suggestion that probationers at the Western General Hospital who had completed three years training should be transferred to the Eastern General Hospital during their 4th year as Staff Nurses. At that time there were nine 4th year nurses at the Western General Hospital under an intensive tuition course for State Examination and therefore they could not be transferred. These nurses would shortly leave the service of the Corporation to take other training, so the shortage could not be made up in this way. The Matron at the Eastern General Hospital received applications from two Staff Nurses, one Assistant Nurse and two Probationers. Under these circumstances the Sub-Committee of the Public Health Committee recommended that the Medical Officer of Health should in the meantime engage up to two trained nurses for the Eastern General Hospital at the usual fee.

The nurses' dormitory was originally on the floor which later became B flat, as children's wards, and nurses on night duty slept in cubicles on B flat. There were probably fifty student nurses.

The new nurses' home, completed in 1939, was built for nurses employed at the Western General Hospital. This new building provided comfort, cleanliness and convenience with facilities for sleeping, eating, relaxation — both mental and physical — and instruction in the profession of nursing.

Each sister and nurse had a bedroom to herself; the sisters' bedroom being provided with a small dressing room. There were separate sitting rooms for

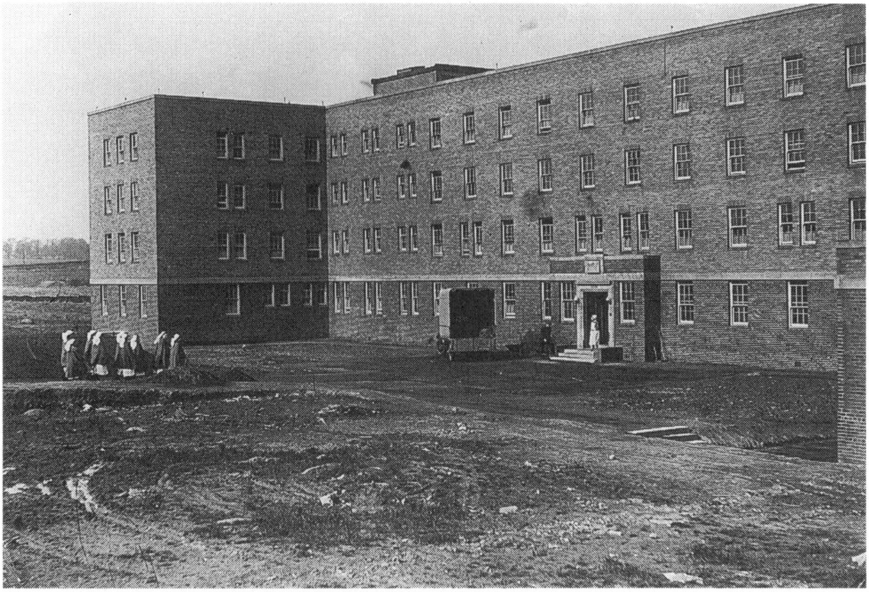

Newly built Nurses' Home, 1937

nurses and sisters with partitions between which could be drawn aside to form one long, large room. On each floor of the home there was a sun roof and sun balconies, and a room specially fitted out with hairdressing appliances where nurses could attend to their own coiffures. There was a teaching department with facilities for the educational needs of probationers. An important feature

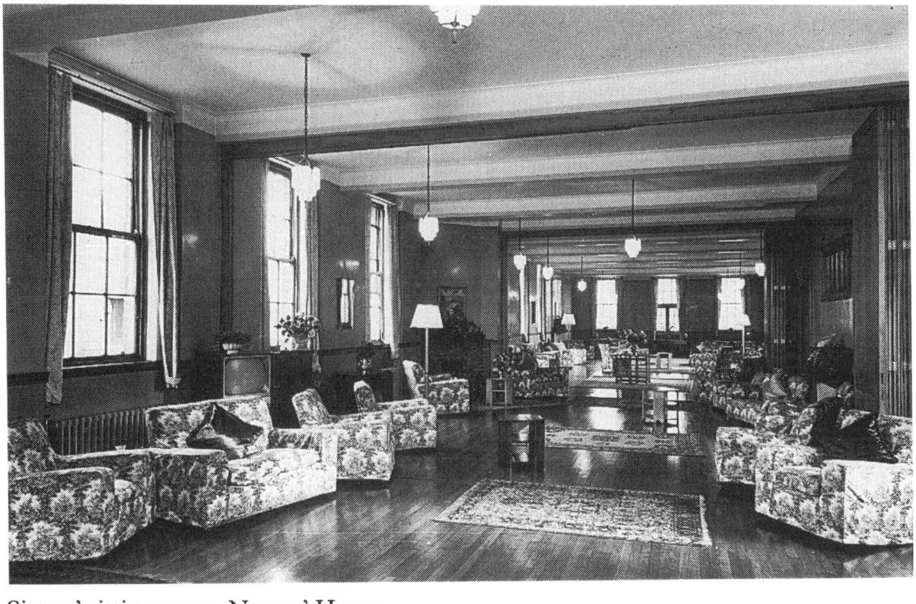

Sisters' sitting room, Nurses' Home

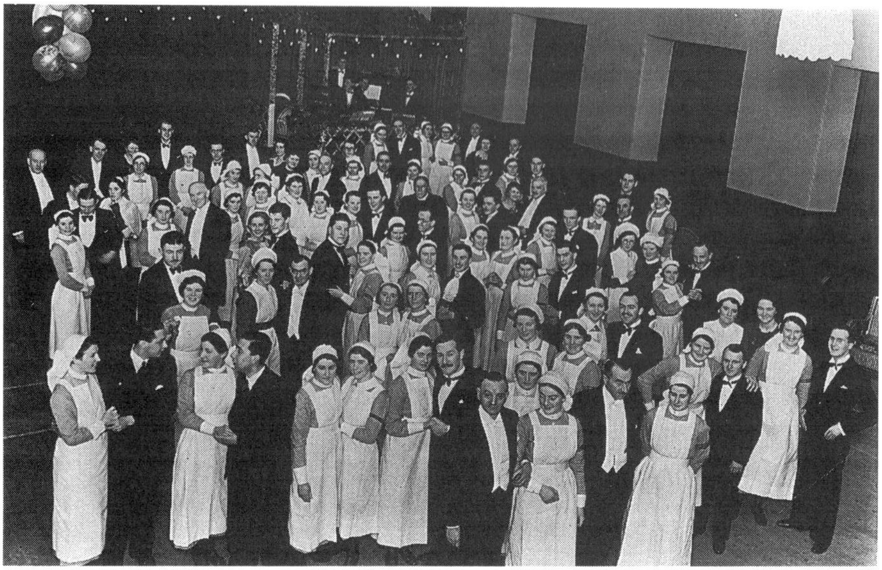

Doctors/Nurses dance, probably late 1930s, in Recreation Hall

was central heating, thick pile carpets and an engaging variety and tastefulness in colour and decoration throughout the nursing quarters. (*Evening Dispatch*, 1939). A hall was set aside as a recreation centre to host whist drives, dances (including an annual ball), parties and there was a facility for playing badminton. Over 200 nurses were accommodated in the new quarters.

By January 1938 the purchase of the following furnishings for the Nurses Home, at a cost of £1,600, was authorised: Mattresses, blankets, linen etc. £1,050; Cutlery, crockery etc. £55; Teaching equipment £230; Epidiascope, projector, screen, films etc. £100; Demonstration kitchen equipment £30; Library £35; Contingencies £100.

Two of the most famous nurses of the pre modern era were Sister Christine Orr who started in 1935 and Miss Margaret Nimmo who started in 1942. Sister Orr was the Sister D2 until she retired, and Miss Nimmo became Matron. Nurses were paid, in 1935, £20 a year. They had to buy: 24 aprons, 12 dresses, 6 pairs of collars and cuffs plus belt, 2 pairs of black shoes and stockings (lacing shoes). These were bought from a shop in the 'Bridges'. They had to buy all their books including a nurses' dictionary.

Student nurses entered the hospital service and went straight on to the wards with no training. They worked a 56-hour week which started at 7.30 a.m. Evenings off started after 6.30 p.m. but nurses had to be back in the nurses' home by 10 p.m.

Miss Teresa Allan was Matron in 1935. The first sister tutor was Sister Levack. The time for teaching available to each sister tutor was limited to the spare hours available. Initially the nurses were taught by the assistant matron for the first year, then by Miss Levack. This was a four-year training school called Western General Training School. The consultants gave lectures and the training was recognised in 1931/32. Sister Graham trained nurses in Craigleith, Eastern General and Western General.

The nurses' uniform was blue and white striped and reached the ankles. The cap had to be pleated, butterflying at the back. The uniform included stiff cuffs, collars and belts, black shoes and stockings, and an apron. Nurses in training wore pale blue, sisters wore darker blue, plain cap and lace frill. Nurses ate in what became the residents' dining room.

C flat was run by Sister Dewart. There were 20 beds — diabetes, cardiac, kidney and the nurses' sick bay. An anaemia cocktail was made by Sister Orr which consisted of scraped liver and pure orange juice. Dr Murray Lyon was the doctor in charge. Diets cooked by the nurses included jellies and cooked chicken. Ordinary diets frequently included rabbit. The menus were: *Breakfast*: Kipper, boiled egg or scrambled egg, porridge; *Mid-day*: Fish or rabbit, stew with carrot and turnip, steam pudding, junket, rice pudding, sponge pudding and cornflour.

Problems arose for the care of sick nurses. There was no sick ward for nurses at the Western General Hospital.

In February 1938 the accommodation and number of nurses required to allow a change from a 54 hour week to a 48 hour week was:

Estimate of nursing staff	132
Nursing staff required for 48 hour week	152
Domestics required for 48 hour week	74
Present accommodation for nursing staff	160
Present accommodation for domestic staff	46
Further accommodation required : domestic	28
: nursing	0

At that time a Staff Nurse salary was to be increased to £70 a year to be in line with other general hospitals.

Development: Other Departments

In 1932 arrangements were made for the bacteriological services of the Municipal General Hospitals to be met by the Bacteriology Department of the University. Such services included the examination of sputum, faeces, urine, blood, cerebrospinal fluid, throat swabs, pus and other materials by smears and cultures. Several thousands of such specimens were examined during the year. Qualitative and quantitative chemical examinations of blood, urine, stomach contents and other fluids was also provided by the municipal section of the Edinburgh University Biochemical Laboratory. 1690 examinations were made during 11 months of the year. A biochemist was appointed in 1934 to work in the Muncipal Section of the University Biochemical Laboratory. In 1936 the Biochemisty Department was transferred from the Edinburgh University to the Western General Hospital and a total of 798 examinations were made.

The haematology laboratory was at the back of the Children's Department. The hospital Pharmacy was in D Block and this was run by John Hall.

In 1932, 267 persons died, and 88 post mortem examinations were made. From 1936 onwards all pathological work for the hospitals was undertaken by the University Pathological Department under Professor A Murray Drennan. The University Department of Bacteriology provided the bacteriology service for the hospitals.

In addition the lay Clinical Assistant made special investigations, including 214 electrocardiograms.

Porters

The Minutes of the Public Health Committee on 13 July 1938, included a discussion concerning the gatekeepers at the Western General and the Northern General. The duties of gatekeepers were such that they frequently had to leave the gates and in their absence their wives were required to answer the telephone and supervise admissions to the hospital. The Medical Officer of Health considered this an undesirable arrangement and suggested that two porters should be appointed at each hospital to undertake the gatekeepers' duties. The Committee agreed to the establishment of the two porters at the usual salary. It was pointed out that there was a degree of urgency in the case of the Western General as the present gatekeeper was due to retire on the 21 August. During the late 1930s a man named Coleman was the head porter who was still working at the hospital in the 1950s. The hospital engineer, Mr Hunter, lived in a cottage at the back, where the present Outpatient Department is sited.

Around 1935 a library service for patients was organised by Mrs Dick (wife of Mr Bruce Dick) on a weekly visit.

The Craigleith Children's Home

In 1930 the Corporation assumed responsibility for the orphans and children who lived at Craigleith Hospital. In 1936 the infants were transferred to a residential home, Bruntsfield House, administered by the Public Assistance Committee. The empty wards were made into a larger and better maternity unit.

Thereafter children were no longer admitted to the poorhouse, but were cared for in the Children's Home, Crewe Road. The number of children in the Home at any one time varied between 59 and 87. Annual epidemics of rubella and chickenpox were prominent illnesses.

During 1932 the commonest problems for which children were treated were skin, respiratory, infectious and parasitic diseases. During the year 141 were surgical cases, 656 were medical cases and 161 were newly-born babies. Some children were boarded out. Many children were sent to the country board during the year for convalescence. The greatest number of children resident in Craigleith Children's Home was 115 and the lowest number 53, the average being 76. The average number of healthy children resident in the Children's Home in 1937 was 95, and 78 children were sent to the country board.

In 1938 the diet of the children in the children's home was:

Older Children's Diets : 2 — 4 upwards

6am	Milk	
8am	Breakfast –	Porridge and milk
		Bread, butter or margerine or bacon fat
		1 egg every second day
		milk
mid morning		milk
12.30pm	Dinner –	Soup
		meat or mince and potatoes
		green vegetables
		or fish
		milk pudding
3.30pm		cocoa
5.30pm	Supper –	Bread, butter or margarine

Cod liver oil with malt every day, jam occasionally.

During the 39/45 war the children were sent to Oxgangs and Strathearn House, Saxe Coburg Place.

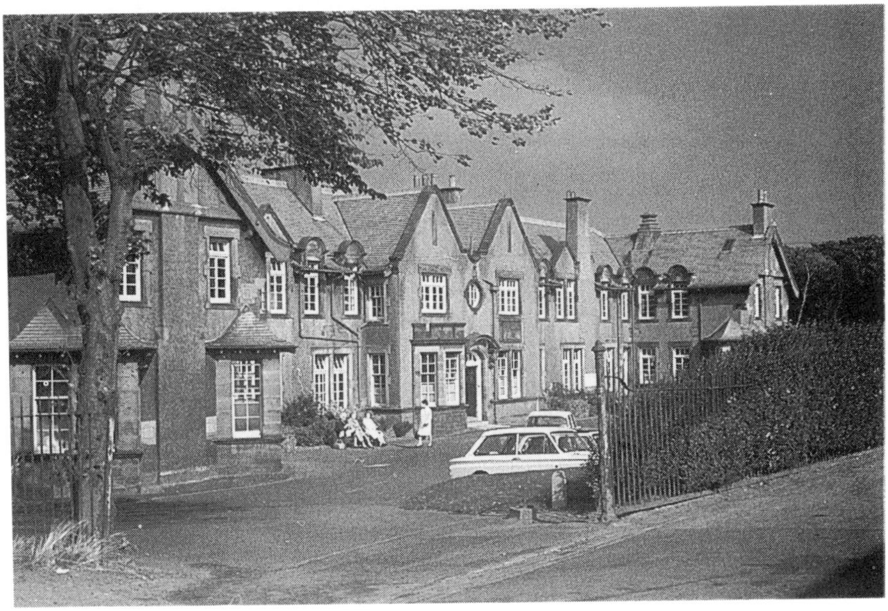

Children's Home/Paderewski Hospital

Statistics for 1938

		Admitted	Discharged	Died
Adults:	Males	952	808	150
	Females	1,918	1,799	122
Children:	Males	806	764	40
	Females	647	641	33

Total number of cases treated		4533	
Cured	2,571	Not improved	428
Improved	1,013	Died	345

Causes of Death	Adults		Children	
	Males	Females	Boys	Girls
1. Infectious and parasitic diseases	12	7	3	3
2. Cancer and other tumours	27	12		
3. Rheumatism, diseases of nutrition and other general diseases	3	8	1	
4. Diseases of the blood and blood forming organs	1	5		
5. Diseases of the nervous system and sense organs	13	10	4	7
6. Diseases of circulatory system	31	31	1	

During the year 978 operations were performed, 563 of them major and 415 minor. General anaesthetic was used in 795 operations and 89 operations used a spinal anaesthetic. 94 were under local anaesthetic.

Classification of Operations

1. Operation on brain, spinal cord, and peripheral nerves	1
2. Operation on lymph glands	108
3. Operation on upper air and food passages	132
4. Operation on breast and thorax	59
5. Operation on abdomen	260
6. Operation on genito-urinary organs	147
7. Operation on bones and joints (including amputation)	80
8. Various unclassified operations	191
Total	978

Urological Department

Examinations: (Cystoscopic and Pyelographic) 210; Bougies 242
Operations: (Transurethral resection of prostate 17
Fulguration of tumours 2)

Dental Department

Total number of patients treated, adults 61; children 66

Ear, Nose and Throat Department

Total number of operations 150, of which 12 were for mastoiditis.

X-Ray Department

Total number of patients examined 1,859, barium meals and enemeta 329, maternity patients X-rayed 62, lipiodol into lungs 37, retrograde pylographies 104, cholecystographies 49.

In the maternity department abortion cases totalled 63 and 26 other cases of complicated pregnancies were not confined. There were nine deaths due to toxaemia of pregnancy, one death from cardiac failure under anaesthesia and one death from pulmonary embolism.

Between 1932 and 1938, the total number of admissions in the Maternity ward rose from 100 to 850 and the total number of deliveries from 75 to 660.

The Special Diet Department looked after 151 patients of whom 39 per cent had diabetes, 41 per cent stomach disorders, and six per cent kidney disorders.

The massage and electro-therapy department looked after 428 patients of whom 284 were cured and improved. The treatments included massage, galvanism and faradism, diathermy, infra-red and radiant heat, ionisation and ultra violet artificial sunlight and re-education exercises.

The range and number of tests in the Biochemical Department included:

sugar	351 tests	urea	397 tests
nitrogen	103	creatinine	153
icteric index	111	Van den Bergh	36
cholesterol	21	calcium	38
albumin	13	CSF: protein	70
sugar	65	chloride	60
faecal fats	29	Urine: sugar	22.

5

The War Years 1939–45

1. The General Hospital

At the outset of the 1939-45 war there was widespread fear of enemy bombing, resulting in large numbers of casualties. Sir Stanley Davidson received a message from the Secretary of State for Scotland. When war broke out it was anticipated that within the first few months, the German Airforce would bomb the large cities. This might destroy the big hospitals in the centre. Therefore a second line of services needed to be prepared, to be known as the Emergency Medical Services (EMS). Hutted hospitals were to be built in the neighbourhood of the big cities of Britain so that casualties from bombing and from the War overseas could be accommodated. The Chief Medical Officer for Scotland, Dr James McIntosh; Professor Mackie, Professor of Bacteriology at the University of Edinburgh and Sir Stanley Davidson were asked by the Secretary of State to be his advisors on the site and construction and staffing of these new hospitals. Six hutted hospitals, each with 1,200 beds were to be built. The expectation was that Britain would win the War and they were built in sites of value to the nation not only during but after the War. These sites included Raigmore near Inverness, Stracathro near Brechin and Bridge of Earn near Perth. In addition Sir Stanley was appointed Professor of Medicine to the new Edinburgh Polish Faculty of Medicine and Consultant Physician to the Norwegian Army in Scotland. A hospital had to be equipped and staffed for the Norwegians. In anticipation of the bombing of Edinburgh and large numbers of casualties, the available Hospital beds and provisions had to be rapidly expanded in Lothian.

The arrangements were included in the Emergency Hospital Scheme. In 1939 Bangour Hospital, the three Edinburgh Municipal General Hospitals and, at the last moment, Gogarburn Certified Institution was included in the Emergency Hospital Scheme. This provided 4739 beds for wartime casualties. An exchange was effected with the Public Assistance Committee whereby the Northern General Hospital became a Home for elderly, infirm patients. Craiglockhart Institute, one of the Committee's Residential Homes for the Elderly, became an Emergency Hospital under the Control of the Public Health Committee, and renamed the Southern General Hospital. From the three Emergency Hospitals the Corporation had call on 500 beds for ordinary civilian sick persons. This was a substantial reduction from the peace time accommodation and entailed careful selection of cases for admission. Dr Kemball, a Dental Surgeon, was appointed to help with casualties with jaw

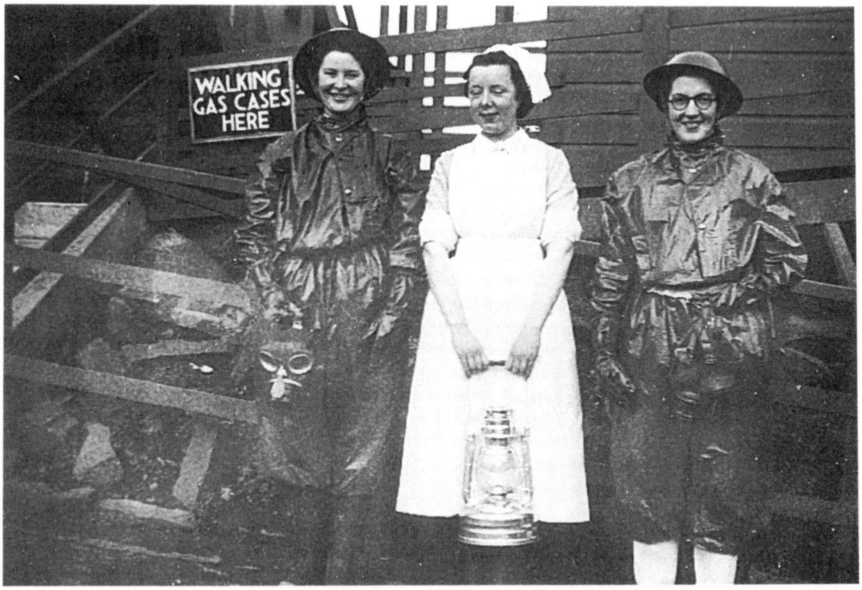

Nurses on Air Raid training (Sister Christine Orr in middle)

and with facial injuries. Dr Slessor was appointed as Resident Surgical Officer in 1939.

In 1944, under the Emergency Hospital Scheme, the Western General Hospital had 260 beds for this scheme, which was reduced in 1944 to 200. The Polish Medical School allocation under the scheme was increased to 150 beds. If British patients were admitted under the scheme, the hospital would be asked to recover such monies as patients could afford and this would be credited to the Emergency Scheme.

The Emergency Hospital Scheme was for the treatment and the reception of air raid casualties. To this end, an extra operating theatre was built in the Western General Hospital. In the event of an air raid, the number of ordinary sick were to be reduced to an essential minimal and priority given to the emergency casualty patients. The Hospital still continued to play its day-to-day role as a civilian hospital with certain beds allocated for military purposes. Patients were admitted to the Municipal General Hospital from the waiting list of the Royal Infirmary. During the War, casualties were brought into Leith from France and usually were fractures, often with the plasters full of maggots. These soldier patients were accommodated in the two previous gynaecology wards. Casualties were brought to the Paderewski Polish Hospital from the Altmark and included German prisoners. As war went on, increasing numbers of civilian patients were admitted.

The Public Health Department was responsible for recruiting and training nursing auxiliaries for the hospitals and in addition civil defence workers. The civil defence workers were responsible for bringing the casualties to the Emergency

Hospitals. Volunteers were also recruited to act as stretcher bearers. In Edinburgh they were paid 2s 6d (13p) for each attendance for enrolling and training. It was agreed that casualties would be brought into a reception ward from the north side of the hospital.

At the outbreak of the war anti-bombing precautions were initiated. The boilerhouse was surrounded by sandbags as a protection against air raids. An important requirement during this period was the covering of all windows with blackout material to decrease the likelihood of bombers finding their targets. In 1939 all the hospital railings were removed for scrap metal for the war effort — 250 yards of the main block, six yards around the kitchen, 12 yards at the gatehouse and 15 yards in the gardens south of the gatehouse.

During World War II the three Municipal General Hospitals in Edinburgh looked after many foreign nationals. After the fall of Poland, Scotland became a refuge for exiled Poles and hospital facilities were needed for treatment. The Western General's Children's Home and Wards D5, D7, and D8 were allocated as a separate Unit for Polish combatants and civilians and named the Paderewski Hospital in honour of Poland's national hero and world famous pianist. This was partly a clinical training school for the Polish School of Medicine and also catered for the Polish population.

The Matron of the Western General Hospital during the Polish Medical School was Miss Teresa Allan who was given the Polish Gold Cross for Merit in 1947. This recognised her work in the provison of nurses for the Polish section of the Hospital during the war.

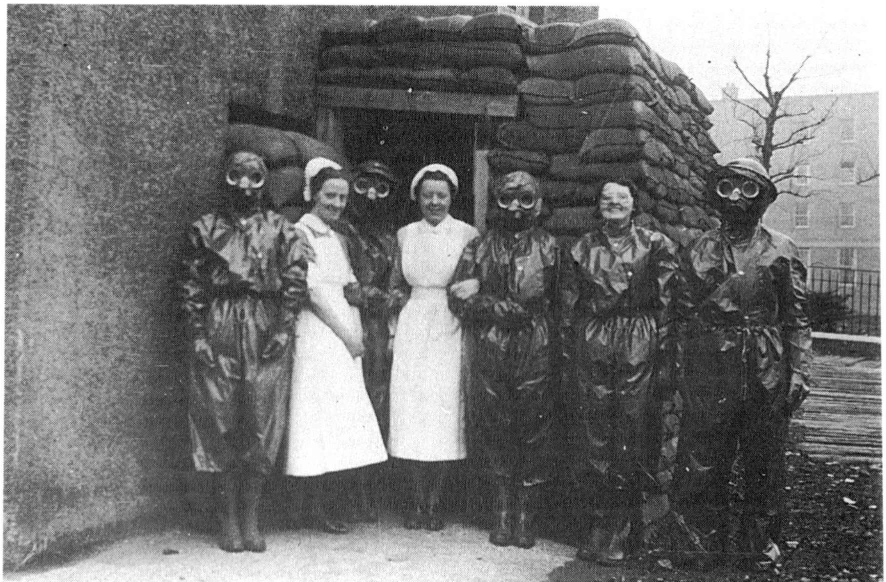

Nurses at gas mask training

The view held in medical circles in those days was that as most of the clinical talent and modern equipment was in the voluntary hospitals they should be used for the diagnosis and treatment of patients who could be cured. Incurable patients could be sent to their homes to be looked after by their family doctor. If the situation in the home made this impossible contact was made with the Medical Officer of Health who was responsible in law for providing such patients with beds in hospitals. Consequently, the Western, Northern and Eastern were occupied to a large extent by incurable medical and surgical patients.

There were some refurbishments of the Hospital during the war period. In 1944 an emergency electrical supply to theatres was installed, electricity was introduced to ward D4 and a telephone was also installed in the Almoner's room. In March 1945 running water was installed in the wards at a total cost of £296. At the end of the war the inevitable arrears of painting and other hospital maintenance work were undertaken by the City Architects Department at a cost of over £29,000. When the Municipal hospitals were handed over in 1948 to the Regional Hospital Board they were in good working order, although the legacy of a chronic nursing staff shortage was inherited by the new administration.

In 1945 The Western General Hospital's average weekly costs were £4 4s (£4.20p) a week for each patient:

Cost of Salaries	%
Doctors and other staff:	41.0
Medicine:	13.0
Provision to staff and patients:	19.0
Heating, lighting & water:	11.0
Repairs:	6.0
Rates:	3.0
Upkeep of ground:	1.0

The money was collected from patients. However 94% of patients paid less than 25s (£1.25p), 76% of patients paid less than 10s (50p) and 40% paid nothing.

In 1944 Mr Logan was appointed as a Thoracic Surgeon at the Western General Hospital with 17 beds and an Anaesthetist was appointed to assist him. Ian Aird was appointed to the Surgical Unit. He subsequently moved to the Hammersmith Hospital in London where he became a highly distinguished Professor of Surgery. Ethna Little was appointed Assistant in Obstetrics and Gynaecology.

The provision of food during rationing was a problem. Nurses had to bring in their own butter and sugar which was rationed. There were lots of rice puddings, macaroni and cheese on the menu.

On the social side, there were regular dances in the Nurses Home. Matron would telephone the Paderewski Hospital and tell the Polish CO that the nurses were having a dance. This continued until one particular occasion when there was 'misbehaviour' and the nursing staff were denied permission to attend these occasions.

At the beginning of the war a large, 7ft water tank was built behind the recreation hall to meet fire regulations in the event of a bombing attack. This proved to be a source of temptation for medical students to push nurses into. Amongst the pranks played was the night when residents painted gentian violet on all the toilet seats in the nurses home.

The grand tradition of giving a layette to the mother of the first child born in the Western General Hospital Maternity Unit at the beginning of each year began in 1944. The money came from the fund for welfare work in the Public Health Department and the layette cost £6. The Lord and Lady Provost were invited on the first day of the year and presented the layette.

One of the problems created by war was an increase in the numbers of illegitimate births. Often the pregnancies were concealed, and the mothers did not enjoy the safety of good obstetric care until late in their pregnancy. In 1944 the number of illegitimate babies who died in institutions numbered 65, of whom 33 died in the Western General Hospital. This reflected maternal health as much as anything.

During the war years chronic nursing and domestic staff difficulties were experienced, particularly in the Eastern and Southern General Hospitals. The problems of recruiting nursing staff was such that in 1944 the grade of Male Nurse/Nursing Orderly was introduced. They were paid 72s a week rising to 78s a week (£3.60–£ 3.90). The position to some extent was relieved in 1945 by the employment of male nursing orderlies who had had wartime experience in the Medical Service of the Army, Navy and Air Force. Training Schools were established at the Western General Hospital to enable them to qualify for State registration.

By 1945 recruitment problems had eased, but housing and other accommodation became a real problem. Additional nursing accommodation in the form of prefabricated huts was built alongside the Nurses Home. These were subsequently demolished to make way for the Alexander Donald Building.

In 1945 the Public Health Committee Meeting was approached by the Medical Office of Health who asked for a Preliminary Training School to be provided for nurses. This was a pre-requisite for recognition of the nurses Training School. The course was to last three months and there would be four intakes with 12–16 nurses a year.

A biochemical technician was appointed in 1945 on a salary between £255 and £265 a year. There was also increased work in the Dispensary. At that time there was one male Pharmacist, and one Assistant Pharmacist responsible for dispensing drugs.

Supplies of tobacco, sweets and cigarettes were given to certain patients who had limited income: for example old age pensioners up to a maximum of 2s 6d per week (13p). The total bill for such largesse in the Western General Hospital was £20 in 1946.

Sir Stanley Davidson described the changes which occurred in the Western, Eastern and Northern General Municipal Hospitals in the *Royal College of Physicians of Edinburgh Chronicle July 1975* In October 1938 he had returned to

Edinburgh to take up the position of Professor of Medicine, having been in Aberdeen University as Professor for the previous eight years. He was also appointed Director of the Medical Wards of the three Municipal General Hospitals — the Western, Eastern and Northern. This was at the insistence of the Lord Provost who was an important member of the University Court who had heard derogatory remarks about the catering, nursing and medical services in these hospitals. Sir Stanley was asked to investigate these problems and write a Report for him and the Medical Officer of Health in regard to the correctness and potential for improvement of these views . The Report was never made but it was felt that the sad state of affairs was not the fault of the medical and nursing staff but the system under which they had to work.

2. Polish School of Medicine, University of Edinburgh

When Poland became an early victim of Nazi Germany many Polish young men escaped by a variety of routes to France where a new Polish army was formed. After the fall of France in 1940 a large proportion of the serving Polish Forces were evacuated to Great Britain by the Royal Navy to regroup in Scotland. Following the occupation of eastern Poland by Russia in 1939 many thousands of Polish men and women were arrested and interned by the Russians and taken to hard labour camps east of the Urals and even as far away as Siberia. When Germany invaded Soviet Russia these prisoners were released in 1941. Some travelled by ship and lorry across the Caspian Sea to Persia (now known as Iran), others walked from Siberia through Kazakhstan to Iran where they met up with the British Army and eventually many came to Scotland. Many of these Polish units who came to Britain subsequently fought with great courage and valour for their country in the Polish Army . There were a number of medical students in these Polish Forces, whose studies were interrupted by the war. There was also a number of University Professors and Lecturers in the Medical Corps of the Polish Army.

The Commanding Officer of the Military Hospital at Edinburgh Castle was Lieut. Col. Professor F.A.E. Crew. He was already well disposed to Poland as a number of Polish students of genetics had worked with him, amongst whom was Dr Kopec who returned to Poland. He was later summarily executed in one of the retaliatory exercises that the Germans were given to. He was aware of the presence in the Polish Forces of a number of medical students, professors and lecturers. He developed the idea of a Polish Medical School in Edinburgh, separate from but integral to the Edinburgh Medical School. This would enable these young students to complete their Medical course, to be of service to their army and, after the war, to Poland: a singular concept in the history of Medicine. In October 1940 Professor F.A.E. Crew presented the idea to the Dean of the Faculty of Medicine, Professor Sydney Smith who agreed, as did the Faculty, Senatus and the Principal, Sir Thomas Holland. A proposal was sent to the Polish Government in exile in London who gladly accepted.

For the Poles the driving force was provided by General W Sikorski. The

Professor of Surgery of Poznan University, Dr Antoni Jurasz was given the job of organising the medical school and he became the first Dean of the School. He was the first surgeon ever to operate successfully on the pancreas. He drained a pancreatic cyst to the stomach, and he ranks with the surgical greats. He was an Anglophile, whose mother was an English woman who remained in Warsaw, and was present during the Warsaw Rising at the end of the war and survived to die some years later. He was born in Heidelberg where his father was Professor of Laryngology. Professor Jurasz and Professor Crew had similar appearances. Some people wondered why one appeared one day in a Polish uniform and the next day in a British uniform and vice versa

Polish Medical School Created

In 1941 an agreement was signed between the Polish Government and the University of Edinburgh in which the Polish Medical School was created. The Polish School of Medicine in Edinburgh was established on the 24 February 1941 as a completely independent but integral part of the University of Edinburgh.

Similar schools were established in the University of Liverpool where there was a Polish School of Architecture and a Polish Veterinary School at the Royal (Dick) Veterinary College in Edinburgh, and a Faculty of Law at the University of Oxford.

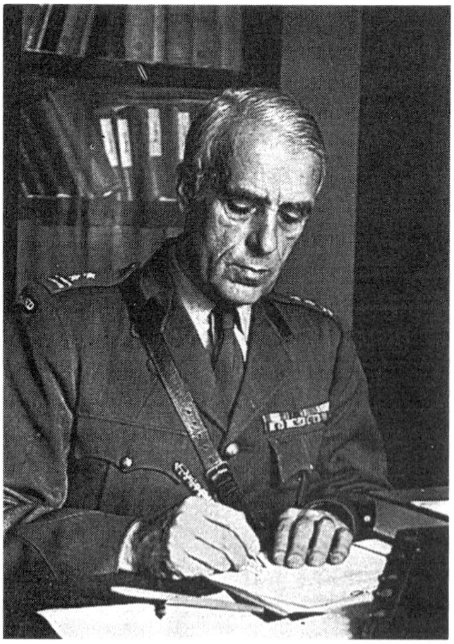

Lt. Col. Professor A Jurasz, Organiser and First Dean of the Polish School of Medicine

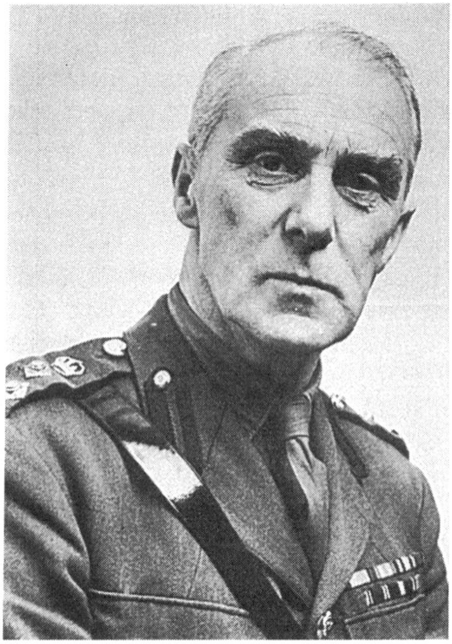

Brigadier Professor F.A.E. Crew, initiator of the Polish Medical Faculty at the University of Edinburgh

The constitution of the Polish Medical School was:

1. The Head of the Polish Medical School should be the Dean with the power of a Rector or Principal of a Polish University;
2. The Faculty shall consist of Polish Professors who have held chairs in Poland, Professors of the Faculty of Medicine of Edinburgh University would teach only those subjects for which Polish professors were not available. The Dean should be one of the Polish Professors elected by the Faculty and approved by the competent Polish authorities after consultation with the University of Edinburgh;
3. The curriculum and standard of teaching, and of examinations of the School shall be the same as those in the medical faculties in Polish universities and as far as possible required by the Medical Faculty of the University of Edinburgh.

The examinations were either in Polish or English, depending on whether the chair was held by a Polish or Scottish professor.

Students matriculated at Edinburgh University. The degrees of the graduates were the same as in the pre-war Polish Universities and were conferred at the University graduation ceremony by the Polish Dean. Subsequently the Medical Practitioners and Pharmacists Act for 1947 allowed graduates of the Polish School to register as medical practitioners in the United Kingdom. Most of the newly graduated doctors joined the units of the Polish Army, Navy or Air Force for the remainder of the war.

In April with the concept of the Polish Medical School established, Professor Jurasz, accompanied by other senior academic staff and Mr Banks, later the Lord Provost, were taken by bus, first of all to view a hospital, opposite the City Hospital, which later became Greenbank Nursing Home. This was not considered suitable. They were then taken to the Western General Hospital and the Children's Home which was separate from the main building on the east of the main hospital and which was considered a suitable building. It was empty, the children having been sent to other homes in Craiglockhart. The hospital had all the necessary facilities and the school opened within six months.

The Polish Medical school was opened by the President of Poland, Mr W Raczkiewicz at a large ceremony in the McEwan Hall on 22 March 1941. The Lord Provost of Edinburgh, and representatives of the British and Polish Governments were present.

At the inauguration the Polish medical teaching staff consisted of 22 Professors and Lecturers, among whom a few women. Seventy Polish students attended the Inaugural Ceremony and were drawn from Polish Military camps in Scotland. They were later joined by medical students from the Polish military units in other parts of the world, mostly the Middle East.

The Polish Professors were J. Fegler, A. Jurasz, W. Koskowski, L. Lakner, B. Nowakowski, T. Rogalski, J. Rostowski, J. Ruszkowski, A. Straszynski and J. Dadlez.

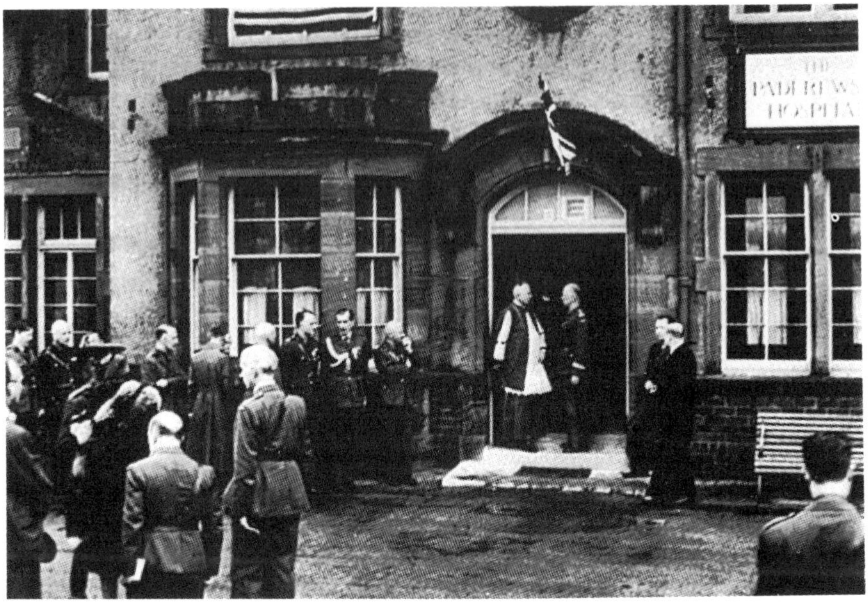

Dedication of the Paderewski Memorial Hospital October 1941

The Edinburgh Professors were Professors Crew, Davidson, Drennan, Johnstone, McNeill, Mackie, Marrian, Sydney Smith, Kellar and Learmonth.

The full Polish Faculty consisted of Sir Stanley Davidson, Professor Murray Drennan, Professor J. Fegler, Professor R. W. Johnstone and then a number of Polish and other members of the Edinburgh Faculty. Dr Tomaszewski, who later became a general practitioner in Edinburgh, was a member of the teaching faculty.

The activity of the school peaked in the academic year of 1944 to 1945 when the number of students reached 220. Over the eight years there were over 330 medical students of whom 227 graduated MB ChB, and 18 graduates received MD diplomas after submitting a doctorate thesis.

The pre-clinical subjects were taught in the appropriate department of the Edinburgh Medical Faculty. Anatomy, histology and biology were taught in a building belonging to the University, in Bristo Street, opposite the McEwan Hall. This was demolished in the 1970s.

The majority of the clinical teaching was in the Royal Infirmary. Some practical instruction in medicine and surgery was in the Paderewski Hospital. Ophthalmology, larynology, stomatology (dentistry) and radiology were taught entirely in the Paderewski. There were also offices and a pharmacy in the hospital. Most of the students lived in a hostel at 5 Grovesnor Crescent.

Among the other teaching hospitals were the Royal Hospital for Sick Children, City Hospital, and the Eastern General Hospital.

The teaching staff consisted of 10 Professors and 27 Lecturers. Aside from teaching they published about 100 research papers. All clinics, hospital wards and laboratories were open to the Polish students and every facility was provided. The Department of Anatomy, Histology and Biology was given use of lecture theatres, tutorial rooms, microscopes, instruments, reagents, slides and films. Separate buildings were provided for offices.

Paderewski Hospital

The Polish hospital was independent of the Polish Medical School. The hospital was opened on the 17 October 1941 in the Nurses' Hall at the Western General Hospital in the presence of the Polish Prime Minister and Commander in Chief of the Polish Army, General W. Sikorski; the Deputy Prime Minister, Mr S. Mikolajczyk;. the Lord Provost of Edinburgh, Sir Henry Steele and others. The Earl of Rosebery officially opened the hospital. At the outset it was planned that there should be 120 beds, the number was later increased to 150. The hospital was named after the Polish composer and pianist Paderewski who earned money in North America by giving concerts to support the hospital.

The Patron of the Hospital was Princess Alice, Duchess of Gloucester.

During the war there were a large number of Polish civilians and members of the armed forces in Edinburgh. Possibly between 2,000–3,000 Poles were living in this part of Scotland, driven there by the war. Patients also came from the Polish navy in Rosyth and civilians came up from London. Injured and ill soldiers were brought from the front to Edinburgh. There were a further three hospitals in Scotland, one being at Taymouth Castle.

There were various Polish institutions in Edinburgh : the Polish School of Medicine, Polish Veterinary School at the Royal (Dick) Vet. College, the Polish church at St Ann's Oratory (still existing) at Randolph Place, a number of military offices, Polish Red Cross, Scottish-Polish House (British Council) at Greenhill Gardens, to name only some.

The budget of the Paderewski Polish hospital was independent of the Polish Medical School. The medical staff were on the staff of the Polish School of Medicine. The Paderewski Testimonial Fund of New York in the United States provided substantial sums for the purchase of hospital equipment which was intended to be transferred to Poland after the war. The Scottish authorities provided the running costs of the building, nursing staff, catering and laundry. Some expenses were taken over by the military and Polish Government in London.

An official coat of arms for the Polish School of Medicine was designed. After consultation with the University authorities and the Lord Lyon King at Arms, the Coat of Arms of the School was finally accepted and authorized in 1942. It consisted of a white cross on a blue field, with the Polish eagle in the centre, medical symbols of rod and snake in the lateral fields, the thistle in the upper field and a castle on a rock in the lower field. This plaque was lost for many years until it was found by Martin Eastwood during one of the Public Service Union strikes in the Health Service in the 1980's. The original is to be seen in the entrance of the Outpatient building of the Western General Hospital. Copies of this are in the Royal Infirmary of Edinburgh and the University of Potsnam and Warsaw.

In 1942 the Duchess of Gloucester unveiled an ornamental commemorative tablet 3ft by 3ft by 2ft in the lobby of the Paderewski hospital:

> This tablet is erected in deep gratitude and sincere appreciation of the generosity of the Secretary of State for Scotland and the Corporation of the City of Edinburgh in making this building available and rendering all possible assistance in the establishment of the Polish Hospital in Edinburgh during the Second World War.

Another tablet of similar dimensions was given in memory of American donors to the Paderewski Memorial Hospital and was unveiled two years later by the wife of the American Ambassador to Britain, Mrs Wyatt. These plaques were stolen after the war during maintenance work.

In wartime the Western General Hospital was certainly the busiest Polish place in Edinburgh. The Paderewski Hospital regularly accomodated 120–150 hospitalized patients (civilians and soldiers) from various parts of Britain (particularly London). The number was increased to 150 with the increase of war activity, the invasion of Europe and during the post war period. The average daily number of outpatients was about 100, attending various departments,

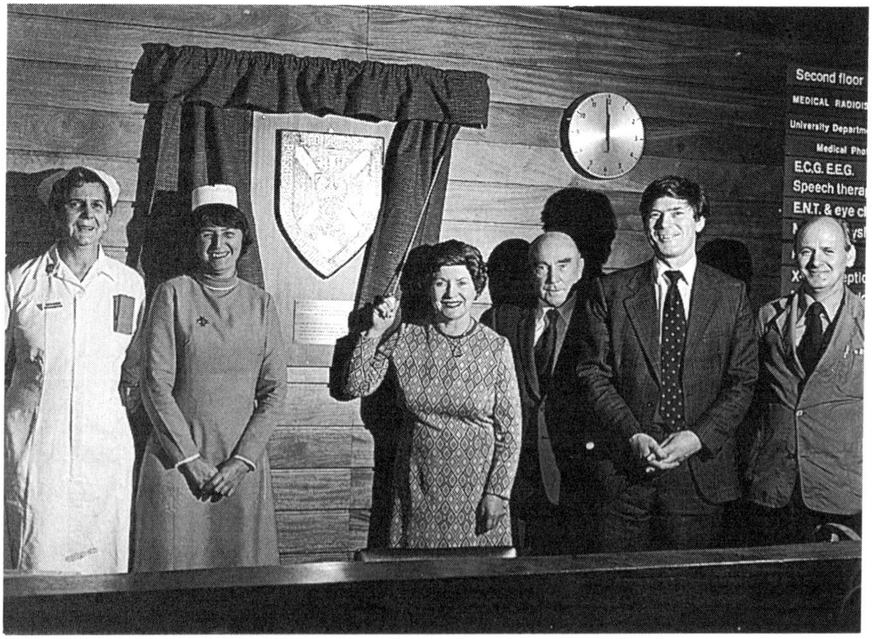

Unveiling of plaque commemorating Polish Medical School 1979; (Sister Trina Wheeler, Outpatient Sister; Miss Helen Griffen, Deputy Matron; Dr W Tomaszewski, Reader in Medicine, University of Poznan and Polish School of Medicine, Edinburgh; Dr Martin Eastwood, Chairman of Clinical Staff Committee; Mr Charlie Wood, Head Porter; at Outpatient Department, Western General Hospital

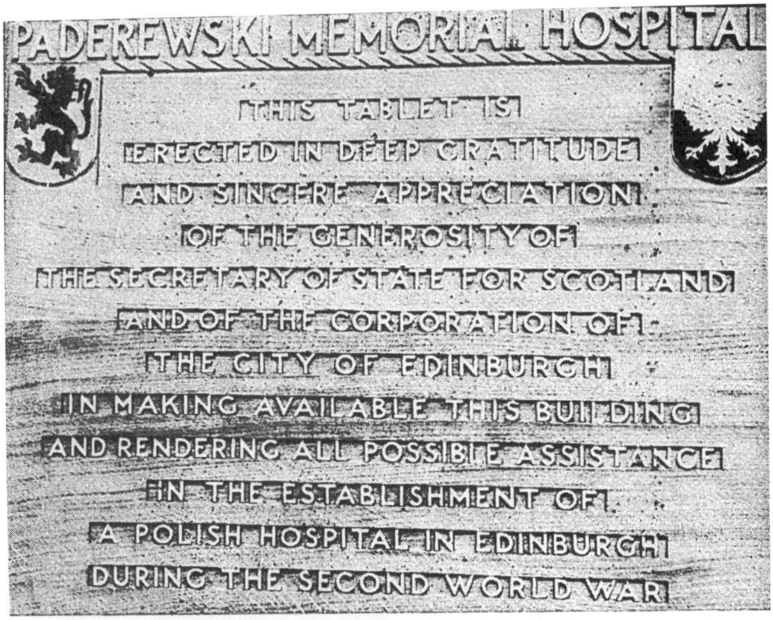

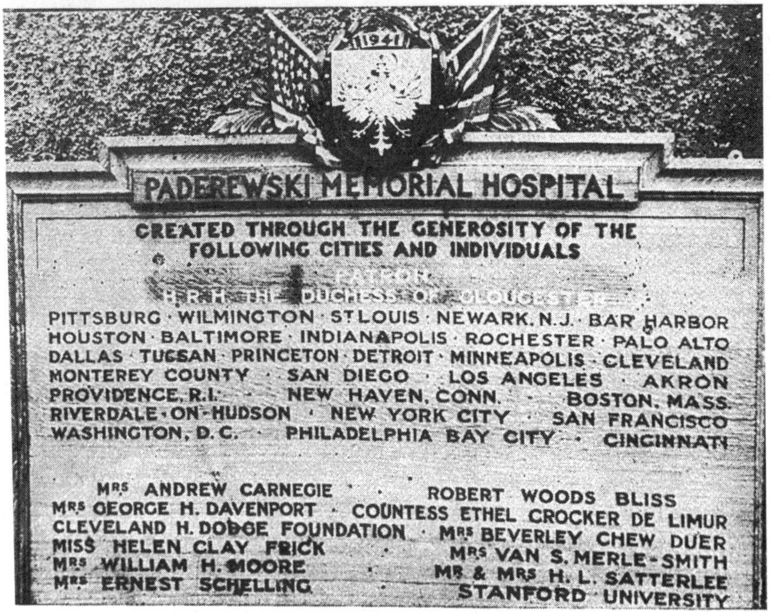

Plaques to the Paderewski Memorial Hospital which went missing during building of Outpatient Department especially stomatology (dental department). The X-ray department had a Polish radiologist on duty.

During 1942 the number of Polish out patients was 12,134 and by 1943 this had increased to 34,129. The number of patients in the wards rose during the same period from 1203 to 1539, largely war injuries. The Polish war cemetery at Corstorphine Hill contains 200 graves of Polish soldiers.

The Polish medical staff, Polish students and Polish visitors to the patients made Polish uniforms a daily sight in the west of Edinburgh. The Polish language was heard widely not only in the Paderewski building but also in other departments of the Western General Hospital. Buses passing Crewe Road brought regular groups of Polish civilians or soldiers to the hospital. Military ambulances brought soldiers daily from the Polish camps to the outpatient departments or for hospitalisation. The Western General Hospital was the place for meeting friends, reading Polish papers and to discuss the current politics or the military situation in other parts of the world.

In general, 'life was like a dream' for these exiles. 'Things happened that could never be foreseen by cool reasoning.' Both students and the teaching staff had crossed hostile frontiers in order to reach the Forces in the West. Here in Edinburgh unique opportunities were presented that opened new chances and never to be forgotten opportunities through the Polish School of Medicine and the Polish hospital in Edinburgh. Students and the teaching staff considered themselves to be in a privileged position. Also the numerous Polish patients who daily entered the grounds of the Western General Hospital felt themselves lucky to be able to converse freely in Polish with their doctors without the use of an interpreter.

Apart from the Paderewski building the surgery and gynaecology/midwifery wards of the Western General Hospital were used by Polish patients in designated rooms. Polish medical students attended the delivery of babies of both Polish and Scottish women. They also took part in emergency obstetric calls to Scottish patients in the town (ambulance) assisting the doctor and the midwife.

The nurses in the Polish wards were Scottish, some of them from the Hebrides who had the Gaelic. They were all liked and were highly appreciated by the Polish patients for their skill and friendliness, sense of duty and humanity. Some of them learned a number of Polish words which they used to the delight of the patients.

The Polish Medical School was established by an agreement between the Polish Government and the British Government solely for the duration of the war. There were to be no new students at the end of the war. However, 37 senior medical students came to Britain, having been liberated from prisoner of war camps. The School had stopped accepting students and they were admitted to a private medical school that stayed open for a further two years. The teachers attached to the official Polish School of Medicine in Edinburgh cooperated in the teaching of the students in the private medical school which ran in parallel with the official school. These unofficial students were given a certificate to show they had concluded medical studies and had passed all the necessary examinations to obtain a medical diploma. This was recognised by the General Medical Council and enabled them to apply for examination in the London Conjoint examination, LRCP and MRCS. Some 15 of the students finished their course and passed their examinations. Some students had completed only the first three years of their course in Poland before the war, were regarded as having the same privileges of returning British soldiers and were admitted as medical students for the standard British courses.

Postwar

After the war the School gradually ran down and the last group of students graduated in March 1949. The completion of the School came when the last Dean of the School, Professor Rostowski, unveiled a plaque in commemoration of the Polish Medical School in the New Quadrangle in Teviot Place.

The plan was that at the end of the war there would be a transfer of the School and the Hospital to Poland. Post war collaboration with the University of Edinburgh was envisaged. This was not to be. Post war realities, the iron curtain in Europe and the Stalinist terror in Poland shattered the dreams. Two visits by Professor Jurasz to post-war Poland was sufficient to convince him of the situation. Disillusioned, Professor Jurasz settled in the United States, where he tried to re-establish a Medical School, without success. He died in the USA in 1961.

Most of the graduates settled in Britain after the war, a few in Edinburgh, others emigrated to the USA, Canada, Australia, New Zealand and France, or joined the Colonial Service. Only 10% returned to Poland.

6

The National Health Service, 1948

The National Health Service

The Administration of the Hospital

All Corporation administered hospitals, including the Municipal General Hospitals, passed out of the control of the Corporation at the inception of the Health Service and were thereafter administered by the South Eastern Regional Hospital Board. These changes in administration resulted from more than two years of discussions.

With the inauguration of the Health Service there followed a period of inactivity while the new administrative bodies found their feet and endeavoured to survey the situation in order to plan a co-ordinated service. This meant that the service had to continue in old and unsatisfactory accommodation, quite unsuitable for modern medicine.

With the introduction of the National Health Service in 1948, the Public Health Committee was renamed the Health Committee, and its membership was reduced to 15, including Chairman. Two standing Sub-Committees were created:

1. Medical Health Services — dealing with the care of mothers and young children, prevention of illness, care and aftercare, Local Authority nursing services, home helps and health education.
2. General Health Services — concerned with infectious disease control, sea and air port sanitation, mental health and the work of the sanitary and veterinary departments.

The National Health Service Bill

The responsibility for hospital services was taken over by the Government. Existing hospitals, voluntary and public were transferred to Government control. The administration of the hospitals were entrusted to Regional Hospital Boards.

The Local Authority and University explained that, owing to the financial state of the country in 1945, 'there was no possibility in the immediate future of financing the building of a new hospital block at the Western General Hospital, which would contain the necessary accommodation for patients with acute and curable diseases, and also the requisite laboratories for appropriate research.'

In order to try and change this Sir Stanley Davidson met with Sir Sidney Smith, Dean of the Faculty of Medicine at the University of Edinburgh, and the Medical Officer for Health of the City of Edinburgh. Sir Stanley felt that the selection of the right medical person was of much greater importance in making a successful Clinical Unit than the bricks and mortar of which it was built or the amount of equipment it contained. Sir Stanley said that if he was able to persuade 12 medical specialists of the highest calibre to accept the challenge of developing six new Units in Edinburgh, then the hospital would progress. In 1945–46 many doctors were being demobilised from the services. Many had yet to decide where they were going to work. Six Teaching and Research Units were established. Two new Medical Units were created at the Western General Hospital, one for the study of cardiovascular diseases and the second for gastro-intestinal diseases. In the Northern General there were to be three new Units, Rheumatic Diseases, Neurological Diseases and Respiratory Diseases. At the Eastern General Hospital a Unit for the Study and Treatment of Tropical Diseases would be continued and enlarged. In each Unit there would be a Senior Specialist paid by the University and a second more junior Specialist paid for by the Corporation who also would pay the junior medical staff salaries. At a meeting between the University, the Corporation and the Board of Management of the Royal Infirmary and other small hospitals, a plea was made that every hospital took a quota of the chronic sick. This would allow the new Units at the Municipal Hospitals to obtain sufficient suitable clinical material for teaching and research.

Many patients were admitted through personal communication with the general practitioner, who would telephone the waiting resident or registrar. Many of the local practitioners were frequent visitors to the hospital and were known personally to the staff. In the poor social conditions of the early 1950's a proportion of patients were admitted unkempt, malnourished and verminous; many elderly patients had no teeth and many did not have suitable clothing and were clad in hospital nightgowns. Many came in terminally ill or dying. The two hospital almoners and their student assistants did what they could with very limited resources.

Medical Residents, as the name implies, lived in the hospital and dined together. The old residency was at the main gate with the porters underneath. This gatehouse accidently burnt down. The resident doctors then moved to the medical superintendent's house opposite D block. As there was no official off duty time, friendly co-operation and sharing of duties were essential. There was a cupboard bar in the mess sitting room and mess parties took place with some regularity. Relations with senior staff both on the medical and the nursing side were more formal than today but on the whole tolerant and friendly and like any community of young people working closely together they knew how to 'temper the bitter things with gentle laughter.' (Horace).

By 1946 problems with catering were identified. The kitchen service was to be re-organised with:

1. A main kitchen dealing with soups, meats, fish, poultry and vegetables. Here would work one kitchen superintendent, one deputy kitchen superintendent, one assistant kitchen superintendent and two cooks.
2. A pastry kitchen dealing with puddings, sweets, scones, slab cakes and fairy cakes. This would be served by one depute superintendent, one depute kitchen superintendent and one cook.
3. A diet kitchen responsible for special diets prescribed by doctors and for the supply of light diets. This would be serviced by a Dietitian and two cooks.

In addition to this there would be one male kitchen porter, one butcher, four vegetable maids and four scullery maids. The accommodation for maids in the attic floor was agreed to be very unsatisfactory.

Only resident staff lunched at the hospital. No meals were provided and people went home. Most of the medical staff lived in Eglinton Crescent, so everything was very local.

There were two telephone operators who worked from 9.00 a.m. to 10.00 p.m. then the service was taken over by a porter who was also responsible for other duties. From 10.00pm a nurse took over and this was regarded as an unsatisfactory situation. The whole system was replaced by three male telephone operators.

During this period the library service was organised and an occupational therapist was appointed at a salary of between £175 to £225 per year.

There was an ambition for a swimming pool at the Western General Hospital after the war. During the war an emergency water tank was built which held 140,000 gallons and was 7ft deep and this was close to the Nursing Home. It was felt that tarmacadam should be put round the tank and a simple form of chlorination used — the total cost £520. After many discussions this was not taken up by the Public Health Committee of Edinburgh Corporation.

The medical superintendent during this period after the War was Dr MacMillan, a Glasgow graduate who worked from D Block and subsequently went to the Taplow Canadian Red Cross Hospital. He was succeeded by Dr Sandy Donald who prior to this had worked in the Medical Officer of Health's office and at the City Hospital.

Doctors in Management

Dr Sandy Donald proved to be a masterly supervisor of the post- war development of the Western General Hospital. He was blessed with a very agreeable personality, a friend to all, and most of all a good listener.He worked in close harmony with the Matron, Miss Estelle Adamson.

During the period after the war, the Western General was very much in the mould of Sir Stanley Davidson's original vision. The staff would encourage the change. The great enthusiams of staff were repeatedly dampened by the inauspicious surroundings. A hospital, based on specialties, had strengths and weaknesses compared to the massive tradition of the Royal Infirmary.

The Medical Staff Committee began as a dining club, a forum for socialising the brainchild of Wilfrid Card. The meetings, if they became at all political, dealt with car parking and other domestic issues. The companionship was in part due to the small number of staff, their agreeable nature in general, and Wilfrid Card's sense of *bon homie*. When Card left he presented a loving cup as a memorial and perpetuation of this social life.

The Medical Staff Committee began to be drawn into a more administrative and managerial role. Initially in Medical Education, with a Staff Clinical Round held each week in the Teaching and Research Unit, where there was very good clinical debate. To encourage clinical research presentation, a Card Lecture was initiated and Wilfrid Card came from Glasgow to give the first lecture in 1984. The type of speaker alternated — one year a senior figure, the next year a young clinician with promise.

Sandy Donald retired and was replaced by Dr Jim Ferguson, a vigorous clinical manager and knew his contemporaries from medical school. He participated in the introduction of new concepts of care, e.g. 5-day and day care surgical treatment. Slowly the management team came into being. Dr Ferguson's successors were Community Medicine Specialists such as Dr Jim Cooper who had more of a medical management style. The clinical input came from the Chairman of the Clinical Staff Committee. The Chairman of the clinical staff gradually adopted a role in this new management process. This was an annual appointment and included Dr Bill Sircus and Mr Ian Kirkland. They became part of the Hospital Management team. This proved to be a task that made intolerable demands on a clinician who continued in day-to-day practice, which was the basis of their contribution.

The initial management team consisted of:

Miss Betty McLean	Matron
Mr Alan Shanks	Hospital Administrator
Professor Bill Duncan	Representative from the Medical Staff Committee
Mr Jim Boxall	Hospital Engineer
Mr Charles Evans	Finance
Mr Bill Scott	Pharmacist
Dr Jim Cooper	Community Medicine Specialist.

This team was active in the development of the Phase I building. The whole exercise was hampered by the lack of adequate statistics — how many staff, what was spent on what, by whom and where did equipment and supplies come from?

When management concepts came along in full with 'efficiency savings' the problems were compounded by industrial unrest. Slowly the team coalesced into a good working system, who in general understood each others problems.

The complexities of the changes had to be explained to medical/nursing and auxillary staff, and other clinical staff, who were unwilling to accept or sometimes countenance the changes. Bill Duncan was succeeded by Dr Martin Eastwood as Chairman of the Clinical Staff Committee in 1984. Initially he had no additional secretarial support and spent many weekends in this administrative role. The continued efficiency savings were a constant problem. Miss MacLean was a very good Unit Manager, who steadily guided the hospital through the vicissitudes of change yet retained a central vision of clinical care. Martin Eastwood was succeeded in 1988 by Dr Brian Slawson, a very able chairman, and thereafter the chairman was Dr John Scrimgeour, who in time became the first Medical Director of the Trust.

The development of the Trust had a considerable effect on the medical staff role in management. The Community Medical Specialist ceased to be an active member of the new management team. The Medical Director, a practising clinician took over. The hospital is divided into Directorates, each with a Clinical Director and a budget; the Clinical Director being a practicing clinician. The morass of the early days of management has now been replaced by clearer lines of financial knowledge. The Clinical Staff Committee has reverted, in part, to a social role, the more frequent meetings of the clinicians being in the meetings of the Directorates. Each Unit is administered by a Consultant with Administrative Responsibility. Clinical management now spreads everywhere. The original small NHS staff of the Western could be viewed, helped and facilitated by one Medical Superintendent. Now with a near ten-fold increase in staff, budgets and technical systems, it is necessary to have a system which keeps equally close to the clinician.

Nurses in Management

Historically, hospitals were run by doctors, with Matrons accountable to the Medical or Physician Superintendent for the provision of a nursing service. In the large hospitals there was a Hospital Secretary who assisted the Medical Superintendent in the day-to-day management and ensured the smooth running of services.

In 1966 there was a Board of Management for Edinburgh Northern Hospitals Group with the Medical Superintendent reporting to it. Matron attended the meetings, and the Hospital Secretary provided what is commonly referred to as administrative support. The detail of Matron's responsibility besides nursing services, included responsiblity for the Nurses Home and the School of Nursing. The Hospital Secretary was responsible for support services e.g. supplies, catering, portering and domestics. The Ward Sister at that time exercised more authority over all non- medical staff working on the ward.

The first major change for nursing emanated from the publication of the Salmon Report in 1966, the remit of the Committee being: 'To advise on the senior nursing staff structure in the hospital service (Ward Sister and above), the administrative functions of the respective grades and the methods of preparing staff to occupy them'.

Pay and conditions of service were outside the remit of the committee. This is an important point because of the way the new structure was introduced. There were mixed reactions from the nursing profession to the proposals outlined in the Report, not least because of the change of titles. Pilot sites were selected (Bangour General Hospital was one) with a view to evaluating the implications of the proposals being promoted. The Salmon Report was considered to be far-reaching as it was promoting clear lines of responsibility and accountability, enabling nurses to work in partnership in the decision-making process of the hospital. A career structure for nurses was outlined with levels of responsibility dependent upon laid-down criteria. Before an evaluation of the pilot sites was available, a decision to introduce the new structure was made as there seemed to be difficulty with salary scales for the new posts.

In 1972 a Chief Nursing Officer was appointed, responsible to the Board of Management for the nursing services in all the hospitals of the Group and the College of Nursing. The Principal Nursing Officer was responsible for four hospitals and in each hospital there was either one or two Senior Nursing Officers.

New faces and new responsibilities meant upheaval, uncertainty and inevitably a field day for the critics. However, even where there was radical change, with a new leader at the Western helm, the team of new Nurse Managers and some who had been in administrative posts before the change, rallied round to ensure that the service to patients was not affected.

It was in the early to mid-70's that there was a national shortage of trained nurses. Therefore, the obvious butts of criticism were the Nursing Officers who appeared to be 'running around with clipboards'. In addition, plans to reorganise the National Health Service were well underway with the 'Blue Band' circulars being issued from the Scottish Home and Health Department in abundance, to clarify the details of the changes from lst April 1974.

While Nurse Managers had been settling down in post and struggling to support hard-pressed Ward Sisters, there were periods when they were away at courses to assist them fulfil their responsibilities more efficiently. This led to further strain on the management of the nursing service.

In 1974 the Lothian Health Board came into being with an Area Executive Group — Chief Area Medical Officer, Chief Area Nursing Officer, Finance Officer and Board Secretary. The Area was divided into three geographical districts, i.e. South, West and North with each district establishing an executive team which replicated the members at Area Board. At the Western General Hospital, therefore, the Principal Nursing Officer was responsible to the District Nursing Officer, North Lothian District, the Administrator to the District Administrator. Financial input was provided from the District offices and the Chairman of the Medical Staff Committee represented the local clinical staff on the Western Management Group. Decision-making was to be by consensus. However, in considering the lines of responsibility outlined, this could and indeed did lead to difficulties.

In 1977, after the promotion of an Integrated Health Service, Community Nurses had been subjected to similar changes in management structure as their hospital colleagues. The nursing service within North Lothian District was changed. Previously the Principal Nursing Officer had been responsible for only hospital services. This changed to three Divisional Nursing officer posts, with each responsible for community and hospital services. The Divisional Nursing Officer (Miss McLean) was based at the Western and had responsibility for the Northern General, the Royal Victoria, Corstorphine, and Beechmount Hospitals. The responsibility extended to community nursing services covering the area from Fettes Avenue to South Queensferry. The responsibility of the Senior Nursing Officers and Nursing Officers within the Western did not radically change at this time. The bringing together at Senior Nursing Officer level of those nurses with responsibility for services outwith the acute hospital was constructive and helpful in promoting two-way communication for the benefit of patient care.

Nurses began to settle down to new management arrangements and make a positive contribution. There were others not so enchanted. This may, in part, have resulted from financial stringencies at a time when medical technology and treatment was advancing apace. There was criticism about cumbersome lines of communication, and a lack of clarity about who could make decisions which resulted in pressures, particularly from the medical profession, for change.

In 1978 a White Paper was published recommending that the District structure should be disbanded; there was to be no intermediate management between Area and local level. Again, turmoil and discussion. The deliberations began again until eventually in 1984 the District structure was disbanded. It should also be said that in the ten years between 1974 and 1984, hospital administrators were becoming 'key' to the service. This was not always accepted by professional groups as being correct in a supposedly consensus management environment.

In 1986 General Management was introduced, firstly by the appointment of a General Manager to Lothian Health Board and thereafter at Unit level. Discussion about the number and size of units was inevitable but the Western General, Northern General, Royal Victoria, Corstorphine, and Beechmount Hospitals remained as a Unit with the Unit General Manager at the head. A Unit Management Team was appointed: i.e. Nurse, Finance Officer, Administrator and Chairman of the Medical Staff Committee. Corporate decision-making and full responsibility for all services were vested in the Unit General Manager who was accountable to the Board General Manager.

While the effect on the Western could be said to have been minimal, there is no doubt that the tide of change continued. This culminated in the NHS Reforms with the introduction of the purchaser, provider arrangements and eventually hospitals having the opportunity to apply for self-governing Trust status.

The Western General Hospital became a Trust from lst April 1994. The voice of nursing will still be heard at Trust Board level as the Director of Nursing has a seat on that Board and is responsible for the development of the nursing profession within the Trust.

Management: 1972 Onwards

The 1972 National Health Service (Scotland) Act sought to establish a high degree of uniformity in the management approach through the powers delegated to 12 mainland and three island Health Boards. The main theme of the Act was the integration of hospital services, primary care and certain health services provided by local authorities. The following management approach was adopted in 1974:

(a) *a three-tier organisational structure:*
(i) the SHHD at the centre, responsible for the development of overall strategy and national resource allocation;
(ii) Health Boards with responsibility for determining the local services provided to the public;
(iii) and, within most Areas, a number of Districts with responsibilities delegated to them from Area;
(b) *a strong focus on professional management:* at Area and District level, the professional hierarchy matched the organisational tiers; senior officers were responsible for professional and line management of their departments or functions (administration, finance, nursing, works etc.), and the provision of their aspect of services; only the responsibilities of the Chief Administration Medical Officer (CAMO) and District Medical Officer were different in nature; they had no professional management responsibilities for clinicians, although the CAMO was the head of the Community Medicine Specialists (CMSs) and line manager for certain paramedical staff;
(c) *a team approach to cross-professional management:* at the Area and District tiers the senior professional officers from administration, finance, nursing and medicine were brought together in the Area Executive Group and District Executive Group respectively to manage certain tasks which crossed professional boundaries; the approach has often been termed consensus management; members of the team were regarded as equals, with no formal leader;
(d) *a strong professional advisory structure:* professional groups engaged in the provision of care or treatment were encouraged to set up committees at all levels to offer advice to the SHHD, Health Boards and local management as appropriate.

The Secretary of State recommended in 1981 and then required in 1983, that the District organisational tier be replaced by Units of management. It was stated that there should be the maximum possible delegation of responsibility, including financial responsibility, top those Units. Units of management were required to be 'coherent and discrete areas of management responsibility, forming a district management level to which substantial decisions could be delegated'.

The significant features of the revised organisational structure were:

(a) the overall responsibilities of the Health Board did not change;
(b) while there was a general guideline exhorting delegation, there was considerable freedom given on where particular management tasks would be carried out;
(c) there was no change in the accent on professional management;
(d) the management ethos was still built around the team approach to cross-disciplinary issues; the team at unit level had to comprise an administrator and a nurse and make arrangements for medical input.

Units were therefore created; and even as they were being established, a further change in approach to the management task was announced — the introduction of general management.

1986: To Date

The Principles of General Management

General management is an approach to the management task at every level in an organisation; it should affect how all aspects of the management task are carried out. The Griffiths recommendations made this clear:

> By general management, we mean the responsibility.....at different levels of the organisation for planning, implementation and control of performance. Absence of this general management support means that there is no driving force seeking and accepting direct and personal responsibility for developing management plans, securing their implementation and monitoring actual achievement.

A number of points emerged from this statement which helped to define the characteristics of general management:

— that general management is, as its name implies, general in nature and about the performance of the health care services provided to patients and to the community;
— that it is an overall approach to the management task, a 'driving force';
— that it extends across the whole range of the management task from planning to implementation and control of performance;
— that it should apply at different levels of the health service.

General management is therefore concerned with those issues which cross professional boundaries and which determine the quality of the total service to the patient and the community.

The starting point in establishing general management principles were:

— *responsibility* for the achievement of an objective should be clearly stated and accepted;
— *authority* to control services and resources should match the responsibility given and the competence of the individual;

— *lines of managerial accountability* should be simple and clear;
— *involvement* of those who make decisions on services and resource use is, therefore, necessary;
— *leadership* is essential to ensure that individual goals and motivations are harnessed to the objectives of the organisation;
— *delegation* should be encouraged to ensure that management decisions are taken as close to the point of implementation as is practicable;
— *information and communication* should enable those responsible to monitor services and resource use.

By encouraging *delegation* of decision-making responsibilities, it becomes possible for those directly involved in the provision of services to base decisions on their more detailed knowledge of priorities and the needs of patients. Delegation does not, however, represent an abandonment or replacement of managerial control and must be accompanied by effective arrangements for monitoring and supervision.

If accountability is to be meaningful, *information and communication* systems will be needed to enable those involved in general management to monitor services and exercise control. Equally, these will be required to enable the Health Board to monitor the performance of general management at unit level.

General management involved a fundamental culture change in the approach to managing the health service. It was not simply about a change in organisational tiers, nor about reallocating management tasks between different tiers, nor about revising management teams or procedures. Rather it was a different management ethos; and its introduction led to changes in all aspects of management.

The first phase of the introduction of general management to the Scottish Health Service was completed by the end of 1985, when Board General Managers had been appointed to all the Health Boards.

The Trust was brought into being in 1994. The members of the Trust were:

Mr Michael Walker, Chairman; Mr John Connaghan, Chief Executive; Dr John Scrimgeour, Medical Director; John Hope, Director of Finance; Mrs Alexandra Harvey, Director of Nursing and Quality; Mr Tom Mair, Director of Human Resources; Mr David Brodin, Director of Corporate Services; Mr Henry Fairweather; Mrs Nan Howe; Professor J. Douglas Miller; Mr William Stewart; Mrs Morag Younie.

Buildings

The Western General Hospital of today evolved from the 1867 St Cuthbert's Parish Poor House building. Each phase represents the needs of that time, so in some respects the building programme illustrates the history of public medicine during the last 130 years. The architecture today is described as conscientious, but mostly at cross purposes, adding up to a tangled makeshift.

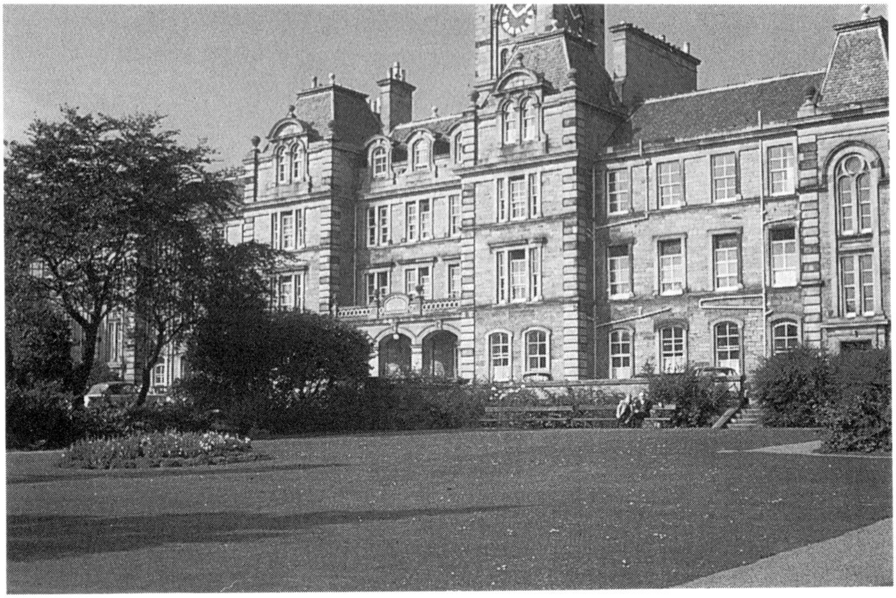

Front of Hospital around 1960

During the 1950s and 60's the Poor House slowly turned into the modern hospital of today. The development of buildings during this period was influenced by John Holt, the then architect to the South Eastern Regional Hospital Board.

In 1950 the visitor approaching the hospital from the Queensferry Road did so along roads bounded by hedgerows with fields on both sides in which sheep safely grazed. Up the main drive, gate posts stood near the present Oncology entrance, along side them a small gatehouse and a boy scout hut which served as the senior staff canteen. Thereafter, grassy slopes led up to the hospital which consisted of the former St Cuthbert's Poorhouse building. On the left of the drive the gardener maintained a large vegetable garden. A crescent of substantial houses, Carrington Crescent, stood opposite Fettes's gate near the present MRC Unit. At the back of the hospital stood the pre-war nurses home, recreation hall and the Paderewski building, originally a children's hospital, later the Polish Medical School, and in 1950 the casualty and outpatient department of the hospital. The residents' rooms were in the former medical superintendent's house opposite the main entrance and also close to the residents dining room in the ground floor of the left wing of the main building. On either side of the main entrance under the Clock Tower were the offices of the medical superintendent and the matron, respectively. The latter, Miss Estelle Adamson, occupied a flat under the clock tower.

In 1946, the first and second floors of the hospital main block were redecorated as private surgical wards, the children's surgical ward and for general purposes. Other areas refurbished included the kitchen and dining room. The outpatient consultative clinic was a wooden hut. This was transferred in 1947 to the building which had previously been the Paderewski Hospital of the Polish Medical School. A follow-up Department was established at a cost of £20,000 and a laboratory over the mortuary established at a cost of £6,000.

In the *Evening Dispatch*, Wednesday, 16 December, 1959 the Western General Hospital was described as dismal old — space-age new. This followed the opening of the neurosurgical block:

Edinburgh's Western General Hospital is a marked study in contrasts. The antiquated Outpatients Department will continue to nestle close to the hospital's space-age Neurosurgical Unit until the latest plans under the £15 million programme for Scottish teaching infirmaries comes to fruition in 1962–63. Many of the wards and corridors had remained undecorated for many years. The dinginess of most parts of the hospital would strike terror into the hearts of the unsuspecting. The corridors are dark and dingy, the lights low in power and inaccessibly high on the ceilings. The patient goes to the Paderewski Outpatients and then has to walk 150 yards, by an open-air walk, to the main building for treatment. Conditions in the Outpatient Department can only be described as shocking. The Waiting Room is small, wooden walled and ill-lit and does not inspire confidence. There is complete lack of privacy in one room, where initial consultations take place — there are three cretonne-covered screens where patients confide their ailments. Each patient can be overheard by the others and the doctor's diagnosis too. Elsewhere in this building are the sterilising and plaster rooms. Next door to the lavatory, the sterilising cubicle remains in the same condition as when the hospital was erected. In one corner dustbins, brushes and mops lie haphazardly.

There were other examples of serious deficiency at the Western — the maternity wards, general medical and surgical wards and kitchens. In the Maternity Unit there and narrow hard benches. There is only one bathroom which combines the sluice room. There are no bedpan washers or sterilisers. The children's ward in contrast, is painted in pastel shades and modern in outlook and in one ward a white budgerigar in a cage swings merrily to and fro. The labour room has three women on three tables in one delivery room and in the first stage labour room no woman can deliver her baby in privacy. The doctors accommodation was awful; 12 share one bath and four washbasins and their individual rooms are small and poorly furnished. In contrast to this is the Neurosurgical Unit which is almost completed. This 60-bed Unit is wide, extremely well lit, centrally heated with day rooms and four-bed wards, each with a locker, wardrobe, prototype beds.

Such comments continue in *The Scotsman*, Wednesday 2 December 1969:

Considerable concern has been expressed about the staff working in squalid circumstances and deprived of the rudiments of modern medicine. Under discussion was the south-east of Scotland priorities for the new building in the 5 years after 1972. Plans had been put ahead for the £7 million Phase II rebuilding of the Royal Infirmary but only £1 million was allocated for the maintenance of services at the Western General Hospital. Phase II of the Western's redevelopment was to be deferred until

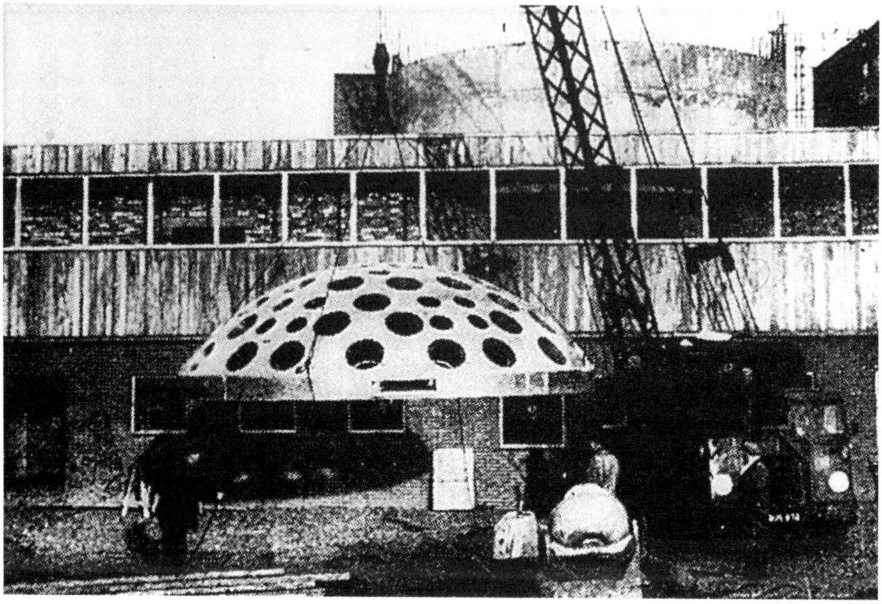

Dome of neurology theatre being placed

the next quinquennium. Clinical staff at the Western General Hospital were concerned about conditions under which they were working. Women patients in D-block had to go through the Gents Toilets to their own toilets, the staff accommodation was poor, staff morale was described as very low and after many years plans for a new hospital were being discarded completely. The Chairman of the Royal Infirmary Board of Management suggested that it was dangerous to make the Western General the first priority without visiting other hospitals in the region. It was also stated that here in the Western are some of the most eminent medical men in their field in Britain working in the most squalid circumstances. Whatever else this Board does, this is an important hospital with an extremely good staff. They do not want to be placated they want to be provided with ordinary standards of working. The Secretary and Treasurer of Edinburgh Northern Hospitals Board of Management, and under which group the Western General fell, said that the Board of Management were unhappy about certain aspects of the old Western General Hospital, originally designed as a workhouse, and not a hospital. The Board had hoped that plans for the new Western General might have been further forward. It is for the general public to decide how much they are going to spend on the Health Service. He also added the staff can still work in tiny wee corners and bring out wonderful results.

By 1982 the total bed complement was 552. There were 20 separate wards and an Accident & Emergency Unit of six beds and a Day Bed Area of 24 beds. The distribution of beds was:

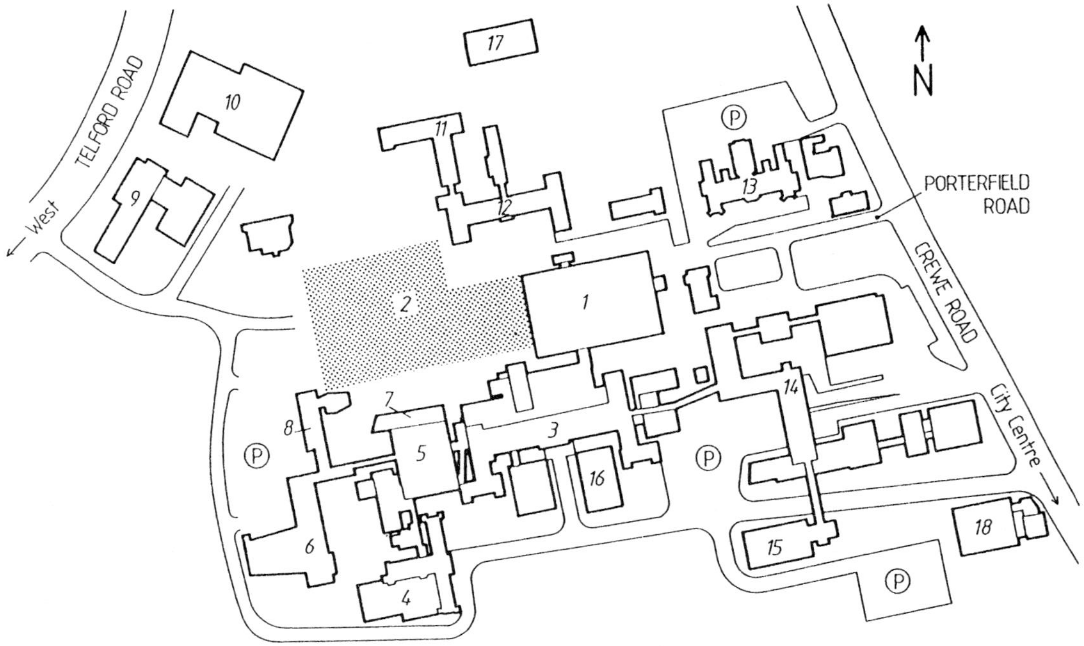

1. Phase 1 - O.P.D, Medical Records, X-Ray
2. Phase 2
3. Main Block - Wards and Depts
4. D Block (Surgical)
5. Operating Theatre
6. Dept. of Surgical Neurology
7. Pharmacy
8. Teaching and Research Centre
9. Microbiology
10. Laundry and Boilerhouse
11. College of Nursing
12. Nurses Home
13. Central Stores and Staff Changing
14. Radiotherapy Unit
15. Transplantation Surgery
16. Clinical Chemistry and Haematology
17. Engineering and Building Dept.
18. Scottish Health Service Centre

Plan of the Western General Hospital, *c.*1970

General Surgery	38	General Medicine and Cardiology	105
Orthopaedic Surgery	13	Metabolic Unit	4
Urology	29	Radiotherapy	111
Neurosurgery	30	Medical Oncology	12
Gastro-intestinal	32	Paediatric Medicine	25
Gynaecology	23	Paediatric Surgery	25
Obstetrics	47	Special Care Babies	14
Nephrology (renal)	8	Renal Transplant	6

During 1982, 17,150 inpatients were admitted, 32,501 accident & emergency attendances were seen and the total outpatients seen including accident & emergency was 115,246.

There were four main laboratories: microbiological, clinical chemistry, haematology and pathology which provided a complete service not only to the Western General Hospital but also to the North Edinburgh Hospitals and Clinics as well as those in East Lothian. A system of specimen collection operated throughout the catchment area using vans that circulated according to pre- determined routes and timetables. Provision was also made for emergency pick-ups when required.

On the south side was the single-storey Scottish Health Service Centre designed by the SERHB Architect's Department in 1969, with a lodge-like E extension of concrete blockwork, 1974.

The Scotsman's report on this building said:

> A £70,000 Scottish Hospital Centre for research into hospital design was opened in the grounds of the Western General Hospital by the Secretary of State for Scotland, Mr William Ross. This was a joint enterprise between the Scottish Hospital Boards and the Secretary of State. The Centre will study ward and theatre design, laboratories, patient care, hospital design, planning and equipment. The director is Dr J. K. Hunter and Mr J. Leithead is secretary. This is a two-storey building containing a model- making room, conference area, offices, reference library and an exhibition hall.

The Nuffield Transplant Unit further along the southern entrance to the hospital 'expresses the isolated mystique of kidney surgery in 1955; a fastidious assembly of smooth (but patchy yellow-coloured) concrete units with a tall ventilation stack and a long access bridge over the roadway'.

The Kidney Transplant Unit of the Western General Hospital, which cost £250,000, was designed by Peter Womersley and Joseph Blackburn and received the first grand project award for 'Architectural Design' in 1964.

> It is an unashamed individual, unorthodox form. It was felt it overcame the problems of long term planning on a restricted site, the organisational complexities of hospital design and the accelerating pace of medical science. It is described as an assertive display of sculptural invention, with the richness and variety of internal spaces wilfully expressed on the external envelope. The north facade of the main block consists of an operating suite, a sterilisation zone and patients' rooms, and expansive areas screen an access corridor from the busy approach road to the hospital. To the south, large

uninterrupted sheets of plate glass reflect patients' rooms, admit views and successfully achieve the interpenetration of internal and external space.

Specifically designed for the transplantation of human organs, the building is technically unique. It is the first building where the creation of a sterile environment has been the primary consideration. The description in *The Scotsman* of Monday 26 February 1968 was:

> Around the core for medical work the architect has dramatically wrapped a peripheral corridor and logically assembled the subservient spaces. In a vigorous essay of exposed coloured concrete, solids, voids, barrel vaults, and curves — all precisely defined — are the basic elements of the building's vocabulary. Few opportunities to exploit three-dimensional form have escaped the architects design plan. Such are the visual qualities of this personal architectural statement — an environment which is essentially one of temporary confinement — that patients may be initially overwhelmed. But even with the brilliantly inventive and imaginative qualities realised in the design one great doubt remains: Is this monumental architecture — so excessively demanding in terms of time — relevant to the rapid development of medical science?

The building was opened by Sir Peter Medawar, Director of the National Institute for Medical Research. Sir Peter, in his opening speech, said that within five years he believed that transplantation of the heart, liver and lung would have become established surgical procedures in much the same way as kidney transplants are now accepted.

On the north side of the road is the modular concrete Cyclotron Unit, built in 1975. The adjoining Radiotherapy Unit and related wards were designed by the SERHB Architect's Department, 1952–6; conventional brown brick walls alternating with white- framed curtain walls of glass and green slate.

The £380,000 Radiotherapy Department at the Western General Hospital was opened in July 1957 by Sir Ernest Rock Carling, Chairman of the International Commission on Radiological Protection. The new building was founded on the reputation of Professor Robert McWhirter. In this building was a four-million-volt linear accelerator that cost £40,000. This was provided for by the Treasury for five areas in Britain. It was also agreed that it was a beautiful building with more than 100 beds and hostel beds for overnight accommodation. The new development accommodated 111 patients with cancer together with suites of rooms for X-ray, diagnostic and therapeutic equipment, operating theatre suite for radium application and a group of research laboratories and dining areas for staff and patients. The building is to the east of the existing hospital. A height restriction was imposed on buildings to the south and an arbitrary building line controlling the shape of the various blocks on the north-east corner of the site. Four-bed wards are placed on both sides of the corridor and based to some extent on the recent Nuffield-type plan to give the wards the best orientation on the north-south access. To meet the total number of beds required and provide isolation wards, a wing was placed at right angles to form the north side of the court used as a car park and ambulance entrance. The high voltage block is placed adjacent to the outpatient department to avoid the need for excessive protection from X-ray radiation.

Temporary laboratories of *c.*1969 and the two-storey steel-faced Library designed by the Common Services Agency Building Division, 1979, obstruct the three-storey frontage of the Paediatric Department (the original Poor House) by Peddie & Kinnear, 1867, enlarged with a Frenchy forecourt by D. and J. Bryce, 1880. Its otherwise bold detail pales beside Peddie & Kinnear's detached W wing (now the Surgical Wards) with a big corbelled arch in the centre block. On the front was a giddy spiral stair of cast iron, recently removed, and to the rear the Wolfson Gastro-intestinal Laboratory designed by Scott & McIntosh, 1966. This temporary building, financed by moneys from the Wolfson Foundation, was intended to be a two-story construction, but the requested allocation only paid for one floor. North of here, behind D- Block, is the old 1914–18 surgical theatres and beyond these the Metabolic Unit.

The residency was originally the Governor's house, completed in May 1902, and consisted of downstairs a parlour, drawing room, kitchen, bedroom, washhouse, w.c., coal cellar and larder and upstairs four bedrooms, a small bedroom or store, servant's bedroom, bathroom and wc. It is not clear when this became the Residency but it would probably be around the time of the Second World War. At the present time it is being refurbished to provide accommodation for patients coming from a distance for invasive cardiology procedures.

The Scotsman, Saturday, 9 February 1963:

> The Western General Hospital is to have a new Metabolic Unit for the investigation and treatment of diseases which include obesity, diabetes, kidney and intestinal troubles and some forms of cancer. The Unit provides accommodation for four patients who would have a room each. Attached to the Unit would be a special diet kitchen and appropriate laboratory facilities.

To the north are the Main Operating Theatres (originally built on legs over the old theatres) designed by Basil Spence and Partners, 1956.

Further west is the five-storey Surgical Neurology block designed by the SERHB Architect's Department, 1952, with stone gable and green slate panelled flanks, and a timber-clad drum over the operating theatre.

The Scotsman, Saturday 2 July 1960:

> Professor Norman Dott, Professor of Neurological Surgery was involved in the design and development of the £500,000 Department of Surgical Neurology at the Western General Hospital. This was opened by the Secretary of State for Scotland, Mr John S. Maclay. It was thought that the Department was the most modern of its kind in the world. The opening ceremony was attended by surgeons representing countries who had been in Edinburgh for a joint meeting of the Societe de Neurochirurgie de Langue Francaise and the Society of British Neurological Surgeons. The Unit was designed to cope with some 1,000 patients a year, with an average stay of 3½ weeks.

To the north is the copper-roofed Teaching and Research Centre by Alison & Hutchison & Partners 1953.

At the north-west corner of the site is the Central Microbiology Laboratory designed by the SERHB Architect's Department, 1959 (their mixture much as before); Boiler House and Laundry by Basil Spence, Glover & Ferguson, 1966, with white steel-clad walls and concrete chimney; Old Boiler House (superseded) by Basil Spence and Partners, 1956, brick with shell concrete roofs; Along the north side is the four-storey brick Nurses' Home designed by the City Architect's Department, 1935; The College of Nursing added to the north by the SERHB Architect's Department, 1958; Then there was a Recreation Hall, like a brick chapel, *c.*1920, demolished in 1994; Facing it are the Outpatient Casualty and Diagnostic block by the SERHB Architect's Department 1966–68; The Pathology block by the City Architect's Department, 1939; The four-storey Human-Genetics block by Alan Reiach, Eric Hall & Partners,1970; Finally, the Old Outpatient Building designed as a children's home by R.M. Cameron, 1912, a harled single-storey pavilion block with jolly red tile roofs and stone dressings, and a house to the east facing Crewe Road (now the Midwifery Centre) to match.

Nursing

Following the inception of the NHS in 1948 and the subsequent changes brought about by a revolution in health care, it was inevitable that major changes would emerge in nursing practice and nursing education.

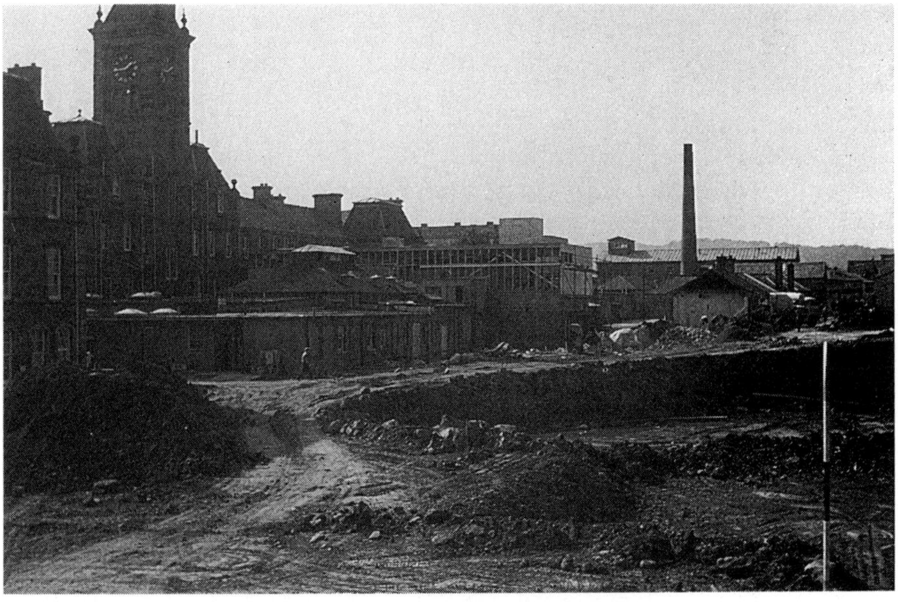

Work in progress for the building of the Outpatients' Department

Some of the significant changes occurred in the middle sixties but the period during the fifties and early sixties were to be the formative years in the lives of many nurses at the Western General Hospital in Edinburgh.

Gradually, as management systems of a new dimension have progressed in the Health Service, so the role of what used to be the Matron has evolved. In many ways the responsibility of the Director of Nursing Services remains the same. The role is primarily that of ensuring that the nursing service in the hospital is adequately staffed both quantitatively and qualitatively. The development of technology within medicine means that the nurses' role is quite different from before the war. Nurses remain the central caring profession. This is in contrast to the diagnostic and therapeutic skills of Medicine and other professions. The present Director of Nursing Services is also responsible for Audit and Quality of Services within the hospital: perhaps an old role in a new guise, but incorporating new skills and techniques.

Matrons

1. 1933 –	Miss Theresa Allan
2. – 1964	Miss Estelle Adamson
3. 1964 – 1972	Miss Margaret Nimmo
4. 1972 – 1974	Miss Elizabeth Edwards
5. 1974 – 1976	Miss J.L.P. Robertson
6. 1977 – 1987	Miss Elizabeth McLean
7. 1987 – present	Mrs Alexandra Harvey

The Matron's office initially was a side room off the main corridor

The hospital was fortunate that, at this important time in it's history, Dr Alexander B Donald was the medical superintendent and Miss Estelle Adamson was the matron. Their remarkable partnership taught both professions the nature of each other's contribution to the overall health care needs and philosophy of the hospital. This mutual respect created a happy and harmonious atmosphere throughout the hospital and this continues in some respect today.

Miss Adamson had trained at the Florence Nightingale School at St Thomas' Hospital in London although she herself came from St Andrews. Those who had the fortune to train as nurses under her influence will never forget the impact that she made, individually and collectively. She not only demonstrated outstanding leadership in nursing generally but she gave nurses a tremendous sense of pride in the hospital and the training school.

Sister Catherine Macgregor went to 'A Flat' as a staff nurse in 1946. She had spent several months in the genito-urinary ward on the other side of the Hospital where Mr David Band ruled supreme and powerfully, with assistance from Mr Sandy Slessor, who was also the Medical Superintendent. Professor Learmonth also occasionally carried out operations.

By comparison with D3 'A Flat' was quite the dullest place. The Hospital was then very much secondary to the Royal Infirmary and it was felt that only their rejects and less interesting cases were received. Dr John Sclater seemed to cover all the medical units in the city apart from the R I E. He visited about twice a week for a ward round. Professor Stanley Davidson also visited on occasions for some undergraduate teaching.

'A Flat' was at the end of the corridor in those days. The radiotherapy unit had not been built. There was a verandah where TB patients were placed in summer. The ward was therefore on both sides of the main corridor with an isolated Maternity Unit at the north end. The Sister of 'A Flat' was expected to conduct deliveries in the absence of the staff midwife. This could happen on a busy waiting day.

Instruments, needles, bowls, catheters were all boiled for sterilisation, dressings were packed in stainless steel drums and autoclaved in theatre. The supply of needles and dressings was strictly controlled — 12 needles for a week while 12 were away for *sharpening* — losing one meant a visit to the Matron's office to explain the loss. The sterile trolleys were set up in the sluice room (just where it is now). These were the days of enamel sputum mugs with a hole in the lid. Nursing staff were surrounded by bedpans and soiled linen so that their vigilance and supervision had to be thorough to prevent contamination.

The nurses' badge was redesigned in 1953. After the Health Service came into being, the Chancellor of the Exchequer had instructed the Treasury to say that Hospital Boards must not use national money to provide badges for nurses. The Sisters of the Western General Hospital agreed that a badge was a most important thing to have. With Miss Adamson, they set about raising money to

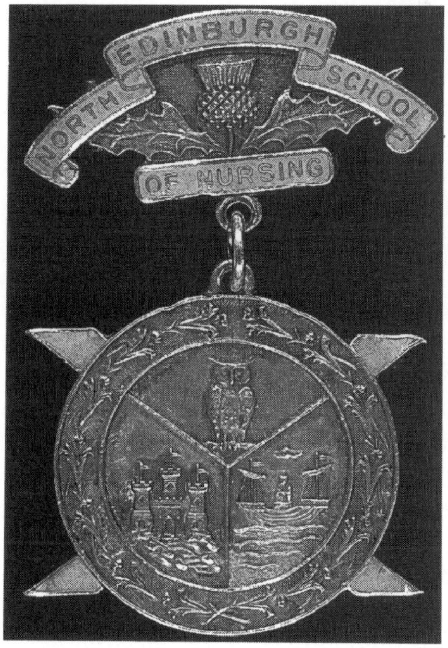

North Edinburgh School of Nursing badge

establish a new nurses' badge for the Western, and they offered the Board of Management a die which was provided by Alex.Kirkwood and Sons in Albany Street (who still hold the die). The price of the badge was met by the nurses themselves. The badge is in silver with a blue enamel scroll around a thistle, and has a circular pendant with the four points of the St Andrew's Cross extending beyond it in blue. The pendant has three divisions within a circle of Florentine irises, which were among Florence Nightingale's favourite flowers. The owl in the top division represents wisdom and recalls Athena, Florence Nightingale's pet owl, given to her in Athens. In one of the lower sections is the 7th century castle of the capital city to remind the nurse of the great traditions and history of Edinburgh. In the other is the Ship of Leith with the Madonna and Child. Unfortunately Miss Adamson did not get permission from the Lord Lyon King at Arms, and some diplomacy was required to avert an embarrassing situation.

A block system developed for the training of student nurses. The nurse training system, which was introduced in the 1950s meant that nurses no longer had to attend lectures while working in the wards or to attend after a 10 hour spell on night duty.

In the fifties and sixties major developments were taking place in clinical medicine and surgery. The hospital was recognised as a teaching hospital, and lovely hospital grounds and tennis courts gave way to major building programmes. The Department of Radiotherapy was followed by the Department of Neurosurgery, and portacabins and laboratories appeared round every corner. The old laundry was demolished. Great plans were afoot for the new hospital.

A new breed of administrator appeared — a hospital secretary, and many of matron's responsibilities were handed over with some relief.

The changes in clinical practices brought about significant changes in the management of patient care: grouping of patients into speciality wards and departments, the development of coronary care and intensive care, the innovative new drug treatments and therapies. All these brought about a greater turnover of patients and greater workload for nursing staff.

The governing body for nursing education, the General Nursing Council, introduced a wider basic training programme for student nurses' training. The student nurses made up a large part of the workforce in the hospital. The students did their clinical placements in the hospital and their educational study blocks in the School of Nursing situated by the 1935 Nurses' Home Building. Student nurses did nine months of night duty during the three year training, three months in each year.

The normal nursing team in each ward consisted of the ward sister, two to three staff nurses and six to eight student nurses. The ward orderly supervised the ward maids. Nursing auxiliaries had not yet been introduced to the Service.

Student nurses had to live in the Nurses Home, certainly during the first and second years of training; one 'late' pass was allowed per week and no student nurse was allowed to be married during her training. The strict rules and regulations brought about a close community spirit and many lasting friendships were formed. The training allowance was small, approximately £230–£280 a year — and with deductions for accommodation, meals and uniform. This gave most students £8–£10 a month spending money.

The backbone of the nursing service was the ward sister and this is still true today. Ward sisters taught by example and, although often feared by students, their professional knowledge and skills were outstanding. Many of these fine women are remembered today with much affection and gratitude. Christine Orr in 'D1-2', Margaret Nimmo 'D5-8', Barbara MacLeod 'C8-18' and Catherine MacGregor in 'A1-6' and many more besides. In the School of Nursing, Marion MacDonald and Jenny Ross hammered home the theoretical and educational skills with much patience and good humour.

The wider basic training encompassed more specialist training and the broadening of the educational curriculum to include psychiatry, obstetrics and community. Student nurses spent less time in their 'parent' hospital but gained wider experience in other hospitals in the north of Edinburgh. As medical developments changed, so did nursing practice. Clinical nurse instructors were introduced to assist the overburdened ward sisters in the practical teaching of nurses at the 'bedside'.

In many ways, although changes were occurring all the time, this period can be remembered as a time of calm before the storm. As the Health Service absorbed a greater part of taxation and trends in society changed, political activity in the affairs of the Health Service increased. The enormous changes in medicine generally brought about significant changes in the manner in which the profession of nursing was to grow and develop. The first Chair of Nursing in the UK was created at Edinburgh University. The importance of nursing education as the foundation of the profession was acknowledged.

Miss Margaret Nimmo, the matron of the Western General Hospital, was a prophet before her time. In 1968 she made the following comments to a national newspaper. She said:

> Undoubtedly hospitals have much to learn from industrial methods of organisation and management, which if applied to the NHS, might increase efficiency and reduce costs. The process of adoption from an era of dedication, selfless service and somewhat muddled, but kindly organisation, to technological expertise is bound to be difficult. Spinsters are vanishing, hitherto ward sisters and matrons virtually ran the hospitals as socially unattractive twins. Their long experience gave stability and a sense of security to other staff and patients. Adverse publicity, hints of disharmony, autocratic attitudes by administration, increase disenchantment. The young today will not respond to organisations lacking in clear objectives, good communication or in just management.

Little did many of us realise that 22 years after she made these comments the government would set about doing exactly what she envisaged so long ago.

The Western General Hospital will always remain for so many nurses a very special place. Organisation and reorganisations come and go but Westerners live on.

7

Development of Departments

Accident and Emergency Department

When the outpatient building opened in 1971, an exciting innovation was the Accident and Emergency Department. Until this time the admission of emergencies was either through the bed bureau or by direct referral from the GP.

In 1986, Dr Colin Robertson was appointed as Consultant in the department. With a background in General Medicine and Intensive Care, he had subsequently trained in the developing specialty of Emergency Medicine. Together with Charge Nurses Sue Rumgay and Douglas Coull, who led the Accident and Emergency nursing team, for the first time in the history of the Western General, the hospital was able to be a fully receiving general hospital.

Unfortunately, the enterprise failed. The Accident and Emergency department was medically under-staffed with insufficient junior staff to provide an adequate level of cover. Despite covering arrangements at both middle grade and consultant level from the Royal Infirmary, it was clear that without appropriate medical and other resources that the Accident and Emergency Department could not fully function. Only a third of the emergencies from the North of Edinburgh came to the Western by the Ambulance Service.

For part of the time the traditional Accident and Emergency Department at Leith also existed and there was strong local support for this established and valued system. The bed system at the Western was defined. The huge aircraft hanger-type of wards at the Royal Infirmary were capable of absorbing everything that a busy, 24 hours Accident and Emergency department could produce, while the small wards at the Western General Hospital were not conducive to a large influx of patients.

The final blow was when the Lothian Health Board decided to rationalise Orthopaedic and Paediatric medical and surgical services and to remove these in-patient facilities from the Western General Hospital. Without these departments providing essential underpinning to the Accident and Emergency department, it could not safely continue. In 1991 the Accident and Emergency department closed and the medical and nursing staff were transferred to the Royal Infirmary.

Anaesthetics

There are few records of anaesthesia in the 1930s and 1940s, although complex procedures in thoracic, gastro-intestinal and urological surgery are known to have been performed. In February 1937 it was minuted that the Public Health Committee resolved, on a representation by the Medical Officer of Health, that an anaesthetist be appointed for the hospital at a salary of £250, rising to £300 per annum; the anaesthetist would attend each forenoon and at other times as required. It was reported on 15 February 1938 that, at this salary, the hospital had been unable to obtain the services of a fully skilled anaesthetist. They had therefore engaged, for a probationary period of six weeks, an anaesthetist at a salary of £16.13s.4d (£16.52p) who attended routine operations, and for major operations the services of a specialist were called in. Over the six months following the start of this arrangement, specialist fees amounted to £31.10s (£31.50p). The committee agreed to the appointment of a resident anaesthetist at £150 a year, the continued employment of a specialist as required, and the annual amount of specialist fees not to exceed £100.

On 26 May 1942 it is minuted that these arrangements were still in force, the resident anaesthetist being a lady, Dr Brown who was appointed on 21 September 1940 when Dr Hoenigsbergen, an alien, had to resign. Dr Brown had no anaesthetic qualification but had attended at approximately 1000 cases a year. Since the end of 1939 specialist fees had amounted to only £9.15/-. Dr Brown was to sit the examination for the diploma in anaesthetics. The Committee agreed that due to the difficulty in obtaining an anaesthetist the annual salary of the resident should be raised to £300 for a qualified person, as a temporary war measure.

Dr John Gillies, in the Royal Infirmary, was the first full-time anaesthetist in Scotland. In 1948, Dr Claude Barrie was the first full-time anaesthetist appointed to the Western General Hospital and placed in charge of anaesthetic services. His registrar was Rhoda Nicol. The appointment was probably in 1953. He was anaesthetist to Sir John Bruce, Charles Falconer, David Band, and Selby Tulloch. Tom McNair, later to be consultant surgeon in the Royal Infirmary and President of the College of Surgeons of Edinburgh, was a registrar in anaesthetics. His duties were to prepare the Pentothal and also the coffee. The anaesthetic was mainly ether.

Dr Dicky Turner, the first cardiologist in the Western, developed the use of cardiac catheters. The first catheterisations were under the most unhygienic conditions, not in theatre, but, with Tom McNair as anaesthetist, they were probably performed in his office accompanied by files all over the floor.

Claude Barrie used ether. One of the problems of ether was that of the potential for sparks. Care had to be taken to prevent static and Claude Barrie developed a spark plug system to test the static. This was developed in the teaching room in the Paderewski. The system was both failure and success in that there was an explosion and the windows of the teaching room were blown out.

Dr Barrie was joined by Dr Gordon Rennie, who later moved to Strathcathro. Dr Alison Ritchie later joined the department, remaining until her retirement in 1966. Dr Archie Milne had sessions at the Western General Hospital between 1957 and 1965, and in 1961 Dr Robert T. Pettigrew joined the staff having already worked at the hospital as a senior registrar since 1957. Dr Barrie retired in 1974 but continued to do locum work in the hospital and abroad until his death in 1979.

In 1960, elective neurosurgery and neuroradiology transferred to a newly-built complex at the hospital, and Drs. Alan Brown and Jean Horton, already in post, became members of the Western staff. This department has expanded to cover the necessary workload in the theatres and in the treatment of chronic pain, the original staff having been replaced by Drs. Dorothy Child, J. Jenkinson and M. Carmichael.

Dr Pettigrew was responsible for the introduction of the concept of a post-operative recovery room: the centralised facilities were the first in Edinburgh, making an important contribution to patient safety. He also performed pioneer studies in the treatment of advanced malignancies by whole body and localised hyperthermia.

In 1966 Dr Brian Slawson succeeded Dr Ritchie and the establishment rose to four in 1971 when Dr Ivor T. Davie was appointed, and to five when Dr James L. Jenkinson came in 1972. In 1974 Dr Barrie handed over the administration to Dr Slawson. After nine years he was succeeded by Dr Nick H. Gordon (first appointed in 1974) who by now had an official title 'Consultant with Administrative Responsibility'. Dr David J. Wright (appointed 1979) took over in 1990 and became the first Director when directorates were introduced as part of another administrative rearrangement.

Junior staff were all first appointed simply to help with the work load, but their training needs have been met by the evolution of a structure which recognises this requirement. Until 1972 there were but two senior house officers; now there are four, who have longer contracts to enable them to rotate through various sub-specialties, which is even more important now that the hospital cannot offer experience in accident and emergency, obstetrics, gynaecology or orthopaedics. Changes in working patterns and in the examination system have also played a part in stimulating change. Twelve who started their careers as SHO's in this hospital are now consultants in the specialty.

In 1972 Dr David Beamish was the first registrar appointed to work in the main hospital department; a rotating post was added in 1975, and since 1979 all registrars have been part of the Edinburgh rotation.

The first part time senior registrar was Dr Jane Freshwater who completed her part-time training between 1975 and 1982; Dr Lynda Rutledge held a similar post from 1987 to 1990. The first full-time senior registrar rotated to the hospital in 1984 and his successors now have colleagues working in Intensive Care and Neurosciences.

The opening of the Day Bed Area, in 1972, increased the scope of work in anaesthesia. A most significant development came with the opening of the Alexander Donald Building with its Intensive Therapy Unit, replacing the Recovery Room Annex wherein Drs Pettigrew and Slawson had initiated the care for very ill patients requiring artificial ventilation. The new ITU was staffed by specialised nurses and doctors, two extra consultants, Dr Ian S. Grant and

Dr Ian R. Armstrong being appointed because of their special expertise in this field. Extra junior staff were also appointed on the closure of Leith Hospital, with contributions from surgery and medicine. The unit staff were in post in May 1988 and the first patients were admitted in June. Since when the scope and quality of this care in the hospital has greatly increased. Significant dates when the scope of the work of the department has changed include:

1987: The department had to cope with increased activity through the closure of Leith Hospital, with transfer of general surgery to the Western General in 1987.
1989: the closure of Bruntsfield Hospital, resulted in an increase in paediatric and gynaecological work in the Western General.
1991: The closure of Deaconess Hospital in 1991, was followed by the arrival in the Western General of the Lithotripsy Centre and the concentration of urological surgery at the Western General.

Finally the Breast Unit transferred from the Longmore Hospital in 1992

The anaesthetists have always been central to life in the hospital. Dr Slawson was the second chairman of the clinical staff to experience the new management structure. He held that post for three years. Dr Gordon has been both secretary and chairman of the clinical staff. Dr Gordon and Dr Wright have been secretaries of the Scottish Society of the History of Medicine.

Edinburgh Breast Unit

The Breast Unit was started by Sir Patrick Forrest in the early 1970s when he was Professor of Surgery in the Royal Infirmary. He found that the management of patients with breast cancer in a busy General Surgical Ward was not appropriate. Longmore Hospital had one ward available on a five day basis for day case general surgery. This facility was under utilised and so he established the Breast Unit at Longmore Hospital. This developed into a multi-disciplinary Unit, with input from various specialties, e.g. Radiotherapy, Dr Alan Roger; Medical Oncology, Professor John Smyth and Dr Robert Leonard, Radiology, Dr Alastair Kirkpatrick, Dr Jim Walsh, Dr B. Muir, Pathology, and Dr T. J. Anderson. The Unit became extremely successful and much liked by the patients. In December 1991, Longmore Hospital was closed as part of a general strategy to close small hospitals to increase efficiency. The announcement of the closure of Longmore Hospital resulted in a public campaign to reverse the decision, or at least guarantee that adequate provision was made for the new Unit. Dr John Baynham (Chairman of Lothian Health Board) promised the public that provision would be made at the Western General Hospital for an integrated Unit in January 1992. Later that year the Unit at the Western General opened having converted a ward in the Radiotherapy block. The adjacent operating theatre was totally refurbished. The offices were on the ground floor close to the radiology facility. What was missing was adequate Outpatient facilities. As an interim measure the Paediatric Outpatient Block was made available for some Breast Clinics, however this proved to be inadequate. For this reason the main New Patient Clinic still continues at the Royal Infirmary. The unit was promised that a new Clinic would be built attached to the Breast Unit, paid for from the money obtained from selling Longmore Hospital. Building of the new Clinic is to start this year.

The Breast Unit sees 90% of the breast cases referred in the Lothians and provides for the assessment of all the screen detected abnormalities in the South East of Scotland. At present there are three Surgical Consultants (Udi Chetty, Mike Dixon and Elaine Anderson). The radiology is provided by Dr Jim Walsh, Alastair Kirkpatrick and Bernice Muir, Oncology — Bob Leonard, Radiotherapy — Ian Kunkler and Lilian Matheson.

The Edinburgh Breast Unit has led the trend to have a specialised Breast Unit providing comprehensive services. These include: diagnosis, counselling, surgical treatment including breast reconstruction, oncology, radiotherapy, psychology and psychiatric backup. All the specialists involved agree with the principle and efficacy of an integrated Breast Unit. The present Directorate structure, where the Breast Unit comes under the Surgical Directorate has made this difficult.

Although its main aim is to offer a first class clinical service, research into the management of breast diseases has been an important activity of the Unit. The unit collaborates with the Scottish Cancer Trials Office which is directed by Dr Helen Stewart. The Cancer Trials Office is closing and its activities are being taken over by the Scottish Cancer Network. There is collaboration with the Scientists in the Imperial Cancer Research Laboratories under the direction of Professor W Millar and with Professor Michael Steel, formerly of the MRC Unit and now in St Andrew's University.

Cardiac Department 1950–90

The Cardiac Department at the Western General Hospital came into being in 1948 when Dr Richard Turner was appointed. On his arrival, he was accompanied by three supernumerary doctors, looking for posts following their war service: — Drs David Illingworth, Ian Grant and George Thomson. Everything changed from that moment. The enthusiasm was infectious, obstacles were easily overcome and no-one was allowed to stand still.

Dr Turner looked round the place and every cupboard was a potential clinic. He worked hard and expected everyone to do likewise. Soon after his arrival the ward sister resigned and Sister Catherine Macgregor was appointed. There was no elaborate selection procedure. Dr Turner went to see the Matron and said he would be quite happy with the present staff nurse; in those days there was only one staff nurse and six students for the 36 beds.

A great breakthrough came when the Isolation Maternity Unit was vacated and two rooms were made available. The steriliser was moved and so a self-contained cardiac catheterisation unit developed.

The patients came from all over, including Whitehaven, from where a steady stream of patients was generated by a colleague of Dr Turner's.

The range and number of investigative techniques progressed. A technician was appointed after a year or two and the cardiac laboratory became a separate unit. The beginnings were small. The present, most impressive, cardiac laboratory had its roots in that little dark room so long ago.

Dr Turner set the tone for patient care, interest and management; it was an excellent training ground for nurses and there was always a waiting list for staff nurses for 'A Flat'. Dr Turner set about organising an ECG service and fluoroscopy for cardiac calcification screening. He initiated cooperation with the thoracic surgeons, and with Andrew Logan in particular. At the surgical unit at the Eastern General Hospital, they created what was to be one of the largest series of cardiac patients treated surgically in Britain. The patients had their operation at the Eastern General Hospital, returned to the Western General ward, and were then transferred to Astley Ainslie and back to the Western again for a final outpatient check-up. At that time the most frequent cardiac problem was rheumatic valvular heart disease and acute rheumatic fever was common in women and children. During the war, tying the patent ductus arteriosus was the first treatment of a congenital abnormality of the arteries and had been successfully performed by Mr Walter Mercer in the Royal Infirmary. In America, Harden and in London, Brock had in a handful of cases successfully performed dilation of diseased mitral valve (stenotic) by the surgeon's finger introduced through the left side of the heart (left atrial appendage). In 1950, Dr Turner had a young woman of 21 in his care who developed intractable pulmonary oedema from mitral stenosis. He persuaded Mr Logan to operate on her, all else having failed. The operation was a dramatic success and this is believed to have been the first intracardiac operation in Scotland. The patient, who had three further cardiac operations, led an active life, including many years as a cardiac technician, and died at the age of 62. Further developments in cardiac surgery rapidly followed. Until the development of bypass surgery in the 1980s mitral valvotomy and ligation of the ductus arterious were the only effective cardiac surgical treatments. The valvotomy operation was made more effective through the use of transventricular dilation, a technique devised by Mr Logan. The surgical series published by Logan and Turner was a landmark in its day. Dicky Turner and his colleagues were to publish many important accounts of their medical and surgical experience. These papers gained Turner and Logan a national and international reputation for results which compared favourably with those at other leading surgical centres. They introduced these invaluable new methods to this area of Scotland, and with peripheral clinics, particularly at Stirling and Inverness. The catchment area increased, so that even to this day the turnover in surgical cardiology at the Western is greater than that at the Royal Infirmary. By-pass surgery was perhaps rather slower to be instituted, mainly because when it appeared, the cardiac surgeons in post had all been trained in the pre-bypass era. It was not until the later appointment of consultant surgeons who had had experience in the USA or in South Africa that this next important step moved onto a firm basis. The surgery was not done at the Western, and thoracic surgery was performed at various times at the Eastern General Hospital, the City Hospital and the Royal Infirmary.

A second consultant with an interest in cardiology, Dr Michael Matthews, had joined the cardiology department from St Thomas's Hospital, London. In many respects he was the traditional cardiologist aware of the value of clinical signs, a great talker and listener, he saw and understood the needs of people who had become patients. Amid the excitement of the necessary technological advances, he remained contemporary in his knowledge but retained the virtues of a physician.

Mike Matthews' contributions were clinical and administrative. As with most clinicians of his generation, he was brought up to believe that all aortic valvular stenosis was on a rheumatic basis. This was what Karsner and Koletsky had concluded in their textbook on calcific aortic stenosis in 1947. In two articles, Smith and Matthews (1955), and Bacon and Matthews (1959) proposed that the disease was often the result of calcification of a congenital bicuspid aortic valve, known to be the commonest congenital abnormality of the heart (between 1% and 2% of the general population), and due to rigidity rather than fusion of the cusps. It appeared that the calcific process was the same as that which occurred at a later age in the normal tricuspid aortic valve. They also pointed out that this process had been described by Paget (1844) and Peacock (1853). This had been forgotten, although Osler's description of the liability of such valves to infection (infective endocarditis) had become generally accepted. At the present time calcific aortic stenosis is recognised to be by far the commoner fate of this congenital fault, and is held to be the cause of the majority of cases of calcific aortic stenosis presenting between the ages of about 50 and 70. Rheumatic disease, now fortunately much less common, brings about fusion of three cusp valves and usually presents earlier, and in old age fatty and calcific degeneration of tricuspid valves is the usual cause of the disease. It is strange that something now accepted to be so common had been to such an extent overlooked for more than 100 years. Mike Matthews was also interested in Q fever, an infection affecting the heart, and more common in rural areas.

Mr Orford, the ECG technician and his assistant Miss Malcolm had a room off the main corridor fitted with four beds. Each was surrounded by a wire cage to minimise electrical interference with the string galvanometer Elmquist machines then in use, which recorded photographically. There was also an upright fluoroscope which Dr Turner used frequently. It was in this room that the earliest cardiac catheterisations were carried out, starting, possibly in 1952/53. The first catheterisations were under the most unhygienic conditions, not in theatre. The anaesthetist was Mr Tom McNair. They were probably done in his office accompanied by files all over the floor. Dr Hugh Fraser assisted Dr Turner in a very dark dingy room in the main corridor — called the ECG room. This room also acted as the hypertensive clinic and mitral valve clinic. This was a hive of activity. It was said that the X-ray screening machine used had been recovered by Dr Turner from an American warship! True or false, much work was done there, with the assistance of the registrars, Hugh Fraser, Ian Grant and Edward Harris. Pressures were measured by saline manometry.

The catheters were boiled and then packed for steam sterilisation. Patients had a sedative, and were monitored on return for bleeding. There is no recollection of any disasters. A separate catheterisation laboratory was established in a room at the north-east corner of A flat. Catheterisation procedures were carried out under fluoroscopy. Instruments were sterilised by autoclave or boiling. Electromanometry was available and Fick principle cardiac output measurements made with Douglas bag air collection, Haldane gas analysis and blood oxygen content measurement. The arrival of a Benedict-Roth spirometer was greeted with relief by registrars and technicians. Mr Ramsay, the senior technician, constructed a variable resistance exercise ergometer from parts of the junior technician's father's bicycle.

At that time cardiac surgery was developing rapidly and weekly clinical meetings with the cardiac surgeons had started. The main emphasis was on valvular heart disease in adults, although congenital disease was also treated. Constrictive pericarditis and pulmonary heart disease were not uncommon. In those days paediatric cardiology was not a separate speciality. The importance of long-term follow-up for proper evaluation of surgical treatment was early realised and new and follow-up clinics for valvular and congenital cases were established.

Hypertension was the other main interest of the department. Newly referred cases were admitted for a few days for extensive laboratory tests including renal biopsy and retinal photography through the co-operation of Dr Stokoe of the Department of Ophthalmology. Dr Turner was soon involved in the treatment of hypertension, inevitably at first with the primitive drugs then available. At follow-up clinics, results of treatment and side-effects using each type of antihypertensive drug as it became available were studied, from hexamethonium to mecomylamine. The treatment of hypertension, if asymptomatic, which, of course, is true of most of those who are found at routine examination to be hypertensive, elicits in the patient what might be called a 'low gratitude index'. Nobody feels any better for treatment, and many feel worse, particularly with the side effects of the earlier drugs. Dr Turner's energy and enthusiasm were put to full test; he had to persuade patients to submit to, and to persist with treatment, because it was known that the risks of hypertension were significantly reduced in this way. There are early memories of hypertensive clinics under crowded conditions, with little privacy, with patients separated only by curtains, and within earshot of the waiting area. They could be heard vying with one another in parading their status symbols in a progression, in some cases, from pills to sympathectomy, and even adrenalectomy! It was Tony Dornhorst, also from St Thomas's, when later Professor of Medicine at St George's Hospital, who used to say to students on occasion: 'Don't just *do* something, *stand* there!' Dick Turner, though trained in the same hospital, was certainly not of that school of thought! Turner was also a local innovator in modern coronary care, and the use of cardiac pacemakers. In his later time he became a spirited advocate in the field of preventive cardiology, not on the basis of his own research in that field, but by the colourful and vigorous publicity which he gave to the findings of others.

In the mid 1970s the hypertension clinic was transferred from the cardiac to the renal department, under Dr Anderton's care. Treatment of cardiac failure in the early days included mercurial diuretics by injection and intractable massive oedema was treated with surprising success by mechanical drainage by Southay's tubes.

In 1964, a third, part-time, consultant appointment was made, Dr Arthur Kitchin, who had sessions in the University Department of Physiology. He subsequently (1970) transferred to full time clinical medicine.

By this time, the A flat annexe had been built, extending eastwards and providing offices, duty room, kitchen and waiting area. The cardiac laboratory was transferred to a new room at the other end of the main corridor and was linked to the X-ray department. With the development of bypass open heart surgery, cardiac surgery moved from the Eastern General to the Royal Infirmary. The new surgical possibilities required new methods of haemodynamic investigation, including catheterisation of the left side of the heart. The new laboratory had image intensification and angiocardiography equipment and much use was made of indicator dye dilution studies of the circulation.

Another great advance of the early 1960s was the tackling of the problem of so-called cardiac arrest. Initial attempts were by direct manual open massage of the heart through a thoracotomy and this was successful, at least temporarily, in one or two cases. Soon electrical defibrillation of the heart through externally applied electrodes became standard practice. Cardiac arrest teams were organised on a rota basis to be available throughout the hospital. Arrhythmia was recognised as the main cause of death in the early period following a heart attack and logically this demanded the setting up of dedicated units where such patients could be continuously monitored and treated. In April 1966 one of the first UK Coronary Care Units was opened, in wards A2 and A4 respectively with separate trained nursing staff and Senior House Officer. Medical supervision was shared amongst the medical teams, with daily rotation of junior staff and weekly rotation of supervising consultants.

An increasing number of patients with cardiac dysrrhythmias were by this time being treated by permanent transvenous pacemaker implantation. This required long-term outpatient follow-up in a special pacemaker clinic. While maintaining a general acute medical service on waiting days, the increasing numbers of patients being referred from all over Scotland led to problems of accommodation. Post operative surgical cases and patients treated in the coronary care unit were quickly sent to the Astley Ainslie Hospital where a cardiac rehabilitation unit was set up by Dr Elizabeth Cay. Dr Turner, with the agreement of the physicians concerned, arranged out-patient clinics for cardiological cases at Kirkcaldy and Stirling and at Inverness for two days every three months. This arrangement has persisted until 1995 when these hospitals appointed their own local physicians with a special interest in Cardiology.

During the 1970s the patients investigated and requiring heart operations greatly exceeded the number of operations possible in the Royal Infirmary so that long waiting lists built up. For several years before surgical facilities were expanded, a proportion of patients were referred for operation to the Brompton Hospital, London.

The proceeds of the sale of a house were left to the cardiac department by the widow of a former patient and this was used to establish the Mackenzie Fund for Cardiac Research. This rapidly grew to allow purchase of equipment and for training as well as specific research projects. Another of Dr Turner's initiatives were the founding of the Edinburgh Cardiac Club which formalised through regular meetings the already good relations existing with the Royal Infirmary Cardiology Department and annual joint medical/surgical meetings with cardiological colleagues in Glasgow and Newcastle.

Initially, treatment of heart attacks in specialised Coronary Care Units was greeted with some scepticism and indeed opposition. When the benefits became obvious better facilities were provided. A new 6-bedded cubiclised unit was built out from A4 on the lawn south of A flat. This was fully equipped for dealing with all cardiac intensive care problems and was staffed by nurses trained in this speciality. An earlier geographic extension was a teaching room provided by the University for clinical teachings; it extended westward on the terrace in front of the hospital. With the completion of the new Out Patient block, 'Phase One' as it was optimistically named, Cardiology acquired a new catheterisation laboratory, seminar room and offices on the second floor. The laboratory was fitted with up-to-date electronic and radiological equipment which greatly facilitated the task of those carrying out complex investigations. Much of the original electronic equipment, as in the case of the coronary care unit also, was designed and built by the Department of Medical Physics under Dr Smith and Mr Duval.

Dr Turner retired in 1974 to devote himself to what had become his main interest, the primary prevention of atheromatous disease and particularly coronary disease. His post was not filled directly, but a new radiology post was established with part-time responsibility for cardiac radiology. This has become increasingly important with cineangiography and echocardiography and more recently CT and MRI scanning. The post is held by Dr Colin Turnbull whose continued active role in cardiac catheterisation ensured that high standards were maintained for all the cardiac X-ray techniques and equipment. Dr Malcolm Merrick developed the radionucleotide studies, in a close liaison with the Cardiology Consultants.

Throughout this period, clinical teaching of undergraduate students took the form of a junior clinique attending daily for instruction, with a few senior students and postgraduates attached for longer periods. Staff contributed to undergraduate lecture series and also to postgraduate courses in medicine and cardiology. Several contributed chapters to medical textbooks. Dr Turner published two small but very popular guides to auscultation and to electrocardiography.

Papers from the Department published in medical and scientific journals include large longitudinal clinical studies of various types of valvular heart disease; of patients treated with a variety of antihypertensive drugs and of patients following acute myocardial infarction; clinical studies of the relation of aortic stenosis to a bicuspid aortic valve; chronic Q fever; Marfan's syndrome, and the pulmonary circulation in emphysema and the effect of oxygen thereon; as well as physiological studies of transport function in the central circulation, continuous ECG waveform analysis and the effect of pituitary hormones on the peripheral circulation. More recently the department has developed an international profile in advanced cardiac ultrasound, and has published papers on interventional cardiology, innovative open access services and heart failure.

Arthur Kitchin had become responsible for continuing the management of Dr Turner's patients when he retired and shouldered a huge burden of clinical responsibility, in particular the investigation of the increasing number of patients being referred for coronary bypass. In the cardiac laboratory, he applied a highly physiological approach to the detailed assessment of patients with valvular and congenital heart disease. In order to achieve precise measurements, the use of the trans-septal puncture and dye dilution curves were part of the normal procedures. The quality of cardiac catheter investigation that he achieved was almost without parallel within the United Kingdom. This earned him the immense respect of all of his referring general physicians. His quiet and unruffled manner, which inspired such confidence in patients, was an essential component of his catheterisation technique. He published many important studies including the long term outcome of patients with coronary heart disease.

Arthur Kitchin erected a very large bushel in front of an exceedingly bright light. Well versed in physiology, having for a time a joint appointment with the University Department of Physiology, and after a useful year with Dr Jeremy Swan in the Department of Cardiovascular Investigation at the Mayo Clinic, Arthur ran a laboratory of world class standard. He was blessed with a capacity for seeing investigations through until the necessary data had been obtained. With a minimum of fuss, in his quiet way, he achieved the maximum of results. Surgeons, accepting patients investigated by Arthur, spoke warmly of the consistent high quality of his work.

Dr Matthews retired in 1982 and his retirement coupled with Dr Kitchin's in 1987 severed the link of cardiology with general medicine. Their successors, Drs Shaw and Starkey, are occupied full-time in specialist cardiology which is increasingly time-consuming and technical with the newer interventional procedures of angioplasty and valvuloplasty.

The decision to create a full-time cardiologist post when Dr T. R. D. (Stuart) Shaw was appointed in 1983 began a new era of investigative and interventional cardiology. Stuart Shaw was an innovator. He enthusiastically introduced Problem Orientated Records in the Department, and used the method to enable a more holistic approach to the patient. An excellent communicator, he readily won the support and co-operation of his patients. Working for some reason best known to himself on New York time in Scotland — one wondered what he would have done in New York — he spent long hours in the hospital, usually far into the night. Technically he was very adept, and those whom he trained spoke enthusiastically of what they had learned from him.

The network of hospitals where Dr Turner had developed follow-up clinics for his valve disease and hypertension patients became an increasing source of cases for cardiac catheterisation and in particular for coronary angiography and the rapidly expanding treatment of coronary artery bypass surgery. The 'outreach' clinics at Stirling Royal Infirmary, Victoria Hospital in Kirkcaldy and Raigmore Hospital in Inverness, continued to support the warm professional links with local physicians which had been a feature of Western General Cardiology. The new cardiac laboratory installed in 1982 and the increasing use of echocardiography in the ECG Department were the trigger for the move of consultants' and junior staff offices from A Flat to the 2 floor of the Outpatient Building. When the Phase 1 Building was designed, it included a large cardiology department area. The Cardiology Department had a modern suite of rooms which initially it struggled to fill. However, the Department of Medicine, under the dynamic leadership of Professor Christopher Edwards, was able to take up the surplus accommodation: this included a basic science cardiovascular laboratory headed by Dr Brent Williams.

In 1983 the first coronary balloon angioplasty was undertaken. The initial patient was a member of the hospital staff who had developed post-operative angina and repeat angiography had shown that her coronary bypass graft had almost occluded. The hospital management, struggling to contain costs within a fixed budget, refused to sanction the new treatment. The balloon equipment was provided from endowment funds. The success of her case — she plays a prominent role in her department some 12 years later — stimulated a radical change in the function of the cardiology department. It was no longer restricted to a diagnostic role but now offered an alternative treatment to cardiac surgery. Interventional cardiology received a further boost in 1987 with the arrival of Dr Ian Starkey whose main interest has been in angioplasty techniques and who has pioneered the use of rotary devices and stents. Ian Starkey is a dedicated cardiologist, curler and Saturday morning golfer and is probably best as a cardiologist. He epitomises the approach of Western General Cardiology. This combines Dr Turner's enthusiasm for active treatment with Dr Matthews' emphasis on individual patient care and Arthur Kitchin's careful physiological cardiac studies: each of these continued to be of vital importance in the case-selection and performance of the interventional techniques. These influences applied when the United Kingdom's first percutaneous mitral balloon valvotomy was carried out at the Western General in 1986 by Dr T. R. D. Shaw. Mitral balloon valvotomy required atrial trans-septal puncture which had been a long-established technique at the Western General Hospital, which has evolved into the Scottish Centre for this type of interventional therapy.

An increasing number of enthusiastic post-graduate fellows were attracted to the Department, often working hard but unpaid, and they provided an essential supplement to the progressively reduced junior staff as hospital medicine became 'consultant-led'.

Dr George Sutherland moved from the Thoraxcenter, Rotterdam, in 1990 as a British Heart Foundation Honorary Consultant. He introduced advanced echocardiography techniques and transformed echocardiography at the hospital, attracting substantial research grants and post-graduate fellows from many countries. The Department rapidly developed the reputation of being one of the premier cardiac ultrasound centres in the world. Dr John McMurray was appointed as an additional consultant in 1993 and introduced his special clinical and research interest in heart failure and Open Access Services. Dr Bill Price always had a special association with Cardiology. He became the Clinical Director for Medicine when the Hospital became a Trust in 1994. He led the plan to install a new cardiac laboratory and to build a new day ward for cardiac patients. During 1995 the department underwent a radical change. In addition to a new digital X-ray cardiac laboratory, a Day Care Ward was opened and associated with hostel accommodation in the old houseman's residency building which became Turner House. Links were also re-established with general medicine with acute cardiac admissions 'triaged' to the care of the cardiologist.

1993 was also the year when A Flat's first cardiac staff nurses, Miss Catherine McGregor, had reached the age when she attended the department for her own treatment of calcific aortic stenosis. She remembered the days when the hospital corridor ended at A Flat, when the sister there would be called on to lend a hand at unexpected delivery of babies in the adjacent Maternity Unit and when the nurses had to account for all the needles with which they had been issued for the week's use.

If Dr Turner were to arrive again, he would find much had changed but he could still engage in a discussion of the same problems he faced when he had only his caravan — a lack of space, insufficient staff, a need for newer equipment, surgery based at another hospital and so many patients needing help. However, the new status of Trust hospital has added a vigor to the development in Cardiology and the plans for the expanded hospital envisaged by the Lothian Acute Services Strategy provide further improvements in the care of heart disease.

In the meantime, the life of the hospital and department has been graced and enlivened by so many personalities of all types of staff: Rickie the porter who really wanted to be a circus clown and gave performances during wheel-chair transport; Yvonne the 'agony aunt' secretary to whom staff brought their troubles; Mrs MacGregor and Jeanette the 'surrogate mother' ward clerkesses; the superb nurses, technicians and radiographers, as well as the blossoming junior medical staff and the consistently eccentric consultants who could diagnose everything except their own eccentricity. Together they have created one of the best cardiology departments in the United Kingdom which continues to serve a very wide area of central and northern Scotland as well as the City of Edinburgh. The advent of Trust hospitals led the appointment of cardiologists at district general hospitals but the friendly links with the Western remain and the new consultants carry out their angiography at the hospital and have become Associate Consultants of the expanded Department.

Clinical Chemistry Laboratory

The original laboratory for Clinical Chemistry in the Western General Hospital was established in 1937 by Dr C. P. Stewart, of the Department of Clinical Chemistry, Edinburgh University, at the Royal Infirmary (RIE). He remained as Biochemist in charge of the Biochemistry service for the group until he retired in 1962. All the specimens from the Western General Hospital (WGH) were initially analysed in his department in the Royal Infirmary (RIE).

In 1946, Dr Elizabeth Gilchrist, who was a member of Dr C. P. Stewart's laboratory in the Royal Infirmary, moved to the laboratory in the WGH which was in a disused wash house. She worked with two technicians. When there were too many specimens, the excess were sent to Dr Stewart's laboratory department. Dr Gilchrist returned to the RIE in 1950 where she worked until retirement in 1955. The chief technician in the WGH was Mr Dennis Smith who retired in 1969. He was replaced by Mr J Pilley who is still in post.

In 1950, Dr Sidney Tompsett a senior lecturer in Dr Stewart's department transferred from the RIE to the WGH. In 1952 Mr William Forshall was appointed as senior biochemist and graduated as PhD in 1958. In 1964 Dr Tompsett returned to Dr Stewart's department in the RIE and Dr Fred Scandrett transferred from the RIE department and took over until 1966. During Dr Tompsett's time the number of technicians increased to six.

In 1956 the laboratory was transferred to the Northern General Hospital (NGH) to accommodation shared with the Bacteriology Laboratory until 1962 when Bacteriology moved to the new department in the WGH. The number of technical staff increased by one a year from 1962 to 1964.

In 1962 Mr William Edwards was appointed as senior biochemist with Dr Tompsett. He retired from the WGH in 1993.

The Research and Teaching Centre was established in the WGH in 1958 by Edinburgh University and the South-East Regional Hospital Board to give research facilities for the academic staff of the WGH. Dr Stewart, Dr Wilfrid Card and Dr John A. Strong were the originators of this idea. This laboratory was initially supervised by Dr Christine Thomson, a lecturer in Dr Stewart's department and three technical staff.

By 1962 it was accepted that the Clinical Chemistry laboratory, staff and equipment should be upgraded. The laboratory returned to the WGH from its temporary accommodation at the NGH.

After discussions it was agreed that

1. a service was required for the whole of the Northern Group of Hospitals;
2. there had been a failure to provide suitable facilities for the rising demands,
3. and to increase the number of senior personnel and provide trainees;

4. laboratory accommodation was inadequate;
5. the equipment had not been updated or replaced by mechanised instruments
6. that research and development facilities were not available;
7. no quality control was carried out.

It was agreed by a Clinical Staff subcommittee that there should be a transfer of the laboratory to the NHS from the Edinburgh University, the establishment of a Principal Biochemist post and improved secretarial services.

In September 1966, Dr David B. Horn was appointed Head of Department. He came from the Royal Victoria Infirmary, Newcastle upon Tyne, where he had been the Top Grade Biochemist with Professor Latner. This established a separate clinical chemistry department in the north of Edinburgh independent of the Royal Infirmary.

From then onwards considerable developments were made in Clinical Chemistry in the Northern Group. This started with the new laboratory in the WGH. The only available site was the front lawn on the Southern side of the hospital, which many members of staff were sorry to see disappear. Delays in the completion of the building meant that occupation took place on 21 October 1968, approximately four months later than planned.

From 1 September 1966 to 21 October 1968 the work in the laboratory was upgraded. In 1966 the staff included Dr Horn, a senior grade biochemist, William Edwards, a chief technician, Dennis Smith, and one senior and six junior students. In 1966 a new principal grade biochemist was appointed, Dr Raymond Heyworth, who transferred to the RIE in 1978. He was succeeded by Miss Shirley Stein who retired in 1983 and replaced by Dr Heather Barbour who had been principal grade biochemist in Dundee. She left in 1993 and was succeeded by Dr Phillip R. Wenham already a member of the department.

Dr Horn's colleague was Dr Gillian Blundell who was appointed to the department in 1977. Dr Blundell became Head of the Department following Dr Horn's retirement in 1987. Dr Peter Ashby, was appointed as Top Grade Biochemist at the end of 1987. Improvements from the NGH-based laboratory included an increase of staff of four additional biochemists, nine technicians and a secretary. The volume of work also increased with the analyses per year rising in a regular and massive manner. The accuracy of the estimations was greatly increased as a result of Quality Control. A very considerable amount of methodological development work was undertaken and increased after the move to the WGH. In the period from 1967 to 1973, a research project was undertaken with Dr MacGregor on the effects of Clomiphene and pergonal on the fertility of women and involved the estimation of urine oestrogens and pregnanediol. Another Research project transferred by Dr Horn from the Royal Victoria Infirmary, Newcastle upon Tyne, was the estimation of blood ammonia.

The Department served five hospitals, i.e. Western, Northern, Eastern, Leith Hospitals and Musselburgh Maternity Hospital. Following the 1974 reorganisation of the National Health Service, the hospitals served increased to eleven, i.e. WGH, NGH, EGH, Leith Hospital, Roodlands, East Fortune, Belhaven, Edenhall, Herdmanflat, Corstorphine and Beechmount and General Practitioners in the North Lothian District. To facilitate this extended service, Dr Horn and Dr Gould established a Laboratory Van Service from the NGH. This provided an efficient collection and delivery system for hospital and GP specimens and results to and from the hospitals and to the laboratories. In October 1979 the biochemistry service for the Royal Victoria Hospital was transferred from the Royal Infirmary to the WGH.

In 1968 the number of estimations was 90,000. The workload was 391,000 tests in 1972 which increased to 555,000 tests in 1974. The range of tests was increased after 1972 with Maternity, Paediatric and General Practitioner Services being extended. The on-call commitments increased very considerably.

In 1968 there was a very serious crisis as the Department was actively involved in the handling of blood and urine specimens from the Nuffield Transplant Surgical Unit at the WGH during the hepatitis outbreak. Some fifteen deaths occurred in clinical, nursing and laboratory staff. There was no hepatitis infection in the biochemistry staff but very considerable care was necessary for specimen handling. Much of the experience gained was subsequently used by other laboratories throughout Britain and assisted in the development of methods for the handling of 'High Risk' specimens.

From 21 October 1968, the laboratory progressed in the development of automation, the handling and rapid estimation of large numbers of varied and complex biochemical fluids and reporting to the clinical wards of these results. The ponderous flame method for sodium and potassium determinations from the NGH was used for a short time and then, in sequence, spectrophotometers, atomic absorption spectrophotometers and autoanalyser equipment were used. Micro-technique systems, which gave accurate results using a minimum quantity of specimen, were introduced. Whereas volumes of the order of 3–5 ml had initially been required for various estimations, the new system carried out the same estimation on quantities of roughly 50 μl, with a much higher degree of accuracy.

The improvements included the construction of a specimen reception area. A system was evolved which extended from the request form to the logging and manual recording of the patient data onto record cards. Rotadix card masters were also introduced, each hospital having a different colour card. This was a lengthy and demanding procedure, which called for detailed checks for accuracy.

There was a special excreta analysis laboratory. The faecal specimens were collected by the patient in paint tins; after delivery to the laboratory they were mixed with water and homogenised on a paint can shaker. A very unpopular measurement for patient, nurses and laboratory staff. This is no longer used.

In the main laboratory, Technicon Autoanalysers, produced in America allowed rapid and accurate automated analysis for the estimation of sodium, potassium, chloride, carbon dioxide and urea, glucose, creatinine, uric acid and phosphate, working at sixty specimens per hour. The accuracy was increased by the use of the developing science of quality control.

Another automated recording, previously unheard of, was quantification of protein by the scanning of protein electrophoretic strips on the chromoscan, which is important in the diagnosis of liver and cancerous ailments.

A recording spectrophotometer, the SP800, was also introduced and was used mainly for enzyme and barbiturate analysis.

Blood gas analyses were made on capillary blood samples instead of the 2ml arterial sample normally used. Specimens were dealt within 5–10 minutes and a rapid service was provided not only in the WGH but also to the other hospitals in the group if taxi delivery was made. Chromatographic analysis for amino-acid, sugars and indoles in plasma as well as in urine. A steroid analysis laboratory in the department provided an oestrogen analysis service as a diagnostic aid in the control of therapy and for pregnancy induction. The laboratory also estimated plasma cortisol and urinary steroids.

The remaining section of the laboratory was used mainly for research and development which included ammonia studies, steroid and amino-acid investigations. In 1976 a study looked at the control of coronary heart disease risk factors in general practice and also for plasma renin activity in diabetic autonomic neuropathy.

Shortly after the new department was opened in the WGH it was anticipated that there would be increase in the work of Clinical Chemistry with population screening, patient profiles, intensive care area and in providing a rapid service for all areas including paediatrics and out-patient departments.

In 1970 a worksheet preparation was set up with a computer working off line and this was effective by 1972. The first computer obtained was an Elliot 903, from the Computer Unit (DSN) at the WGH with the assistance of one of its staff. The equipment was upgraded in .1972 when a new autoanalyser with sixteen channels was introduced. Results as peaks created by the analytical machines were transmitted to the computer. The abiding philosophy was the development of rapid, accurate results using internal standards as the reference: for serum alkaline phosphatase, bilirubin, digoxin, etc.

In 1975 it was decided that all clinical chemistry results would be reported in the International System of Units (SI units) and this system has been continued ever since.

The range of tests continued to increase. Continuing development of an effective and economical off-line data-processing system was applied to the greater majority of the tests handled in the department.

The annual workload in 1967/77 had increased to 702,703 tests for patients and by 1977/78 this had climbed to 730,680 tests. This rise was due to the introduction of enzyme-linked immunoassay techniques and a service for methotrexate, barbiturate and the anti-epileptic drugs. The staff was increased with ten graduates, 33 medical laboratory scientific officers (MLSO), four full-time members of the clerical staff and five part-time members. Laboratory hand books were given each year to all doctors in the hospitals and to all the

GPs. The handbooks identified the 75 analyses available, the nine plasma drug assays, the three cerebrospinal fluid, the 48 paediatric analyses available and the 22 urine assays.

In 1979 there was a further large increase in the workload due to the introduction of the Alpha-fetoprotein (AFP) programme for the Lothians, Fife and the Borders. The AFP measurement was very effective for all pregnant women at 16 to 18 weeks gestation as a screening procedure for open neural tube defects; anencephaly, open spina bifida, exomphalos, twin pregnancy, threatened or missed abortion, feto-maternal haemorrhage, congenital nephrosis and severe epidermal defects.

In 1979 there was a continuing development of the computer system with the introduction of the 2050 system including disc facilities.

The increases in emergency biochemical measurements continued to increase. This was restricted only by a request that the on-call service was to be requested solely by a consultant or a senior registrar to the biochemist on standby.

In 1981 the workload again increased, to 986,700 patient tests. In 1981–82 the purchase of two Rotochem centrifugal analysers greatly improved the efficiency of the department.

In January 1982 a multichannel analyser and computer (SMAC) was bought to replace the existing analyser and from August 1982 eleven analysers were carried out on the system. This proved to be a very effective analyser and lasted until 1991.

In 1982 Dr Horn began the development of an upgraded computer system, providing an excellent opportunity to assess the benefits of the use of this technology within a laboratory department. The Lothian Health Board agreed that a laboratory information computing system would be developed by the department with a locally based company, Digital Equipment Company Limited (DEC). DEC had been suppliers of hardware for many years but had only recently entered into the software field. The development was given the name HORLICS (after Dr Horn its principle developer; Hor(n), laboratory, information, computing, system). It was intended to be the standard system in the Lothian Region. A very considerable effort had been expended within the NHS on laboratory computing facilities but the transfer of systems between laboratories did not prove easy. The DEC system allowed ready and speedy input of patient information and test requesting details. This lead to the production of worksheets for the numerous tests carried out in the department. These tests were carried out on other equipment, much of which involved high technology, and the results were transferred by a variety of means into the main computer. There they were collated and presented in a cumulative form for visual checking and validation of clinical acceptability by the biochemists. Reports were then generated in a cumulative form on A4-paper, giving all the results obtained from any patient over a period of ten different requests days in columnar form. This facilitated the interpretation of results by biochemists and clinical staff. The introduction of this data-handling system greatly decreased the amount of time spent reporting results manually. It also lead to a more efficient use of staff and cost saving.

As more and more of the repetitive and routine tests were handled mechanically and by micro-processors, a greater proportion of time was spent in applying scientific skills to the advancement of knowledge and patient care.

In April 1983 the new system was set up and Mrs Dorothy Coulter, an administrative assistant, was, and remains very active in the control of the computer with the clerical staff. Interest in this system extended well beyond the confines of Edinburgh

More recently the instrumentation has extended to the very efficient Kodak analyser. Two Kodak analysers have been used for about four years and the Monarch analysers and the SMAC II have been taken out of use.

The current staff, with Dr Blundell as head, consists of six biochemists, 19 MLSO's and seven whole-time and part-time clerical staff. The number of analyses continues to increase and this is due to the efficiency of the analysers and the upgraded Horlics computer system.

Medical Oncology

Medical Oncology or cancer medicine is still a relatively new sub-specialty of internal medicine and was only officially recognised during the late 1970s. This specialty has a strong academic basis, principally for research and for training. Throughout the United Kingdom the specialty has been established by the creation of University Chairs, almost all of which have been established by the cancer charities. The Imperial Cancer Research Fund created the first Chair of Medical Oncology at St Bartholomew's Hospital and subsequently endowed a Chair at Guy's Hospital in London. By 1978 their funds were sufficient for them to establish a third Chair in the United Kingdom and their Chairman of Council Professor Sir Eric Scowan suggested Edinburgh University as the most appropriate setting. In 1978 the first Professor of Medical Oncology was therefore appointed to Edinburgh. The post was taken by Professor John Smyth who at the time was a Senior Lecturer at the Royal Marsden Hospital in London. John Smyth was appointed to the Chair on 1 April, 1979 and came to the Western General Hospital in October of that year. At that time the Western had an internationally recognised Department of Radiation Oncology headed by Professor William Duncan and provided all of the non-surgical oncology needs for Edinburgh and the south east of Scotland. The siting of medical oncology within the Medical School aroused controversy. Although there was agreement that medical oncology should be based at the Western General there was considerable debate as to the departmental affiliation. John Smyth argued for the need to have a close working relationship with radiation oncology. It was important to remember that Medical Oncology was a sub-specialty of medicine. For the sake of trainees it was important to be part of the overall Department of Medicine at the Western General. By 1980 it was decided that there should be a new University Department of Clinical Oncology containing two Units, one of radiation and one of medical oncology, each headed by a Professor. The staff of the Medical Oncology Unit could also be members of the Department of Medicine, at that time under the Chairmanship of Michael Matthews. Considerable building alterations were made to house the Medical Oncology Unit and this again was not without its problems. Initially beds were borrowed from the Radiotherapy Unit. The location for the department was in what had previously been the top floor dining room, which had been a very popular facility. This was re-allocated to provide inpatient accommodation (12 bedded ward), and a day patient facility. During 1981 further funds were obtained from the ICRF to establish an extra-mural Unit within the University Department principally to provide a laboratory and laboratory funds for staff and ongoing research. No strangers to the concept of temporary buildings, the Western gave permission for a prefabricated laboratory to be built on the lawn opposite the Superintendent's house. By the end of 1980 the Medical Oncology Unit was in full operation with a core laboratory staff, new hospital accommodation and the beginnings of an excellent working relationship with colleagues in radiation oncology. In 1984, following the resignation of Professor Alan Emery, the top floor of the MRC building became vacant. The medical oncology academic accommodation moved from the, so-called, temporary laboratory to the top floor of the MRC building where it remains to this time. Over the 15 years of its existence, the Medical Oncology Unit has expanded its clinical activities considerably. It now provides a regional medical oncology service to Edinburgh and the surrounding districts with Consultants providing regular outpatient sessions at Kirkcaldy. Joint clinics are held in a number of disciplines with colleagues from the Royal Infirmary, St John's and the Eastern.

The main area of research activity has been to try and identify less toxic forms of cancer therapy and to develop new anti-cancer drugs and regimens. The Western can be proud of its achievements in this regard. This is reflected by over £11 million of research funding that has been raised and the international reputation that the Unit now holds for its research productivity.

Of paramount importance to patient care is the concept of the quality of service given. Equally important is the approach of medical and nursing staff to patients recently diagnosed as having malignant disease. Much of the research activity that has been conducted has looked at these issues. They form a major part of the training programme which concentrates on attitudes to patients, to the need for adequate exchange of information with patients and wherever possible their active participation in the programme of therapy for them. Collaboration with clinical psychology has been seen as very important. The Unit has received international recognition for its work in what is now called psycho-social oncology. A number of people have progressed to Consultant appointments, some needing to go as far as New Zealand. A notable success was the first Lecturer, Dr James Carmichael, who is now the Professor of Medical Oncology in the University of Nottingham. The range of challenges in medical oncology is wide. One of our former trainees, Dr Michael Cornbleat, is now Director of the Fairmile Marie Curie Home. A recent Research Fellow,

Dr Jeremy Kean is now a Senior Registrar in Palliative Medicine at St Columba's Hospice.

The advent of Trust status with its emphasis on providing cost-effective health care is a particular challenge for medical oncology. Treatment is frequently intensive and expensive and results are far from satisfactory in terms of survival. There will always be a need for research to improve on these results. The Western General can be justifiably proud of the way in which it has developed a Medical Oncology Unit with a truly effective working relationship between the National Health Service, the University and the major Cancer Charities.

Clinical Research Centre

The Clinical Research Centre was established in 1990 in a five-year collaborative agreement between the University of Edinburgh, Syntex Pharmaceutical Company, and the Lothian Health Board. The agreement was supervised by a Management Committee which included the then Dean of the Faculty of Medicine, Professor Cairns Aitken, the subsequent Dean and Provost of the Faculty of Medicine, Professor Christopher Edwards, and the Head of Clinical Pharmacology, Professor Michael Lee. This new research unit is based in the clock tower building at the Western General Hospital, within the original medical wards of the hospital. The wards were refurbished to provide a fully functional 20 bedded clinical trials unit. Given the interests of the partners in this venture, the emphasis was placed on academic research in a clinical environment, and space and time were specifically allotted to academic clinical research and patient care. In addition, the relationship gave Syntex the possibility of performing high quality cardiovascular research, and develop new drugs for the treatment of heart disease, in the academic setting of a teaching hospital.

The Director, Dr David Webb, was appointed in January 1990 and took charge of the unit in March 1990. He also held responsibilities as a senior lecturer in the University Department of Medicine and as a consultant physician within the hospital. By the time of the official opening, by Lord James Douglas Hamilton in October 1990, there was already a small but active team of researchers working in the Clinical Research Centre. Over the next 5 years there was a rapid expansion of both academic and pharmaceutical research activity, with similar increases in staffing. When activity reached a peak, in 1994, the University was employing three full-time doctors, two administrative secretaries, and seven full-time nurses to perform clinical research in the unit, with an annual budget in excess of £1M. Over this period, the unit gained an international reputation, and attracted substantial grant income, for its work on the endothelin family of local hormones and for its innovative use of a wide range of cardiovascular techniques. In acknowledgement of this work, in 1994, Dr Webb was awarded the SmithKline Beecham Foundation Prize for Research from the British Pharmacological Society and Dr Haynes, his lecturer, was awarded the Derek Dunlop Prize in Clinical Pharmacology from the Royal

Society of Medicine and an Advanced Training Fellowship from the Wellcome Trust. Over this time, the doctors within the unit made a substantial contribution to patient care on the medical wards, to the Hypertension clinic and to clinical teaching. Dr Webb and his lecturer, Dr Haynes, also ran the cardiovascular module of the undergraduate honours course in pharmacology.

In 1994, Syntex Pharmaceutical Company was taken over by the Hoffman-La Roche Company of Switzerland, as part of worldwide amalgamation and streamlining within the pharmaceutical industry. It soon became clear that the five-year agreement would not be renewed after its completion in March 1995. As the number of pharmaceutical research studies reduced, the number and range of academic studies increased. The Clinical Research Centre has become a major base for cardiovascular research within the Western General Hospital, developing close links with cardiology, renal medicine, intensive care and diabetic medicine. Moreover, by this time the Clinical Research Centre had built up sufficient reputation to be able to continue to attract high quality research and related monies, and maintain an independent existence within the University.

In early 1995, Professor Michael Lee announced his retirement. The University had decided to achieve complementarity between the Royal and Western as part of its response to Lothian Health's Acute Service Strategy. One consequence was an independent assessment of the strengths of clinical pharmacology in 1994. On the basis of this report, and the academic success of the Clinical Research Centre, the Faculty of Medicine decided to move the Clinical Pharmacology Unit and its staff to the Western General Hospital. In addition there is to be a new Chair, to take advantage of the potential for high quality clinical research provided by the facilities and expertise within the Clinical Research Centre. Dr David Webb has been appointed to this Chair. It is envisaged that Clinical Pharmacology and Therapeutics will have a bright future in its new surroundings, and that close research links will be established with the Molecular Medicine Centre.

Geriatrics, Royal Victoria Hospital

As a memorial to Queen Victoria's Jubilee in 1887, the Victoria Dispensary for Consumption and Diseases of the Chest was set up as an out-patient clinic initially in Bank Street at the top of the Mound. A plaque in the wall above Christie's the jeweller commemorates this. In 1894 Craigleith House was rented to provide in-patient care for patients with consumption (tuberculosis) and so the Victoria Hospital was born. The hospital was officially opened on the 22 November 1894 by Moir T. Stormont Darling. The visitors book from that occasion is available and makes for interesting reading.

In 1899 Craigleith House and its grounds were bought for £1000 per acre. Four years later three pavilions were built to increase the capacity of the hospital for the princely sum of £11,000. These Y-shaped wards (later described as butterfly wards) were the most up-to-date design at the time. In 1907 two further butterfly wards were opened in addition to an administration building. Royal patronage was given by King Edward VII in 1904, and the hospital became the Royal Victoria Hospital for Consumption.

Most people know of the arched entrance to the hospital and this East Lodge was built in 1908. In those days the two large doors were closed at night using a large wheel in the lodge above the archway. The wheel no longer exists and the doors are not closed at any time. As recently as the 1960s, the gates were closed and kept closed for a month following heavy rain, as a large puddle had formed just inside the gate. A mallard duck and drake decided to nest and rear their young on the 'pond' and despite complaints from some members of the public, the gates remained closed until the ducklings were reared and flew to more suitable surroundings.

About this time when the five butterfly wards were operating, Craigleith House was converted to the Nurses Home and remained so until 1952 when settlement and dry rot forced the nurses out into new buildings — Stewart and Raeburn Houses. This was not before the basement of Craigleith House was used somewhat unofficially as a store for the sale of second-hand furniture and jewellry. Before it was demolished, one could see through the walls destroyed by the dry rot.

At the time that the butterfly wards were built, a number of chalets were also constructed. These were made of wood but had only three walls. They were also on rails with the open side facing the sun. They could be moved round on the rails during the day to follow the sun. Patients with Tuberculosis were nursed in beds in these chalets. Imagine the uproar today if a patient was left in an unheated chalet with only blankets and maybe a hot water bottle during the winter snows for days and nights on end? This was the only 'treatment' available in those days — freeze the organisms to death! Despite many adverse comments from the public, most of the patients were very happy with the personal chalet. It was often difficult to get them to agree to going back into the butterfly wards. Apparently a number of the patients who survived and went home had chalets built in their own back gardens. Dr Roger Smith, the current Clinical Director of the Royal Victoria, remembers the last chalet when he first came to the Royal Victoria in 1973.

Over the years there have been a number of very famous doctors involved in the Royal Victoria Hospital, including Sir Robert Philip, who was responsible for setting up the first clinic in Bank Street, and more recently, Dr Christopher Clayson and Professor Sir John Crofton. It was the latter's revolutionary treatment of tuberculosis using a combination of drugs rather than one drug which led to the virtual eradication of tuberculosis in Edinburgh. This happened in the mid 1950s and as a result there were fewer and fewer patients needing care at the Royal Victoria Hospital. Working with Sir John Crofton at this time was a young chest physician called James Williamson. He saw that following the decrease in tuberculosis patients, the new 'problem' for the Health Service would be the elderly. As a result the Royal Victoria Hospital changed its clients to those elderly people requiring long term nursing care. There was also a need for assessment, rehabilitation and a day hospital.

Two of the butterfly wards were demolished in 1987 and a new building housing 90 beds was built. In 1971 a day hospital, out-patient department, X-ray suite, dental department and office accommodation were added. With a singular piece of foresight, a combined geriatric and psychogeriatric service was started with Dr Williamson and Dr Robinson leading the two specialties respectively. In 1978 a purpose built 30-bedded long stay care ward was built to commemorate the origin of the hospital. This was named 'Craigleith House'. It now looks after respite patients. In 1984, with the increasing number of elderly people in the population, a further 180 beds were added in an extension to the existing 90 bedded building. This gave 150 geriatric beds and 120 psychogeriatric beds in addition to the 30 beds in Craigleith House. Regrettably, the three remaining butterfly wards had to be demolished to make room for the new extension. The administration building which incorporates the Board Room, still remains. The Board Room which used to be the WRVS cafeteria until the extension was built in 1984 has had a facelift and this beautiful room will become the Trust Board Room — a much better place for meetings and interviews than Meeting Room 1 in the Western General Nurses Home!

James Williamson was appointed Professor of Geriatric Medicine in 1976. He made an incredible change to the care of the elderly. No longer were the elderly to be disregarded. They had the same illnesses as the young and some of their own. These were all to be carefully treated.

The Western General Hospital was visited by Geriatricians from the Royal Victoria. In 1990 a geriatric assessment unit was opened in Wards F1–3. In this area the elderly can be assessed and their ability to return home, to cope with their previous way of life, or to move into more supervised care identified. The team consisted of physicians, nurses, occupational therapists, physiotherapists, social workers and geriatric psychiatrists.

The physician in charge is Dr Roger Smith who belongs to the new breed of geriatricians, trained in the specialty of the primary care of the elderly. The result is a service which is central to the smooth running of the hospital.

Gastro-intestinal Unit

The Gastro-intestinal Unit was established in 1948, founded as a joint venture by a physician, Dr Wilfrid Card, and a surgeon, Mr John Bruce, who had been friends in the 14th Army in Burma under the command of Sir William Slim. The Unit pioneered the combined care of patients suffering from gastro-intestinal disease by both physicians and surgeons. Card had been appointed as a physician to St Thomas's Hospital in London, where great consternation followed his resignation to come to a Poor Law establishment in North Edinburgh.

Several factors favoured the development of combined care.

1. The increasing understanding of gastro-intestinal diseases. Advancing technology and procedures made gastroenterology difficult for the general physician;
2. The concept of a surgeon as a 'physician who operated' was untenable as surgical technological demands increased;
3. The philosophy that medicine and surgery were different was beginning to be challenged;
4. The influence of the visionary Professor Stanley Davidson who encouraged the development of new departments staffed by full time specialists with considerable experience and skill and no private practice.

In 1951 Card and Bruce began the experiment. Patients with gastrointestinal diseases were admitted to a ward service under 'joint and equal' clinical control. The beds in wards D1 (male) and D2 (female) were neither medical or surgical. The patients were under the care of a consultant physician for diagnostic procedures and investigations. Their treatment was decided by the physician except for surgery which was defined by the appropriate surgeon. The surgeons decided the nature and timing of the operation, and postoperatively were responsible for care except for nutrition and fluid balance. They took as much interest as they wished in cases with no evident surgical requirements. A House Officer cared for the patient whether the problem was medical or surgical and who was supported by surgical and medical registrars. There was one full-time senior medical registrar and two part-time surgical registrars.

Each week there were separate meetings between the surgeons, physicians and radiologists to review investigations and consider diagnoses and treatment; with the pathologists to review morbid anatomy and microscopy, and the social workers and psychiatrists to explore psychosocial areas. There was a joint weekly ward round attended by the entire medical and surgical staff, overseas and other clinical fellows and by researchers. A journal club met every two weeks and a research reporting group met.

Typical of the vision of the unit was the meeting of the British Medical Association in Edinburgh in 1956 when a highly professional demonstration of the combined approach to the management of ulcerative colitis was mounted. Card employed professional artists and photographers which the clinicians paid for from their own resources. The result was a magnificent display, at a time when these presentations were usually 'in house' and amateurish. Also in 1956 more publicity was received when the unit provided a half-hour programme on Peptic Ulcer in the BBC television series *Your Life in Their Hands*. This was a repeat as the first patient died on the table.

As the number of individuals attached to the unit and the volume of work grew, there was a constant shortage of office and laboratory space. Wilfrid Card had offices in the attics at the western end of the main building. Bill Sircus persuaded the Health Board to buy a secondhand caravan as an office for himself and secretary at the unit entrance.

A disadvantage of the GI unit was a reluctance to admit emergencies.

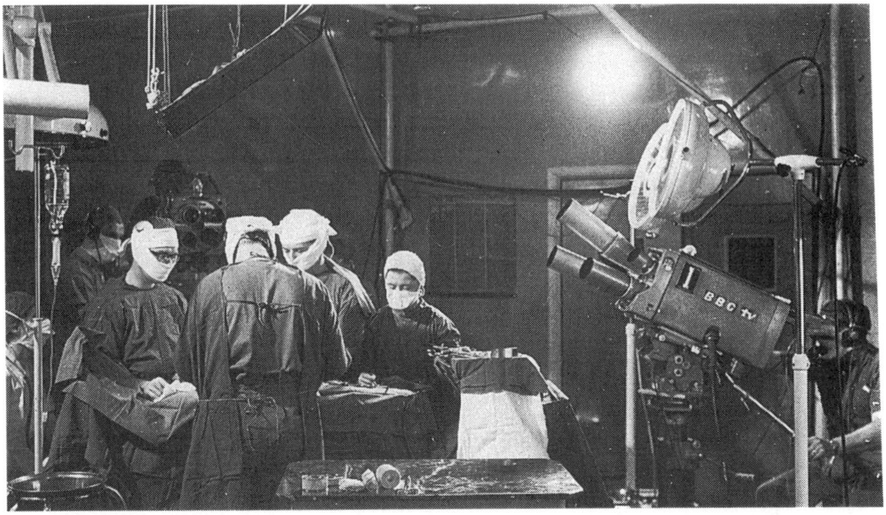

TV programme 'Your life in their hands', with Mr WP Small facing, Mr C Falconer back to camera.

Attempts were made to identify beds for emergencies, but they were seldom available. The surgeons in the general surgical unit saw more of the emergency admissions.

In 1950–51 Charles Falconer was appointed as a consultant surgeon to the Gastro-intestinal Unit. In 1954 William P. Small was attached as a third surgeon to general surgery. All three surgeons were members of the general surgery unit, with John Bruce and Charles Falconer part-time in the GI Unit. Bill Small had no contact with the GI Unit for the first years of his appointment to the Western. His first acceptance to these jealously-guarded wards came when the whole GI staff, medical and surgical, went to a seminar in York. He was left to provide cover and only fully entered the unit in 1958 or 1959. Adam Smith joined the Unit in 1959 as lecturer and in 1961 he became a senior lecturer.

In 1954 Wilfred Sircus was appointed as assistant consultant physician for six sessions a week (the annual salary being £1100). Bill Sircus secured four sessions as an external member of staff of the Medical Research Council. Laboratory facilities were provided by Sir James Learmonth in the Wilkie Surgical Research Department at Teviot Place. Research fellows from both the medical and surgical teams of the unit studied gastrointestinal physiology and pathophysiology with Bill Sircus over many years.

By the mid 1960s Card had left for a new appointment in Glasgow, and John Bruce was fully occupied in his Regius Chair in the Royal Infirmary. The loss of Card was unnecessary and very painful. He was a victim of the natural wish to see the Western General as a clinical academic department in its own right. Admired as a clinician and scientist, his credentials to become Professor of Medicine at the Western General was obvious to the fair minded. This was not to be, he resigned and moved to a chair in Glasgow. Card was a massive influence on the development of the Hospital. He introduced, with others, the concept of gastroenterology as a clinical scientific endeavour. In addition he designed the GI unit coat of arms, approved by the Lord Lyon King of Arms. This is embossed in the form of a medal which is given to all long-term members of the unit on leaving 'for bravery in the face of gastroenterology'. The Medical Staff Committee was his idea. This committee represents the clinical staff and has evolved from being a dining club to an integral part of the new management structure. He was a deceptive man to meet; tall and reserved, he would walk through the hospital with his eyes fixed on the next vision. One day he passed two of his registrars, and instead of walking past, he said 'Hello', prompting one of the registrars, an Australian, to comment: 'My, he's chatty today'. It was his practice to write a scientific paper and keep it in his desk for a year to mature before sending for publication. Yet the whole medical social organisation of the hospital was his plan. Socially he was very skilled and his company was very agreeable.

When one looks back over the operative notebooks, one can see that John Bruce did a tremendous amount of work. Subsequent senior surgeons rather reduced his importance but his endeavour has to be recognised. He was a larger than life man and in his way he was as visionary as Card. A *bon viveur*, his style was more openly outgoing than Card's. His approach was somewhat gruff and sometimes hid his very formidable intellect. The bluffness is indicated by the story of when he drove from the Western to the University he would cross the Mound/High St intersection ignoring the policeman on duty and waving his stethescope — probably the only time he used it. This pattern was abruptly changed when the policeman waved his handcuffs back. Whatever his faults, he worked hard at the Western, supported Wilfrid Card and maintained academic contact through Adam Smith. It might have altered the history of surgery in Edinburgh and the history of the Western had he held the Clinical Chair at the Western, allowing Woodruff primacy for the Chair of Surgical Science at the Royal Infirmary.

During the early 1960s there was a great stramash when the lions outside D1 and 2 were stolen by unknown individuals. Miss Adamson, the matron then, made it very clear that they had to be returned. They had been buried for some two to three months before they were replaced from their grave in a vegetable plot.

In 1966 Dr Card was succeeded by Dr James P A MacManus who had been both registrar and senior registrar in the unit. He had worked with both Sircus and Card on developing acid secretion tests. He previously worked in Boston, USA and never really settled in Edinburgh after his time in North America.

Bill Sircus took over administrative responsibility of the unit which began it's second phase of development under his leadership. In 1969 the role of the rotating chairman was established amongst each of the surgeons and physicians. This change in leadership was established at an oft-quoted and disagreeable weekend meeting at Peebles Hydro. This arrangement and the associated

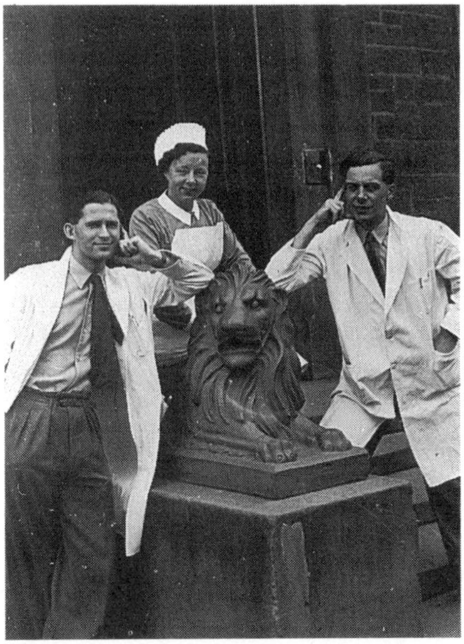

Outside D Block: Sister Orr, two resident doctors and one resident lion in the 1950s.

turbulence continued until the late 1980s when eventually the combined unit system finished.

Bill Sircus too had a visionary approach. He was a clinician of impressive insight and a skilled, innovative endoscopist. He had an ability to attract fellows from abroad and was a renowned teacher of clinical practice. His ward rounds involved shrewd clinical decision-making in addition to teaching. They were very popular for their educational value.

A number of other physicians had a very real impact on the unit. Gerry Crean, a Dublin graduate, was a first-class clinician and research worker. He worked as a registrar and then locum consultant, conducting important studies relating to the histology of the stomach mucosa in patients with complicated duodenal ulceration. Eventually he moved to the Southern General Hospital in Glasgow. His worth was recognised by his election to the Presidency of the British Society of Gastroenterology. John Nimmo, a Physicians' Physician, was a locum consultant for a year, before moving to the Eastern General Hospital in Edinburgh as a consultant.

Many outstanding nurses have worked and trained in the unit. The Sister in charge of the gastrointestinal unit between 1948 and 1977 was Sister Christine Orr. She had a powerful influence on nurses, medical staff and patients and her ability to comfort patients was a model for generations of nurses. The stories about her abound. Her approach was to know everything that happened and she was particularly expert in counselling ulcerative colitis patients who came to ileostomy. She was awarded the MBE for her work.

Sister Orr was succeeded by Sisters Aurea Amos and Betty Sutherland, each in their way worthy heirs. Both were disciplinarians and controllers of colourful registrars who required to be kept on the straight and narrow; housemen were knocked into shape. Since then Sisters Fiona Petrie and Noleen Murray have continued this tradition.

There were a number of overseas doctors attracted to the GI unit including Professor Olga Henriques from Brazil and Dr David Byrnes from Sydney, Australia, Dr Marks from Capetown, Dr Kamal Jalan from Calcutta, Dr John Goy from Melbourne, Dr John Lennon from Dublin and Dr Mahmud Husan from Bangladesh A significant number of fellows, medical, surgical and scientific were able to undertake research work which led to PhD's. Many of the research and clinical fellows have become distinguished contributing gastroenterologists around the world, several appointed to Chairs, and this applies both to the surgical and medical fellows.

A plan was developed for a substantial pre-fabricated building for research laboratories and office accomodation. The Wolfson Trust gave £45,000 towards the project. A long dormant period followed during which Wilfrid Card and John Bruce tried to attract additional money from the Health Board. Plans for a two storey building were drawn. In 1969 the Wolfson Laboratories came into being on the lawn at the west side of the ward block. The distinguished architect miscalculated the amount of money needed to build the laboratory and only one floor was possible. A Clinical Director for the laboratories was funded by the Health Board and the University to carry out GI research. In 1969, Martin Eastwood, an Edinburgh Medical graduate, was appointed from a lectureship post in the Royal Infirmary of Edinburgh. The next and important development was the recruitment of nurses specifically trained in the basic technology of the GI investigation procedures, gastric and pancreatic function tests, motility investigations, small bowel biopsies and others. The scientific staff of the laboratory were led by skillful senior graduate biochemists. The first of these was Derek Mitchell who eventually moved on to St Thomas's in London to be succeeded by Gordon Brydon.

There was a continued need for modern custom-built premises for the rapidly expanding endoscopy service and this was met in the new outpatient building. The new facilities in the day bed area allowed for the reception and preparation of patients and a well-equipped endoscopy theatre.

Bill Sircus was keen to replace the now ageing caravan office, with offices for the physicians and a custom-built investigation suite for clinical investigations. The opportunity came when an elderly Jewish antique dealer in his care in the ward called him over to her bedside and pressed into his hand an old brown paper grocery bag. 'You are to use this for your unit,' she told him, 'and when you come on your next ward round there will be another.' Inside the bag were bank notes of various denominations amounting to £6000. The second bag duly received had a further £4000. With this as a catalyst, Bill Sircus was able to persuade the hospital board to match the gift. The clinical investigation suite — semi-prefabricated — was planned and built just outside the entrance to D block.

During the period 1951 to 1980, patients with ulcerative colitis, Crohn's disease, other malabsorption states, morbid obesity, post resection malnutrition, cystic fibrosis, and malignancies of oesophagus and rectum, were subjected to prolonged in-patient care. Three weeks was the average in-patient period. The introduction of new drugs and procedures and the growth of outpatient facilities reduced the in-patient time and the need for the original number of beds.

There was considerable development of endoscopy from the early days. The first endoscope introduced to the Unit came from Switzerland. Restrictions in those days did not allow transfer of equipment but this instrument was imported illicitly. John Bruce was a director of Hibernian Football club, and following a European Fairs Cup match, the endoscope came back in the dirty laundry basket. Originally only the stomach and duodenum were examined by the endoscope and there was much collaboration between radiologists and pathologists regarding the endoscopic findings.

The Maximal Histamine Test was the standard method of assessing gastric hydrochloric acid output in patients with duodenal and gastric ulcers. The philosophy was 'no acid — no ulcer'. The acid output test was subsequently called Kay's test, but owed its beginning to Wilfrid Card. The type of operation prescribed for the duodenal ulcer was based on the use of this test. Although the whole concept later proved flawed it meant that each patient was individually assessed and in consequence very few were subjected to radical gastrectomy. The standard operation at that time was partial gastrectomy. The plan was for patients with relatively little acid production to be treated by gastroenterostomy, since this was a much less radical operation and the capacity of the stomach was not reduced. The high acid secretors needed additional protection from recurrent ulcer by vagotomy. Selection for ulcer surgery was based on the idea of 'earning'. Surgery was a last resort, not to be embarked upon until many years of suffering had been endured. As a result many patients were denied treatment. The experience of the GI unit showed this attitude to be wrong and that with proper investigation and overall assessment, treatment did not depend on time and length of symptoms. The number of cases operated on each year soon rose to about 150, which is in striking contrast to the present era with less than 20 for the whole of Lothian.

In the earlier years, the most important scientific contribution was the acid secretory studies by Wilfrid I. Card and Francois Martin. This very mathematical study resulted in a paper on the gastric parietal cell mass which became a classic. Another paper written by Sircus and Card redefined achlorhydria. A series of papers looked at blood group substances, secretor status, gastric acid secretion and peptic ulcers in order to try and identify why some individuals developed duodenal ulceration and others did not.

In experimental surgery, C. Hudson and Roy Preshaw worked with Bill Sircus in studying the role of the endocrine system in the secretory responses of the stomach and pancreas. Subsequently Card led another series of outstanding studies on the newly-discovered hormone gastrin, assisted by Gabriel Mahklouf and Jim McManus.

The problem which dominated gastroenterology above all others in the next three decades was peptic ulcer disease and its complications. In those days medical treatment consisted of bed rest, the milk drip, antacids and anticholinergics. Surgery was the mainstay of treatment and was fraught with complications. Short term and long term sequelae were common, and some, such as early and late dumping, bile vomiting and diarrhoea could be dramatic in presentation and readily diagnosed. Others such as anaemia, metabolic bone disease and recurrent ulcer could be more insidious in onset and more difficult to diagnose. The side effects of surgery could become manifest many years later and present in surreptitious ways. For some of these problems, the treatment was medical, for others surgical. The need for combined medical and surgical care and for long-term follow-up was recognised early. It was natural, therefore, that a special interest in duodenal ulcer disease should develop in this, the first such combined Unit in the British Isles. The introduction of vagotomy (the surgical division of the vagus nerves) in the late 1940s had raised the possibility of a more physiological approach than sub-total gastrectomy for acid reduction — considered at that time to be the key to healing peptic (especially duodenal) ulcers. This offered the prospect of a less radical operation with lower operative mortality and hopefully none of the problems of long term anaemia and osteomalacia. 'Tailoring' meant offering radical surgery only to those with aggressive ulcers or with high acid output. Other patients had vagotomy or even gastroenterostomy alone. The results of this trial needed to be assessed.

Dr Card put forward a proposition to the Health Board that patients treated by gastric surgery should be followed to define their long term outcome. As a result, Bill Small established a gastric follow-up clinic with accompanying ancillary staff. This was based upon the Visick Clinical Classification grade, then the best validated approach. The aim was to try to prove the benefit of the tailored gastric operation policy. The problem was that data were retrospective, without control patients who had a standard operation. This proved to be a fairly insoluble problem. Nevertheless, Bill Small was able to show that the post operative symptoms of dumping, bile vomiting, weight loss and the psychiatric factors could be considered independently. Each of these symptoms was evaluated in a series of patients, thus achieving some outcome measure and establishing the follow-up clinic on a firm basis. When Bill Small retired he was succeeded by Iain Macintyre who retained the philosophy but replaced the previous card index system by a computerised record system. Although peptic ulcer is now rarely surgically treated, the Gastric Follow-up clinic continues to flourish. In recent years the follow-up clinic has concentrated upon the long-term results of colonic cancer.

Bill Sircus established the epidemiology, natural history and management of aphthous ulceration of the mouth. Carcinoid and Zollinger Ellison syndromes were studied by Adam N. Smith, Ian G. Cleator, Christine Thomson, Roy Preshaw and Bill Sircus. Later Jack Zeitlin and Adam N. Smith made important studies on the Kinein systems.

Biliary surgery was improved by the use of intravenous cholangiography with the support of Hunter Cummack the consultant radiologist. Great clinical benefit came from the weekly combined X-Ray meetings where all cases were discussed.

The revision of previous peptic ulcer surgery became an increasing commitment of the Unit. This produced a heavy burden, particularly for Charles Falconer, who could spend eight hours or more in theatre, unravelling and re-doing surgery which had not settled the patients' symptoms. Before the advent of the combined unit, the care of patients suffering from ulcerative colitis and Crohn's disease suffered from a fragmented approach. A combined approach met that need, the more so when better treatment, including steroids and salazopyrin, were established. The unit established Stoma care and later revisional surgery with pouch formation and re-anastomosis. Ulcerative colitis cases were reviewed by Kamal Jalan in a series of papers assessing the influence of smoking and contraceptive drugs on Crohn's disease; toxic dilation of the colon; pseudopolyposis in ulcerative colitis; faecal stasis in ulcerative colitis; solitary ulcer of rectum; arthropathies in ulcerative colitis; steroid therapy in inflammatory bowel disease and long-term outcomes and the effect of colonic surgery on bile metabolism. Unfortunately these papers are now rarely quoted and those from Leeds, Oxford and London are better known.

In the period 1969–72 Martin Eastwood and Kiron Das defined the metabolism of salazopyrin in inflammatory bowel disease. Kiron Das was awarded a PhD for his work. He moved on to New York and became a world famous immunologist, studying colitis.

In 1971 the Unit was officially designated as the Gastro-intestinal Unit of the University of Edinburgh. From 1951 to 1980 the Unit had 32 beds with a ward for each sex. With this academic state came a lecturer post. Amongst the lecturers were: Michael Ward now in Brisbane, Richard Logan in Nottingham, Jack Gillon in Edinburgh and Roger Barton in Newcastle.

From 1969, the research interest of Martin Eastwood steered the laboratory towards nutrition, colonic physiology and the effect of dietary fibre on symptomatic diverticulosis. The nutritional studies looked at dietary fibre in the colon, the fermentation of dietary fibre and methods to predict the action of dietary fibre. Methods to identify bile acid malabsorption, a cause of diarrhoea, were established. There developed a close collaboration between Martin Eastwood and Adam Smith to develop methods to study the effectiveness of dietary fibre on the spasms associated with chronic diverticulosis. This led to studies of the intraluminal effects of fibre as a bulky, water-holding agent which altered the flora, biochemistry and the transit function of the colon. The tensile strength and physical parameters of the colon from Scottish and African subjects with and without diverticular disease were measured. This required a visit to Uganda during active military action. Later studies in collaboration with the University Department of Biochemistry used X-ray diffraction and chemical analysis to show the altered collagen structure in diverticular disease. An epidemiological study in Scotland showed that often surgery for diverticular disease was necessary most commonly in elderly women.

Adam Smith studied resection and myotomy for diverticular disease. He established a team to perform pressure and other electro-physiological tests for faecal incontinence and intractable forms of constipation. The bowel problems of spinally injured subjects was a matter for special collaboration with the Spinal Injuries Unit. Concurrent with these studies of anorectal function, Adam Smith introduced to Edinburgh the Park's pouch technique for ulcerative colitis and did the first 20 of these initially with Gavin Browning. He was also the first to do post-anal repairs in Edinburgh.

Martin Eastwood ran the assisted nutrition teams of the Hospital, for Total Parenteral Nutrition and Endosocopic Gastrostomy, for many years.

In 1975, Anne Ferguson was appointed as second physician/senior lecturer when Dr McManus returned to North America. Anne Ferguson's interests swung the clinical and research work of the unit towards malabsorption states, mainly the morphology and immunology of coeliac disease. The longstanding interest in inflammatory bowel disease of the Unit was extended by Anne Ferguson whose interest in mucosal immunology led to a greater understanding of Crohn's and colitis. She developed non-invasive biochemical methods to classify the extent of inflammation in the intestines of patients with inflammatory bowel disease. This was complemented by studies of the epidemiology of Crohn's disease in Scotland, particularly among adolescents. Her overall strategy was to assess the long-term treatment of inflammatory bowel disease in young people. As the realisation developed that duodenal ulcers were associated with helicobacter pylorides infection in the stomach, she and Gordon Brydon established the 14-Carbon urea breath test which has become the modern basis of diagnosis. She became first a Reader, then the first woman Clinical Professor in the university, and subsequently Chairman of Department of Medicine.

In 1985 Bill Sircus retired and was succeeded by Dr Kelvin Palmer. He graduated from Sheffield University and later trained in London and in California. He also had a reputation as a formidable squash player. For many years Kel Palmer and Martin Eastwood, with others from the Unit, ran the Langholm Toun eight mile run. He and John Saunders, the surgeon, introduced a new series of endoscopic skills, in particular the use of laser therapy in treatment of inoperable carcinoma of the oesophagus, stomach and to some extent the colon. They introduced advanced diagnostic and in particular therapeutic ERCP which examines the common bile duct and pancreatic duct which is important in the care of patients with cancer of the pancreas and with impacted gall stones. They also introduced a service for colonic polypectomy in which benign polypi in the colon which may become cancerous are removed by a colonoscope, an important exercise in preventing cancer of the colon. Kel Palmer established a Lothian-wide endoscopic treatment for bleeding ulcers which has saved many lives, especially amongst the elderly. His endoscopic skills have radically changed the approach to many problems in gastroenterology, previously treated by surgeons, or not treatable at all. He has also captained a very strong Cricket Team which repeatedly beats the Royal Infirmary.

With the introduction of simple medical therapies in the treatment of duodenal ulcer, the work of the unit became very much that of the treatment of inflammatory bowel disease in the form of Crohn's and colitis, the treatment of hepatobiliary disease endoscopically and also an interest in irritable bowel syndrome.

Over the 45 years of the unit many books have been written or edited by the physicians and surgeons, all contributed to multiauthor volumes throughout the world. The number of publications from the unit comes to over 1,000, about half of which were joint efforts.

Sir John Bruce became President of the Royal College of Surgeons. Dr Wilfrid Card was President of the British Society of Gastroenterology, 1970. Wilfred Sircus was President of both the British Society of Digestive Endoscopy 1975–78 and Gastroenterology 1978, Vice-President of the European Society of GI Endoscopy 1980–82 and President of Organisation Mondiale Endoscopie Digestive (OMED) 1985–88. Adam Smith became Wade Professor of the Royal College of Surgeons of Edinburgh and its Vice-President and this thus continued the association of the hospital with the Royal College of Surgeons which was at its height when Sir John Bruce was elected President of the College whilst working at the Western General Hospital.

People work for many years in the unit. Long-serving staff include: Doris Roland the clerkess, Jenny Lawrence the domestic. Edith Palmer, Olive Hart, Mary Wilson, Anne Jenkinson, Aileen Stewart, Phyllis Dickson and Alison Barnes who have each worked for many years as secretary or clerkess.

Dr Card had prophesied that the G I Unit as a group activity had been useful

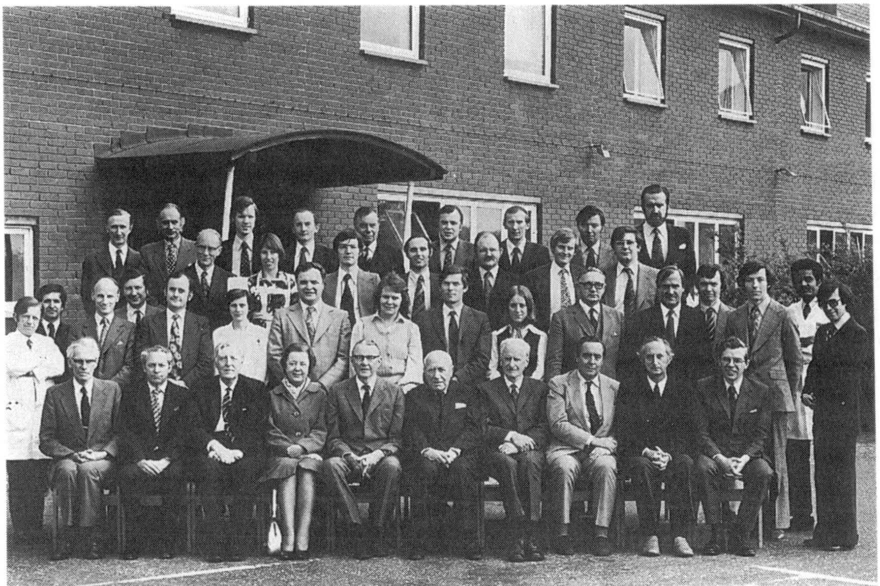

Twenty-fifth Anniversary of Gastro-intestinal Unit 1975

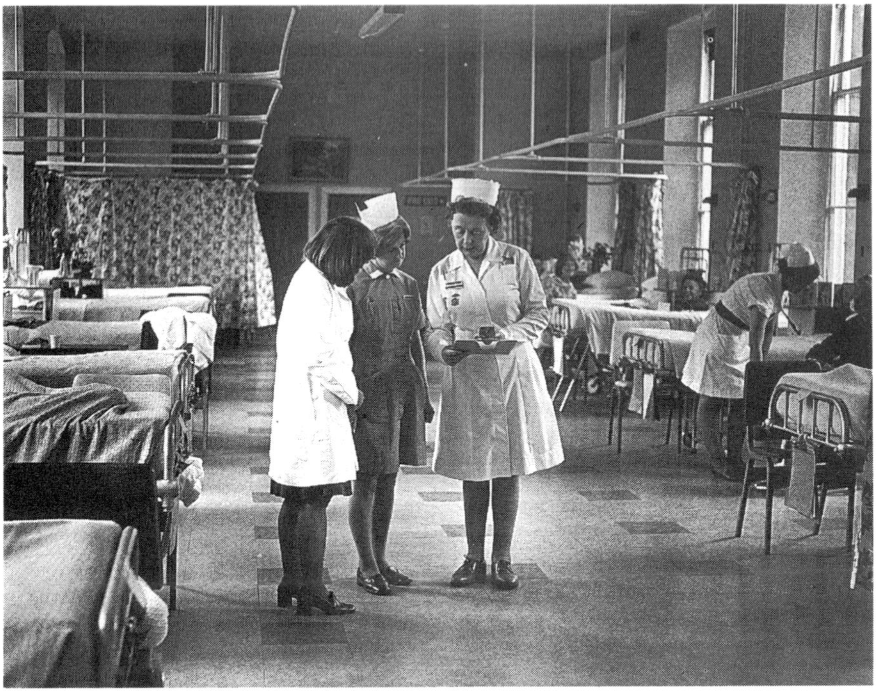

D1 in the 1970s after the removal of the central fireplace.

in its day and had been necessary for the development of gastroenterology. The unit in the Western had been the first of its kind but, being a realist, he anticipated that one day the Unit would come to an end and in a sense his prophecy has come true.

The success of the treatment of duodenal ulcer by newer forms of pharmacological agents has reduced elective surgery of peptic ulcer almost to zero. Even very safe, highly selective vagotomy operations did not prevent a recurrence of duodenal ulceration. It has also been shown that helicobacter infection is a previously unsuspected factor in the aetiology of duodenal ulceration which could be eradicated by antibiotics. The interest has switched away from the mere acid control treatments. The surgical creation of ileoanal pouches has revolutionised the surgical treatment of ulcerative colitis. The dangerous condition of toxic dilatation has almost disappeared. Another change has been the advent of laparoscopic surgery which has increased surgical independence. Regular meetings between the medical and surgical grouping of staff became difficult to sustain in the face of many other administrative matters. Soon the surgeons and physicians held separate meetings. General surgeons in the Western General Hospital moved to the new Alexander Donald building. Thus the old idea of a shared gastrointestinal unit diminished in its importance.

In 1993 the GI unit was moved from wards D1 and 2 to the Alexander Donald building. The gastro-intestinal unit had been in D1 since 1950. This move resulted in a loss of beds. The unit had built its reputation on the orderly investigation of complex problems. This had to be abandoned in the rush and tumble of a ward system where emergency care is all important. Whether this is the end of the G I Unit remains to be seen. Perhaps in the new hospital building the physicians and surgeons will work together.

The General Practitioner Attachment Scheme

Origins and Background

In 1969 a General Practitioner Attachment Scheme was set up at the Western General Hospital. At that time the Health Service had yet to experience any of the reorganisations that were to take place over the next 25 years. In 1966 a working party appointed by the South Eastern Regional Hospital Board, Scotland, had made recommendations about the involvement of General Practitioners in the work of the hospitals with a view to closer integration of the two major parts of the service. One proposal, later to be implemented at Bangour Hospital and to involve the General Practitioners in Livingston, was that 'facilities on a scale to be determined should be incorporated within general hospitals to enable General Practitioners to undertake the in-patient care of their own patients'. Another suggested the 'possibility of allocating for use by selected General Practitioners a limited number of beds from within the existing specialised units'. At the instigation of Sir John Brotherston, then Chief Medical Officer, the Consultant Physicians of the Medical Unit at the Western General Hospital, Drs E. B. French, J. G. Macleod, M. B. Matthews, W. H. Price, Professor J. Strong and Dr R. W. D. Turner agreed to examine methods for putting this second suggestion into practice.

After discussions with a number of General Practitioners, Drs D. G. Illingworth, J. D. E. Knox, G. B. Mackinley, R. C. Macnair and D. E. Williams were appointed for two sessions a week within the Medical Unit. It soon became clear that it would not be practical to designate beds for the exclusive use of the General Practitioners as they would not be able to take as much time from their practice duties as the care of these patients required. Alternative practitioner roles were considered but it was recognised that the most important need was to foster General Practitioner hospital contacts in order to introduce into the hospital a greater awareness of the needs of the patient in the community, particularly at the time of hospital discharge. The presence of General Practitioners on ward rounds undoubtedly increased the sensitivity to these aspects of medical care amongst hospital doctors. The General Practitioners benefited by becoming more familiar with current methods of investigation and treatment. The vocational training schemes in general practice had not yet been initiated so these early experiences with the Attachment Scheme proved to be mutually educational. Regular encounters and exchanges of ideas highlighted deficiencies in communication between the two parts of the service and ways of overcoming these problems were considered. These included computer links between group practices and the hospital but these ideas were never implemented through lack of funds. Personal communication about mutual patients increased with patient care benefiting. In its early stages there were frequent meetings between participants in the scheme. From these meetings grew a number of collaborative projects concerned with the anticipation and prevention of disease. The scheme provided valuable opportunities for teaching undergraduates in the community. Particularly as the majority of the medical students would take up careers in general practice.

By the end of the first year it had become obvious that the scheme was a success. The scheme was extended for a further four years and by the end of that period it included the Surgical, Paediatric and Psychiatric Units as well as the Department of Medicine. The number of available General Practitioner sessions remained the same but in some instances the two sessions were shared so as to increase the number of attached General Practitioners.

A working party recommended the indefinite continuation of the scheme and the appointment of a secretary to assist with the day to day running and organisation. It was agreed by the SHHD, the South East Regional Hospital Board, the University, the Local Medical Committee and representatives from the Western General Hospital, that the General Practitioners should be drawn from the North Lothian District. Especially as they made most use of the Western General Hospital. The objectives of the scheme would be to continue to foster the contact between General Practitioner and the hospital. Individual participants should remain free to explore a variety of GP/hospital consultant relationships depending on personal interests and initiatives.

During its lifetime the scheme has seen the development of vocational training for general practice. Early in 1970 the Board of the South East of Scotland Faculty of General Practitioners established a widely representative committee to establish in Edinburgh a vocational training programme for general practice. The scheme at the Western General Hospital was used to develop a joint vocational training programme. Subsequently vocational training along these lines was adopted for the whole of the region.

From very early on it was clear that the scheme held considerable possibilities for collaborative clinical research. Projects which assessed the pattern of hospital out-patient practice, the value of counselling patients susceptible to coronary artery disease and the use of a general practice population for drug trials were undertaken. With the assistance of the MRC Unit at the Western General Hospital, five practices developed computerised age sex registers containing approximately 35,000 patients. These registers were used for identifying and screening at risk groups and for immunisation. Pilot studies were designed to explore various ways of collecting clinical information to create centralised cumulative personal records available to both hospital and General Practitioners. The scheme subsequently became a focus for combining the resources of several practices in joint projects such as the audit of the Hospital, General Practice Interface. The use of hospital and general practice facilities to identify disease risk factors is an ongoing activity of the scheme as illustrated by the study of Coronary Heart Disease risk factors in two sections of the North Edinburgh population.

The first attached General Practitioners foresaw opportunities for creating a greater awareness amongst hospital doctors of aspects of disease in patient management which received more emphasis in general practice such as the quality of a patient's life and the need to offer advice to patients on lifestyle management. These aspects of the operation of the scheme attracted the attention of a team of Physicians and Students from the Department of Community Medicine at Mount Sinai School of Medicine, New York. They saw parallels between the aspirations of the scheme and their objectives for the Health Insurance Plan (HIP) which was then in its formative days in Manhatten. Exchange visits provided opportunities for observation and discussion of problems which were common to both cities. One New York problem which at that time had not yet been encountered in Edinburgh was drug addiction. A Physician from the Mount Sinai Hospital, a guest of the scheme, spoke of the problem of drug addiction in New York and predicted that it was only a matter of time before it became a problem in Edinburgh.

Since its inception the scheme has seen many 'reorganisations' in the Health Service and has adjusted to the new opportunities. In the present day, General Practitioners with attachments to the new Western General Hospital NHS Trust still participate in the hospital's clinical activities and in joint hospital, community research projects. They also provide valuable contacts between purchasers and providers. Throughout this time the scheme has been guided and supported by Dr Bill Price, who has been responsible for much of the success of these arrangements.

Haematology

Haematology came late to the Pathology service. Until the late 1940s the subject was no more than a side room service provided by the house officer. The Scottish tradition of the ward-based clinical haematologist is a continuation of these side room origins. The range of tests rarely included more than a haemoglobin, white cell count, ESR and occasionally a blood film. All housemen, regardless of how busy the emergency intake had been, were expected to have the blood results for the chief's round later that morning.

The haematology service began in 1948 in a bathroom on C Flat, staffed by two untrained technicians. Two years later, improved accommodation was made available by the Department of Clinical Chemistry in the hospital's old bath house. This small room was to remain the home of the haematology laboratory until it moved into the new accommodation in March 1969. This is adjacent to the Dining Room. This small building then became the blood bank and still functions as the major storage area for Haematology. Staff draw lots for who has to go over there in the winter to collect stores as there is no heating.

Whilst there was no formal consultant haematologist in the Western General for many of the early years, slides were examined by Dr E. B. French.

He was a doctor of many talents which included morphological haematology.

The introduction of a haematology laboratory service in Edinburgh originated with Professor Sir Stanley Davidson. Dr Howard Davies established the concept of a modern laboratory service in Edinburgh in the Royal Infirmary. This was not an easy development and met with considerable opposition. It was not until the appointment of Dr Norman Allan in 1968, that the process of creating a comprehensive clinical and laboratory service was addressed.

The new temporary laboratory and interim academic accommodation was opened by Sir Michael Swann, Principal of the University of Edinburgh in 1969. The new Haematology Department was comprehensive, with laboratory facilities and also four beds in the medical wards and outpatient clinic. It was intended to provide patients with an integrated clinical and laboratory supervision. There was also a University component with a lecturer and a technician for teaching and research.

A blood transfusion cross-matching service was started in 1955 but this was discontinued in 1965 because of lack of space and staff and restarted in 1969.

Between 1967 and 1969 there was a three-fold increase in staff following the appointment of Dr Norman Allan. Norman Allan had previously worked in University College Hospital in Ibadan in Nigeria from 1960 to 1967, first as a Senior Registrar, then lecturer and finally Senior Lecturer. He was seen as somebody who was kind and caring to staff and patients. When he left, his patients spontaneously asked for an opportunity to give him their own send-off and a large number came to the hospital to wish him well. The new staff in 1968 included a senior registrar in haematology, shared with the Haematology Department at the Royal Infirmary, registrar, University lecturer, 24 technicians, one being University, one secretary, three clerkesses and two glasswashers.

The senior MSLO since 1975 has been Mr W. Allen. He typifies the excellent technical service which the laboratories have enjoyed. The path has not always been easy, not the least to respond to continual change in the science and technology whilst enduring an ever-increasing clinical workload.

Undoubtedly the most unhappy time was the tragic death of a young clerkess, Pamela Scott, during the outbreak of hepatitis in 1969.

Despite the humble surroundings of the Haematology Department, some of the trainees have gone on to hold important posts as Consultant Haematologists: Professor Grant Prentice of the Royal Free, Dr Goldstone at UCH and Dr Barnard at St James' all did their spell on the Registrar bench.

Haematology beds were in C Flat. The promise was a move to a fully refurbished A Flat, but this never happened. It took quite a time to get two of the rooms on A Flat and another year or so to move into the present accommodation centred on the old Coronary Care Unit. The window sills have yet to be renewed and repainted.

In 1980 Dr Allan was joined by Dr George Stockdill who moved to the Borders General Hospital in 1986. Dr Michael Mackie replaced Dr Stockdill. When Dr Allan retired in 1993 he was succeeded by Dr Peter Ganly.

The Haematology clinical practise has been built up over the years. More recently *autologous* peripheral blood stem cell and, indeed, *allogenic* bone marrow transplantation have been developed. The use of the Day Bed Area facilities are important in facilitating the outpatient treatment of a large majority of patients. Following review at the Clinic, patients go down to the Day Bed Area, have their chemotherapy. In this way assessment and treatment are over at one visit. Long before the hospital had a specimen transport system, there was a tube system to transport specimens from Outpatients to the Haematology Laboratory which facilitated the review of patients waiting for chemotherapy. In fact, it was Haematology that pushed for the tube transport system for the whole hospital.

Over the years the number of tests performed have grown at a huge rate. This has now 'slowed down' to about seven per cent a year. Despite the increased workload, the staff required for such tests has been reduced. Not only have the general tests increased but also specialist areas have been developed such as immuno-phenotyping and, more recently, cryo preservation of stem cells from the marrow and peripheral blood. The laboratory is the Regional Centre for immuno-phenotyping, covering not only Lothian but also Fife and the Borders. These extra tasks were taken on without increased staff. The laboratory has taken on a great technological change with computerisation which has been overall a considerable benefit. More recently, laboratory staff are expected to become costing experts. This was the first laboratory in Scotland to go through the formal accreditation process laid down by Clinical Pathology Accreditation UK Limited. This unconditional accreditation was achieved at the first attempt following the visit of the accreditors in November, 1992. There has always been a close working relationship with the MRC, particularly as regards the Cytogenetic Service. This is now funded by Lothian Health Board. The MRC however is no longer able to accommodate the Cytogenetic Unit, which has moved into Haematology. This again places a strain not only on space but also on staff.

The resourcefulness of staff in the laboratory is impressive. Life has involved continuous change and this pattern is accelerating. The survivors are presumably those who thrive on chaos. Staff have adapted to the many changes demanded of them. It has been possible to run for a number of years on flexi-time to help deal with the out-of-hours commitment. A year ago, as with other laboratories, a fixed payment system was agreed for out-of-hours working to provide a 24-hour service. For years the quality of the fitments in the laboratory, such as the benching, were below Health and Safety standards. More recently there was a problem with the main flooring developing a number of holes. These were slowly repaired, and illustrate the problems of working in temporary buildings.

The department has always provided a fair share of teaching both to undergraduates and postgraduates. The Friday morning morphology session, i.e. looking at slides and bone marrows, has for many years been a trademark, particularly of the laboratory part of the Haematology Department. This was started by Dr Allan with an old microscope which projected onto a sort of silvered surface. At the beginning of the sessions the first 10 or 15 minutes were spent trying to get the microscope to project onto the silver surface and to clean the silver surface etc. Usually this involved Dr Allan having to speak to the machine to try and get it to project properly. Dr Mackie, as a brash newcomer, pointed out 'that nowadays there was television projection of microscope images and we could have a multihead microscope for around 10 people'. Grudgingly the brash young man won out and a multiheaded microscope system linked to a television is available for these sessions. The basic importance of the session in terms of teaching and discussing problem cases remains. Doctors sitting their Haematology examinations find these sessions very helpful near to the time of the exam.

Another teaching innovation started by Dr Mackie was a Haematology Seminar on a Friday afternoon. This has been well attended, by the medical students over the years and is much appreciated. Norman Allan has been the co-ordinator for the MRC trials in chronic myeloid leukaemia for most of his working life. This involved considerable work, most afternoons of the week, in the MRC building at the Western General Hospital. The most recent trial ran for eight years, and was a particularly important one. Interferon was shown to be of benefit in chronic myeloid leukaemia. Pat Shepherd has helped with this and is continuing with the continued analysis of the trial. Dr Allan was also involved in the Scotland and Newcastle Lymphoma Group from its beginning in 1972. This collaborative scheme eventually encompassed the whole of the North of Britain.

George Stockdill started research projects on chronic lymphatic leukaemia and co-ordinated work with Alan Maddie at Kings Buildings. This work resulted in a number of papers. When Dr Mackie first came to the Western, he continued this work and three or four papers resulted. This work is in abeyance for the time being. Dr Mackie also undertook a three year project working with Fiona Scott (on an MRC Training Fellowship) to look at drug resistance in myeloma.

The most recent history takes haematology to the Oncology Department because of the major clinical workload with inpatients with malignant haematological diseases. It has been decided as part of Lothian Health's Acute Services Strategy that all Clinical Haematology Services for adults in Edinburgh be centralised at the Western General Hospital. Plans are being made for a large dedicated Haematology Ward and new Day Chemotherapy Unit to be shared with other oncology patients and appropriate outpatient facilities to be completed at the beginning of 1996. It is also planned to establish a Chair of Haematology with dedicated research laboratories so that Edinburgh Haematology should be at the forefront of its discipline for the next millennium!

Human Genetics

In 1957 William Court-Brown established the MRC Clinical and Population Cytogenetics Unit at the Western General Hospital. This introduced genetics to the hospital for the first time. During the next decade there were a number of developments, particularly in cytogenetics. In 1967 it was felt appropriate to introduce genetics teaching to medical undergraduates at the University of Edinburgh. The Faculty of Medicine created a foundation Chair in Human Genetics and appointed Alan Emery from Manchester University. Emery developed a Department with three lecturers, initially housed in the bottom floor of the Haematology Block. As soon as he arrived, the University Department and the MRC Unit jointly created the new Genetics Building, the top floor of which was to house the University Department, and in the basement a pattern recognition group from London. The Genetics Building was completed in 1972 and opened by the Duke of Edinburgh shortly thereafter. It had been agreed that the MRC Unit would be devoted to cytogenetics while the University Department concentrated on more clinical topics. Professor Emery founded the first Genetic Counselling Service in Scotland. He spread the gospel of genetic influences in disease to other hospitals in the region. The appointment of Dr J. A. Raeburn as Senior Lecturer in Clinical Genetics in 1982 strengthened the clinical care of patients with genetic diseases in the region. In the early 1970s, Professor Emery created the first Genetic Register in the United Kingdom. This was to be a model for other genetic centres in the United Kingdom. One of the more significant developments was by Dr David Brock in the new Department. He started alpha-fetoprotein screening for foetal neural tube defects. This was an initiative which was to have profound impact on antenatal screening. The early death of William Court-Brown in 1969 meant that the MRC Unit had to seek a new Director, and H. John Evans was appointed to the post in 1970. He presided over a considerable growth in the research interests and directions of the MRC Unit. At the end of the 1970s it was the largest MRC Unit in the United Kingdom. In 1983 Professor Emery took early retirement and the University Department was re-organised as a Unit within the Department of Medicine at the Western General Hospital. The re-organised Human Genetics Unit was accommodated in temporary accommodation and headed by Professor Brock. In 1989 Dr J. A. Raeburn moved to the Chair of Medical Genetics at Nottingham University. The Lothian Health Board created a NHS Consultant in Clinical Genetics (Dr Mary Porteous). The service of clinical genetics was further strengthened in 1994 by the creation of a second Consultant post (Dr David Fitzpatrick). Funds were raised through a variety of research charities for the creation of a new Molecular Medicine Centre linked to the MRC Unit. In 1995 the academic and NHS components of human genetics were reunited under the same roof. Professor John Evans retired in 1994 and was replaced as Director of the MRC Unit by Dr Nick Hastie.

Intensive Therapy Unit

The emerging speciality of intensive care was not formally represented in the Western until 1988 when an eight-bedded Intensive Therapy Unit was included in the Alexander Donald Building. However, on a more informal basis, intensive care has been practised from the earliest days of mechanical ventilation. At the

Respiratory Unit at the Northern General, Dr I. W. B. Grant and Dr John Marshall were amongst the first to successfully ventilate patients with poliomyelitis in 1953. Ventilation continued in the Northern General until the ITU opened in 1988, with patients suffering from asthma, chronic bronchitis and neurological disorders such as myasthenia gravis and Guillain–Barre syndrome being the major treatment groups. Within the Western itself, the annexe of the Theatre Recovery Room was used for many years (from 1974) as a two-bedded assisted ventilation unit, and patients also received mechanical ventilation in the wards of the Department of Surgical Neurology. Until the Western ITU opened in 1988, Edinburgh had only four general intensive care beds, in Ward 19 of the Royal Infirmary. This was woefully inadequate in comparison with other major cities, and one can only speculate about the consequences of this under provision.

Dr Nick Gordon, as Chairman of the Department of Anaesthesia, was responsible for the establishment, staffing and equipping of the ITU. He successfully achieved funding for sophisticated modern monitoring, ventilators and other therapeutic equipment. Two new consultant anaesthetists were appointed to undertake the major clinical responsibilities for establishing and running the unit. Dr Ian Grant, son of Dr I. W. B. Grant who introduced mechanical ventilation 35 years earlier at the Northern, moved from a consultant post at Ninewells Hospital in Dundee to take up the post of Medical Director. He was ably supported by Ian Armstrong who came fresh from intensive care training as a senior registrar in Australia, and David Wright who was very much involved with ventilation in the old recovery room annexe. Junior staff was provided on a multidisciplinary basis with trainee surgeons, physicians and anaesthetists rotating through the unit. Most importantly of all, a team of 32 trained intensive care nurses was brought together under Mr Iain Buchan's leadership to provide the high standards required in modern intensive care.

After a hectic month of preparations, ITU opened on 2 June 1988 and within two hours had its first two patients. Initially only six beds were opened and the first six months of operation were relatively quiet with only 95 patients. However, referrals from the Eastern General, Bangour General, City Hospital and hospitals in Fife, led to a steady increase in workload and expertise in the management of a wide range of clinical conditions such as sepsis, Acute Respiratory Distress Syndrome (ARDS) and multiple organ failure was built up. In June 1991 the closing of the Accident & Emergency Department and the transfer of the regional head injury service to the Western led to a major change in the pattern of the workload. Neurosurgical intensive care became a major clinical interest, and there was a significant increase in the overall workload with 360–400 patients being treated each year. The remaining two beds were brought into use but by 1995 increasing pressure on space makes the provision of additional intensive care beds inevitable. The aggressive intensive care of management of patients with severe head injuries, introduced by Professor Douglas Miller in Ward 20 of the Royal Infirmary in 1981, had already led to a substantial improvement in outcome, and this approach led to further improvements following transfer of the service to ITU at the Western. Mortality over 14 years has reduced by 40% and this intensive approach to monitoring and intervention is now being directed to patients with intracranial haemorrhage.

The Lothian Area Acute Services Strategy will expand acute medicine and surgery at the Western, and bring Infectious Diseases into the hospital. These will all contribute to an increasing demand for intensive care, and allow the ITU to build on the substantial reputation already gained over its short history.

Maternity & Gynaecology Department

Following the 1929 Local Government Act Scotland, Craigleith Poor Law Hospital was taken over by the Public Health Committee and in 1930 officially became the Western General Hospital which included provision for maternity and gynaecology patients. In 1932 the Western became associated with Edinburgh University. Maternity services at the Western really started in 1932 when Professor R. W. Johnstone established a maternity service here. Sister Ruth Christie was in charge of the labour ward as Sister from 1932 to 1953 and was succeeded by Sister Gladys Blunn. Sister Christie was a small, plump lady who was a charmer with dark brown eyes, full of fun. The maternity beds were always in the same wards on the first floor under the clock; some on the ground floor were kept for puerperal fever cases.

Professor R. W. Johnstone was the Director of Obstetrics and Gynaecology, assisted by Dr Robert Traquair Thin. In 1937 the Unit was recognised by the Central Midwives Board as a training school for midwives.

Dr W.I.C. Morris came in 1937 having previously been the whole-time obstetrician in Ayr County Council. In 1939 he had been invited by Professor Robert Kellar to take on the maternity beds in the municipal hospital at the Western. Previous to that, Robert Traquair Thin ran the Unit for Professor Johnstone. The appointment of consultants in those days were made entirely by the 'chiefs'. Robert Traquair Thin had been briefly RMO before moving to the Simpson Memorial Maternity Pavilion. He worked as a GP as well as an obstetrician. Dr Morris's job included lecturing and the reporting of gynaepathology. He took over the Maternity Unit, after a short meeting with Professor R. W. Johnstone in the room immediately to the right under the clock; a room where everybody met. There were approximately 30 beds for maternity and six gynaecology beds. The system was not well organised and the gynaecology patients were referred from the Royal Infirmary. The surgeons operated on a Saturday morning in the general theatre by D-Block. Patients from Granton and Pilton were often small, very tough and rough and often unwilling to come in; sometimes they were concerned about husbands selling the furniture for alcohol. Rickets was a problem, although less so than in the west of Scotland. Complicated rickets and a contracted pelvis often led to a need for caesarean sections. Large babies were a problem. There were also a number of congenital abnormalities, double uteruses, vaginal septa and considerable problems. They were seen along with the middle-class patients, in all a good social mix.

Ante natal clinics were held in the Western. An appointments system was used which owed its origins to the one used by a grocer in Stockbridge who hated queues. When people came in they were given a label with a number on it and then you could go away and do other shopping and were taken when your number came up. The ante natal clinic was run in a similar way.

During the era of the Polish medical school, the Polish women were also looked after. The district midwifery service was run from the Western General Hospital in the Paderewski. Sister Martha MacMillan was in charge of this service, she knew all the Polish patients by Anglicised names. The Polish patients were attended by two obstetricians, Dr Uhma and Dr Jialinski. Dr Uhma supervised the clinical teaching of the Polish Medical School in the Paderewski Building. Dr Uhma subsequently returned to Poland; Dr Jialinski went to Oldham as a GP.

The grand tradition of giving a layette to the mother of the first child born in the Western General Hospital Maternity Unit each year began in 1944. The money came out of the fund for welfare work in the Public Health Department. The Lord and Lady Provost were invited to visit the hospital and hand over the layette on the first day of the year and the layette cost £6.

One of the problems created by war was an increase in the numbers of illegitimate births. Often the pregnancies were concealed, and the mothers did not enjoy the safety of good obstetric care until late in their pregnancy. In 1944 the number of illegitimate babies who died in Edinburgh hospitals were 65 of which 33 died in the Western General Hospital. This reflected maternal health as much as anything.

The medical hierarchical system was: chief, junior chief and clinical tutor. The clinical tutors were in post for five years. Many of the clinical tutors expanded their income by coaching for the fellowship. John Forfar was the paediatrician in 1950. Prior to this Professor Richard Ellis was very interested in the Western General Hospital.

After the war a number of doctors were at a loose end and did not have a substantive post. There were re-training appointments at house officer or registrar equivalent level. These were often prolonged appointments but by 1949 this scheme came to an end. Many became consultants but others were less lucky.

The unit also had a monthly audit meeting and the registrar organised this along with the sisters and GPs. This continued until the unit closed in 1991, precipitated by a financial crisis at Health Board level.

In 1947 the National Health Service made it a statutory duty for the local authority to provide a domiciliary midwifery service. The Corporation decided to build a full time unit. In 1947 the Western General Hospital was recognised as a training centre for Part 2 of the Central Midwife Board Certificate when a District Midwifery Service was established in the Hospital. The first step in the formation of a full-time municipal service was taken when the Sister and four midwives involved in that hospital's district work were transferred to direct employment by the Corporation in July 1948. Five midwives operated from the domiciliary midwives home at Crewe Road, 12 from the maternity hospitals and 22 acting maternity nurses from the Queen's Institute. At that time health visitors went to interview mothers six weeks after the birth of their children.

In 1946 at the end of the war, Dr Morris was appointed consultant with 30 maternity and six gynaecology beds. Dr Morris was appointed to the Chair in Manchester University in 1949 and Dr Archie Duncan became obstetrician in charge with Dr Tony Anderson as fellow consultant. When Dr Duncan was appointed to the Chair in Cardiff in 1952 his place was taken by Dr Thomas N. MacGregor. By this time the maternity wards, situated on the first floor under the Clock Tower, had increased to 47 beds and the gynaecology wards on the second floor to 23 beds. The Unit in the 1950s and 1960s became increasingly clinically busy with 1200–1400 deliveries per year and was active in teaching medical students and pupil midwives. Dr MacGregor's special interest was in gynaecological endocrinology. Dr Anderson was a pioneer of cervical cytology smear screening in this country. A new purpose-built labour ward suite was added to the Unit in 1965 to replace the previous cramped accommodation. Teaching films were prepared of Caesarean and forceps deliveries and gynaecological operations.

In 1968 Dr Ronald Clark was appointed Consultant on the retiral of Dr MacGregor and in 1973 Dr John B. Scrimgeour was appointed as Consultant on the retiral of Dr Anderson. Under their leadership in the 1970s and '80s the referral rate to the department was high. The maternity beds were constantly fully booked and 1400–1500 babies were delivered each year. The Unit continued to be a popular choice for the training of medical students and pupil midwives. Clinical research had a high priority, the main long-term project at this time being a study of the early diagnosis and prevention of foetal abnormalities under the direction of Dr Scrimgeour. In 1988 a third Consultant, Dr David I. M. Farquharson was appointed whose special interest was gynaecological oncology. The maternity and gynaecology departments have always had a dedicated midwifery and nursing staff. In the post-war years the midwifery superintendents were Miss Martha McMillan, Miss Gillian Cruickshank 1953, Miss Betty Rowles 1958, Miss Norah Stephen 1961, Miss Sheila Fleming 1984 and Miss Joan Spence 1988; the senior midwifery tutors Miss Catherine Mackinnon 1947 and Miss Elma Scott 1967 and senior labour ward sisters Sister Ruth Christie, Sister Gladys Blunn 1953 and Sister Hutcheon 1970.

In 1990, faced with increasing financial difficulties, the Lothian Health Board carried out a policy of reorganisation. This meant a closure of many effective units and sadly included the Maternity and Gynaecology Department at the Western General Hospital. The disbanding of this well-regarded Unit was strongly opposed by the local general practitioners and by the signed petitions of many thousands of women in North West Edinburgh. Despite this the gynaecology wards closed in December 1990 and the maternity wards in January 1991.

Three Decades of General Medicine

At the inception of the Health Service in October 1948, the responsibility for providing the staff of Edinburgh Northern Group of Hospitals lay with the University of Edinburgh Department of Medicine, under the direction of Professor Stanley (later Sir Stanley) Davidson. At that time, the only senior medical staff excluded from general medical duties, were those working in the designated specialist Rheumatic Diseases Unit located at the Northern General Hospital and staffed by two physicians, Dr J. J. R. Duthie and Dr J. Sinclair. However in the early years after World War II it rapidly became apparent that general medicine alone would be insufficient to satisfy the aspirations of most physicians and at the same time to develop the quality of the hospital service that patients would expect and indeed deserved.

There was the further important objective of ensuring that the standard of undergraduate and postgraduate education was maintained and promoted in order to satisfy the expectations of students. The Postgraduate Board for Medicine provided for an almost insatiable demand for clinical teaching for Commonwealth and UK postgraduates. Most of whom regarded the need to obtain the appropriate diploma from the Royal College of Physicians as inescapable.

Professor Davidson regarded the facilities available in the Northern Group of Hospitals as suitable and necessary to broaden the resources available in the Royal Infirmary. This in turn was crucial to the maintenance of the reputation of Edinburgh for teaching and training in clinical general medicine and in established and emerging clinical specialties. The plan was initiated by the appointment to Western General Hospital, between 1947 and 49, of Richard W. D. Turner, Cardiology, John G. MacLeod, General Medicine, John A. Strong, Metabolic Disorders, Edward B. French, General Medicine and Wilfrid I. Card, Gastroenterology. The initiative was unusual in that Dr Turner, Dr Card, Dr French and Dr Strong, all came from London, only Dr Macleod was an Edinburgh graduate. The last four had beds on C flat. Dr Card, in addition, shared clinical beds with Mr John Bruce in D1 and D2, which formed the joint Gastro-intestinal unit.

Two units were established at Western General Hospital, the consultants to the first being Turner and MacLeod and to the second, Card and Strong. French had a general medical unit at the Eastern General Hospital and out-patient clinics and teaching responsibilities at Western General Hospital. He had, as will be seen, a crucial part to play in the development of this teaching hospital. No further appointment of any physician whose main interest was general medicine was made at the Western General Hospital for the next three decades covered by this account.

Three units were developed at the Northern General Hospital in respiratory medicine, rheumatic diseases and neurology. The clinical roles of the general physician progressively decreased over the next 30 years. During this time an increasing number of their patients were elderly and many had psychiatric problems. Accordingly there was a need for close liaison with geriatricians and psychiatrists whose specialties were growing apace in other hospitals in the City. While it was excellent to have so much readily available expert advice, there was a danger of medicine becoming fragmented into separate specialised units, however successful. This was balanced by the organisation of regular clinical meetings, by the unifying effects of the University, the Health Board and the Royal College of Physicians. There was a shared interest in teaching of undergraduates and postgraduates and in the physical development of the Western General Hospital.

The physicians with their chosen specialties available to staff the Northern Group at the end of 1948 are named below:

Dr J. Alastair Bruce	General medicine
Dr Wilfrid I. Card	Gastro-enterology
Dr John J. R. Duthie	Rheumatic diseases
Dr E.B. (Ted) French	General medicine
Dr John G. Macleod	General medicine and rheumatology
Dr H. N. Robson	Haematology, part-time, from the Dept. of Medicine, Royal Infirmary
Dr J. G. Sclater	General medicine and rheumatology
Dr J. Sinclair	Rheumatic diseases
Dr Malcolm Smith	General medicine at Leith Hospital
Dr John A. Strong	General medicine,endocrinology and diabetes
Dr Richard W. D. Turner	General medicine and cardiology.

Those physicians who had a declared interest in a specialty additional to general medicine had a substantial clinical obligation to honour. There were virtually no facilities other than the ward clinical side-rooms for any type of investigative or research work. The clinical laboratory for the hospitals in the Northern Group was staffed by Dr Elizabeth Gilchrist and was housed in what had been the laundry. The hospital group and medical staff were fortunate in having Dr Alexander Donald as medical superintendent. He was sympathetic and supportive, in so far as extremely limited resources permitted, in promoting the development of facilities for research at a largely clinical level, and gradually allowing for the initiation of some relevant laboratory studies.

Over 30 years, the physical developments at the Western General Hospital were under constant discussion with the Health Board and the University. Many plans were made, accepted and rejected. Frustration, depression and rage had often to be soothed by the benevolent administration of Dr Donald who embodied the spirit of the hospital. The first new building to be erected was the Teaching and Research Centre which provided a much needed focal point and a theatre for clinical meetings.

For many years the consultants who worked in the medical units at the Western General Hospital were restricted to a small hut for the examination and investigation of outpatients. Often patients were seen on one of the wards or in strictly limited auxiliary ward accommodation. This was a most serious bar to the development of a very important branch of clinical medicine, namely outpatient clinical care. Initially it was the inevitable practice to admit patients for studies which could well have been undertaken in a suitable outpatient department, had it existed. During the first three decades there were about 50 beds in each medical unit, about half of which were General Medical. Approximately 75 beds were on C floor (Card, Strong, MacLeod) and 25 on A floor (Turner).

The clinical meetings were organised from the outset by Dr French whose wide general knowledge and critical mind ensured the highest standards of discussion. All physicians were responsible in turn for presentations and the exchange of information was invaluable. Individual units, of course, held their own meetings to which others were welcome. Ted French's Monday evening meetings continued to be one of the highlights of the week for three decades. Dr French was also an outstanding clinical teacher and stimulated others to follow his example. This was most appropriate because of the demands of a new curriculum for undergraduates and because of the post-war influx of postgraduates mainly from overseas.

In the 1960s the University recognised the need for a Department of Medicine based at the Western General Hospital. One of the functions of which would be to coordinate the clinical teachers in the hospitals north of Princes Street. This department differed from the old established one at the Royal Infirmary by having an elected Head, in which capacity Dr MacLeod served for seven years. He was an outstanding chairman, not as an academic, but as a respected general physician who had a keen nose for what was sensible and valuable in the rapidly evolving medicine. In many virtues he was in the tradition of Sir Stanley Davidson. The subsequent chairmen included Dr French, Dr Michael Matthews and Dr John Strong. With the retirement of Professor Strong from a personal Chair, there was a strong movement for the establishment of a permanent Chair of Medicine at the hospital, and the first appointee to this Chair was Dr Christopher Edwards in 1980.

The two Hospital Departments of Medicine were linked through the Faculty of Medicine. The fledgling was given much support by a succession of Deans and in particular by the Executive Dean, Professor Archie Duncan who oiled the academic wheels.

Another educational project in which the general physicians participated from the outset was *Davidson's Principles and Practice of Medicine*. MacLeod took over its editorship from the 11th to the 15th editions when this was handed over to Professors Christopher RW Edwards and Ian AD Bouchier, forming another link between the two departments of medicine. MacLeod also edited *Clinical Examination* until its 7th edition when Dr John Munro and Professor Edwards succeeded. Both textbooks acquired an international reputation and were translated into many languages. This success was due to the cooperation of many physicians and others but the influence of French was paramount. He scrutinised all the later editions from cover to cover and provided innumerable constructive suggestions. His specialised colleagues did not always agree but French was usually right and when he was not the discussion was stimulating.

The 1960s saw other moves towards staff cohesion and cooperation. A clinical staff committee was set up with an elected chairman; annual dinners were instituted. The non-resident staff, medical, scientific, paramedical and nursing, enjoyed a splendid dining room in the penthouse suite of the then new Radiotherapy Unit with panoramic views over the city. Such a simple measure as this did much to foster an *esprit de corps*.

Although they tried, the general physicians could not compete with their specialist colleagues in the research field but they had other local and national responsibilities. French lectured in medicine at the Dental School and MacLeod served on the Council of the Professions Supplementary to Medicine for 16 years and on the Specialist Advisory Committee on General (Internal) Medicine for four years.

In general medicine there were no longer the giants of student years but the general physicians saw and admired the ever-increasing growth of the specialities; as renal transplantation, medical genetics, oncology and others were added to the originals. The view was that they were indeed fortunate to work in such a stimulating environment which itself was a tribute to the original vision of Sir Stanley Davidson.

The first, in 1948, of the physician incomers was Dick Turner, a graduate of Cambridge and St Thomas's, who was brought in to meet the wish of Stanley Davidson, to institute a Department of Cardiology in primitive medical wards. These were to stay almost unchanged while he was in post at the hospital.

The next Londoner to be appointed was Wilfrid Card, who helped to institute the first combined medical and surgical unit in the field of gastroenterology. His contributions in this field, and later in the application of computerised methods to diagnosis, was a major factor in putting the Western on the international medical map. He was a natural leader, and this was realised and indeed acclaimed by his colleagues. If he accepted himself in any sense as 'primus' he would never fail to observe that it was 'inter pares'. A tall and imposing figure, his capacity for being deep in thought made him often seem remote, and indeed as seen from across the city he was nick-named De Gaulle. But in a social situation he was capable of warm friendship. He had the capacities both for enlightened vision, and of carrying his colleagues harmoniously with him. Among his other innovations were the achievement of a building to meet the needs of teaching and research, with research facilities available to all whether University whole-time or part-time. He never failed to play down the distinction between the two, achievements being of much greater importance to him than status. He and his colleagues felt that they had little real contact either with the Professor of Medicine, or with the physicians in the University department at the Royal Infirmary. Under his leadership and after very careful consideration, a memorandum was presented to the faculty which sought their support for the institution of a separate Department of Medicine at the Western General Hospital. An innovation unique in Britain at that time, though not of course elsewhere, of a rotating chairman elected by the department, rather than a professor appointed in charge, with the chairman serving on faculty and in other ways much as the appointed professor in the existing University Department. On the whole this worked well. Wilfrid Card, modelling himself in this respect on William Harvey, was anxious also that the staff should cement their relationships with regular dinners where with good food and wine this was certainly achieved. When he left the Western to take up an appointment as Professor of Mathematics with Relation to Medicine in Glasgow — a sad blow to the Western — he gave his medical staff colleagues a very beautiful modern silver loving cup.

John Strong, the next recruit and later to become a President of the Royal College of Physicians, was a Dublin graduate, a man of high intelligence and total integrity, and a much admired member of the staff who naturally attracted able young colleagues to his team. He, with Pat Jacobs, was to describe, as a world first, a particular genetic fault as a cause of a known familial disease, Klinefelter's Syndrome. He created an active metabolic unit, and instituted the management of diabetic and metabolic diseases at the hospital.

Ted French, coming from Guy's, was an outstanding 'Physician Naturalist' in the tradition of John Ryle (Regius Professor of Physic at Cambridge), and many of his predecessors at that hospital. He was a true generalist, and his skills were the result of occupations which were becoming increasingly unfashionable. Listening intelligently to what a patient had to say, and looking at them in detail and with insight. He was a living embodiment of the aphorism attributed to a Boston radiologist, 'You only see what you look for, and you only recognise what you know.' Many of his colleagues had the humbling experience of his spotting from the end of the bed what was wrong with a patient who had so far eluded a diagnostic label. One remembers a young man with a puzzling heart whose diagnosis Ted achieved from 30 feet away. His only remark on arrival at the bed was 'Please lift your head off the pillow' which the patient was quite unable to do. He had recognised the premature baldness, and the heart problem was instantaneously explained as a known association of dystrophia myotonica. Or, in the 'specimen room' where he said 'that urine looks like stout', and it actually was. The patient's physician thought that stout with his meals might make the old man feel better. The patient, who did not like it and was too polite to say so, poured it into his urine bottle without the stout being processed in the more usual way. A generation of students will remember Ted's capacity to make students think for themselves rather than to learn by rote.

John Macleod, as the only Edinburgh graduate among the physicians, put a brave face on life with so many immigrants. He was to achieve eminence as successor to Stanley Davidson as editor of a textbook of medicine which has sold more copies, and been translated into more languages, than any textbook of medicine in the English language. He showed patience and good humour in a relentless process of keeping contributors up to date as one edition followed another.

Dr Michael Matthews' memory of the Western was of a happy ship. In the cardiology wards, the comradeship and co-operation with a series of excellent ward sisters is a particular cause for gratitude. As an immigrant, there were problems, but they were not serious, such as puzzlement at a patient who said that she was short of breath and could not think why because she was 'only carrying a few messages ...' all that handshaking at the new year ... the fewer decibels required for laughter. If there was suspicion of all these foreigners coming in, it was well concealed. They were all given their share of committee and other responsibilities as if their 'foreignness' was not too significant. The subcommittees of medicine of the medical education committee had an importance which physicians born and bred in Edinburgh could hardly have guessed. It was at these termly meetings that one could attach faces for the first time to consultant physicians at the Royal Infirmary who had hitherto been only names. There was of course this bond at the Western from what Wilfrid Card called common suffering. Common suffering from the lamentable provisions in a hospital which was in the process of being all too slowly upgraded from an old-fashioned community hospital to a teaching hospital worthy of a medical school with a long and noble tradition. It was largely Stanley Davidson who had the vision to see the possibilities which could follow the invasion of these hospitals by University Staff. And then, in a sense, the immigrants had the locals outnumbered. How well Michael Matthews remembered being taken by Dick Turner to meet Sandy Donald, the medical superintendent, and to find that the matron and the assistant matron were already in the room with him. Both of them, and Dick and Mike Matthews, had all come from St Thomas's Hospital, London. Another vivid memory is that when he was appointed as a Physician and Cardiologist in 1954 he was much surprised to be asked by the Chief Administrative Medical Officer of the then South-Eastern Regional Hospital Board whether he would like to see the model of the new hospital. As it turned out, the new outpatient department, quite different from the model, was to not be opened until much later, and the new medical wards, also different, were to be opened in the year after he retired 28 years later.

One curiosity of that era was connected with an annual photograph of the consultant staff. This photograph was taken by a technician, who, as was the wont in that period, wore a brown coat. One year he came to take the photograph wearing a white coat. The camera was set on a timing mechanism and the technician joined the group on the back row. Shortly after this he resigned his post to live in Canada. The next news of him was his imprisonment. He had used the photograph as his evidence of belonging to the medical profession. He had been employed as a doctor on the basis of this 'qualification'.

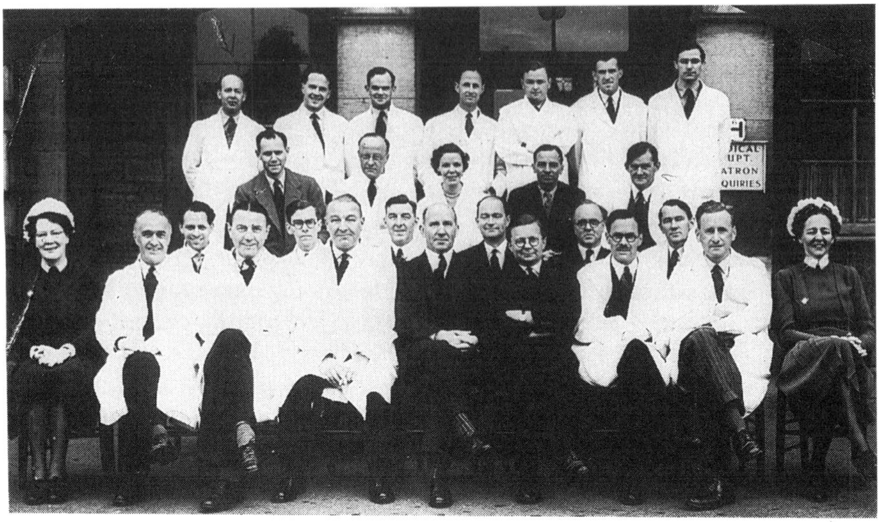

Physicians, Surgeons, Lecturers, Senior Registrars and Matrons. Front row: Miss E Watt, Deputy Matron; JM Mason Brown; Wilfrid Card; David Band; Sandy Donald; Dick Turner; John Forfar; Hunter Cummack; Miss Estelle Adamson (Matron); Second row: Bill Sircus; Bill Small; Charles Falconer; John Macleod; Mike Matthews; Jim Drennan; Third row: ?; Claude Barrie; Rhoda Nicol; Tony Anderson; Selby Tulloch; Fourth row: Urology technician who posed as a doctor in Canada; remainder are registrars.

These physicians can be regarded as founding fathers of modern Medicine as a specialty. Gradually they were replaced by a new generation. The first of these was Dr Bill Price, a Cardiff graduate who came to Edinburgh in 1962 as a Research Fellow in the Department of Medicine. He also was new in that he was the first of a new breed of Physician, the physician scientist. Whilst continuing a tradition of medical care they were scientists in their own right. He had previously been a Registrar at the Eastern General Hospital before moving to the National Heart Hospital. He came back to Edinburgh from Newcastle as an Honorary Senior Registrar and worked in the general medical wards and in the outpatients of Dr French. He then was appointed Senior Lecturer and Honorary Consultant Physician in 1969 at the Western. He developed a Migraine Clinic in which the research interest was the evaluation of new therapies for this condition. His major contribution was in genetics and cytogenetics with a clinical interest in patients with cytogenetic abnormalities, delayed puberty, male and female hypogonadism, growth abnormalities and Marfan's syndrome. The cytogenetics element of the research was in conjunction with the Medical Research Council Unit. Dr Price's contribution was in the clinical, laboratory and epidemiological aspects of cytogenetics. He initiated a prospective mortality study of patients with sex chromosome abnormalities. In 1980 he became involved in the application of new techniques of molecular biology to clinical genetics. He was one of the first to study the X-link form of retinitis pigmentosa. He also studied the molecular genetic aspects of haemophilia and agammaglobulinaemias. The techniques of molecular biology were also applied to the genetic component of coronary artery disease. He also ran a Lipid Clinic in conjunction with the Royal Infirmary and St John's. Bill Price, Arthur Kitchin, Philip Wenham in Clinical Chemistry, and general practitioners looked at a study of premature coronary heart disease and its predisposing factors in men in the North of Edinburgh. This was started in 1985. They showed that in Leith over 70% of the men were native to Edinburgh and in Cramond less than 30% were born in Scotland. Mortality from coronary artery disease was significantly higher in Leith than in Cramond. There was also a significant influence of family history on premature coronary heart disease in first degree relatives. This was evident amongst the Leith men but not in the Cramond group. The predisposition to familial coronary artery disease in men in Leith was associated with specific genetic characteristics and also with an abnormally low level of plasma HDL cholesterol which has been associated with risk of coronary artery disease. In 1992 Dr Price reduced his commitment to the MRC Unit and became the first Clinical Director of Medicine in the Western General Hospital. His contribution to the literature extends to more than 90 papers.

In 1970 a new specialty was added to the Department of Medicine, namely Nephrology or Renal Medicine. The Western General Hospital had long provided an excellent Urological Service but there was little provision for the specialty of Nephrology. In the 1960s Sir Michael Woodruff had pioneered renal transplantation at the Royal Infirmary and obtained funding from the Nuffield Trust to build the Nuffield Transplant Unit at the Western General Hospital. This was opened in 1969 and it became clear that it would require the services of a Renal Physician. In 1970 Dr John Anderton was appointed as Renal Physician to the Western General Hospital to provide support to the Renal Transplant Service and to develop a nephrological service in the Western. The splendid facility of the Nuffield Transplant Unit was available and at the same time the Urological Ward had expanded into a new Department which was called Ward D3. Nine renal medicine beds were incorporated into this Department providing a comprehensive Surgical and Renal Medicine Service.

In the 1970s a new form of treatment for chronic renal failure became available, chronic haemodialysis. Initially this was provided in the corridor of the Nuffield Transplant Unit but it became clear that a proper facility would be required in due course. A public appeal was launched and over a quarter of a million pounds was raised. In this raising of funds Dr John Anderton was the important leader and Mrs Maida Fairbairn was the Kidney Unit Appeal Secretary. The fundraising included the sponsoring of John Anderton running marathons — his best marathon was three hours 11 minutes. Patients and friends were particularly active in raising money. The Chronic Dialysis Unit was eventually opened by the Princess of Wales on 6 October, 1986. The Western has therefore been able to provide facilities for the management of a wide range of renal conditions with a comprehensive renal and surgical service.

In addition to the Renal Unit commitment, John Anderton joined the medical team in the Department of Medicine and was paired with Dr John Macleod in C8–18 from 1970 through to 1984 when John Macleod retired. At that time Leith Hospital closed and David Boyd joined the medical team replacing John Macleod.

Paul Padfield was appointed as Consultant Physician in July 1981, as an Endocrinologist. His general medical sessions were officially in Leith Hospital. Professor Edwards, who had been appointed as Professor of Medicine the year before invited him to share his general medical intake at the Western. At that time they had a system where each worked six weeks on and six weeks off in general medicine. There were 25 general medical beds on C Flat, C1–5. By modern day standards the wards were not very good. The toilet facilities were undoubtedly poor, this was a concern at that time. They had a Medical Registrar who was shared on rotation with Leith Hospital and a Lecturer in Medicine, who at the time was Colin Feek. Whilst his main remit was endocrinology he also trained in general medicine. Two or three years later Michael Matthews retired. Somehow an agreement was made whereby Dr Padfield undertook the care of Mike Matthews' general medical beds, thereby leaving the commitment at Leith Hospital. Both Professor Edwards and Dr Padfield took on a larger bed commitment, or at least a larger waiting day commitment but continued the business of sharing six weeks on and six weeks off. In truth, general medicine, throughout the 1980s, didn't change much in the sense that the hospital took whatever came in through the door. There was no Respiratory Unit at the Western so occasionally the hospital saw patients with asthma. Obvious infectious diseases, which tended to be admitted to the City, were rarely seen and this was also true of drug overdoses as they were admitted to the Royal Infirmary. So in that time medicine was never truly general. Towards the end of the 1980s, several other things occurred including the retirement of Arthur Kitchin. Arthur Kitchin had been a Cardiologist, although he, unlike Mike Matthews, had done invasive cardiology. He also had general medical beds. Paul Padfield did a lot of the early research in the field of vasopressin and blood pressure. In all the papers he wrote he always referred to a paper which had been published around 1967. This was on the effect of vasopressin infused on forearm blood flow. The paper was by an A. H. Kitchin. Paul Padfield never realised that in fact this was Arthur Kitchin who had been a Physiologist before he had become a Cardiologist. Arthur therefore gave up his general medical beds when he retired and his replacement was Ian Starkey. Stuart Shaw had replaced Mike Matthews, and both of those took on no general medical commitments as they were Cardiologists. This was in recognition of Cardiology as an important specialty to be developed in its proper form. Cardiologists were no longer involved in general medical takes. This was already the case for respiratory medicine, for gastroenterology, neurology and for cardiology in other hospitals. At the same time Leith Hospital closed as an acute hospital. David Boyd, who was coming to the end of his medical career, transferred from Leith to the Western. He took on the general medical work that had been Arthur Kitchin's, with shared beds with John Anderton in what was then C8–16.

General medicine continued to occupy C1–5 and C8–16 in the old building until the opening of the Alexander Donald Building. There was discussion and debate as to who would occupy which of the floors in the new building. General medicine at that time was a strong force and its practitioners argued convincingly that it should occupy the whole of the top floor of 72 beds. The plan was a slight change in that the 12-bedded centre of the top floor of the Alexander Donald Building was to become a medical admissions area. There was some debate with the nursing staff as to whether there should be a high dependency area for acute admissions. Medical East became the admitting ward, which it has remained ever since, allowing a concentration of both medical and nursing staff on admitting days. David Boyd retired before the move to the Alexander Donald Building. There were many casualties from the closure of Leith, which had an established service to a close community. Dr Boyd was a caring physician who was committed to Leith. The move to the Western was not necessarily easy or even happy. In Leith Dr Boyd had a whole succession of Consultant colleagues. Only his last colleague, Mike Ford, really worked hard to support him. The others often had unevenly divided loyalties to other hospitals.

At that time general medicine was changing and Dr Padfield extended his role as a general physician in addition to endocrinology and hypertension. Professor Edward's academic activities and administrative work were continually growing. So Dr Padfield took on a full admitting share in his own right and Professor Edwards started to share takes initially with Dr Bob Leonard. Dr Leonard was a Senior Lecturer and is now an NHS physician in Clinical Oncology. He worked with Professor Edwards in the same rotation as Dr Padfield. The other two admitting teams were John Anderton and Bill Price. Dr Padfield, Professor Edwards and Dr Leonard occupied Medical North, Bill Price and John Anderton Medical South.

General medicine was again to be eroded with arguments that the gastroenterologists could look after gastrointestinal bleeds better than general physicians. The general physicians argued that endoscopy might diagnose the cause of a bleed but did not effect the outcome. Very rapidly it became possible to intervene therapeutically with the endoscope. Almost by default, all bleeders were admitted under the care of the gastroenterologists. This is a recent innovation, as recently as 1991–92, GI bleeds were previously admitted to the general physicians. Only those who were very ill were transferred to the gastroenterologists. At the same time Cardiology increased in its scope, not the least because of developing significant interventional techniques that required beds. There was a tendency for general medical beds to be further exclusively used by cardiology patients. Cardiologists prior to this did not have access to medical beds. Cardiologists, if, for example, they had a patient with heart failure, admitted the patient to the medical beds under the care of the waiting physician of the day until discharge. They were then followed up in the outpatients by the cardiologist. It became clear that this was not a reasonable way of management. So the major step was made that Cardiologists had admitting rights to the general medical beds, initially two or three patients, but as time went on this number grew. Now the Cardiologists tend to occupy maybe a dozen of the 72 beds on the medical floor at any one time. So general medicine was shrinking. The same number of admissions came to the hospital every day under the heading of general medicine. The speed of turnover was increasing and patients were being discharged sooner. In general medicine the average stay time came down from what probably was around eight or more days in the middle 1980s to possibly five days now. There were less bed, faster turnover and constant, even increasing, overall patient numbers.

The Respiratory and Rheumatology Units moved from the Northern to the Western in 1991. This was important for the spectrum of specialties in the hospital but it did impinge again on general medicine. Some of the complicated chest cases which would have come under general physicians previously were now admitted directly to the respiratory physicians. In 1993 GI Unit moved out of the Nightingale wards in D Block, one male, one female, invariably full of patients. The unit moved into reduced accommodation in Medical North. This liaison has never been happy, either for the general physicians or for the gastroenterologists. The general physicians felt that yet another bank of their medical beds had been taken — the gastroenterologists felt that they could no longer rely on beds being available for some of their urgent but not truly emergency type admissions. General medicine remains in Western General Hospital and everybody says that it is important to maintain it. The belief is that general medicine has to be retained as a core for teaching, both undergraduates and postgraduates, but there must be better use of specialist beds. There is almost an inevitability that general medicine can hardly exist in a teaching hospital much longer. The belief is that there is an inexorable move to the American system, wherein the so-called general physicians will simply be those who are involved in acting as a clearing house for acute admissions. General practitioners will still send people in who are unwell and where the diagnosis is uncertain. Less and less will the body system involved be uncertain and most patients will be readily categorised into a specialty.

Another specialty, emerging in the last four years, is stroke medicine. There was a time in general medicine when admitting a stroke patient was one of the most unpleasant aspects of general medicine because there was nothing to do medically for these people. They would be admitted with their stroke, they would survive or not, probably relating to the level of nursing care, and then they would begin a long-term rehabilitation. There would be nothing more to do medically. These patients were not fit enough to move anywhere else and the availability of long-term care was limited. So there was a period through the 1980s in general medicine, when 25% of acute medical beds were blocked with people who truly did not need a medical bed. This is no longer the case, in part due to the emergence of acute geriatric assessment areas three or four years ago, in the major teaching hospitals. This has relieved some of the load of, so-called, social admissions or even patients with strokes who might need rehabilitation more than an acute medical bed. The major change in general medicine at the Western occurred when A & E closed. There was a time when it was considered that all medicine needed was an acute admitting area and that for medicine, as opposed to the rest of the specialties, the Accident and Emergency was less important. This thinking was wrong, and wrong in the sense that no longer were people brought in by 999 calls. For a while there were less acute chest pains, but nor were there the old people who had fallen behind the door and couldn't get up. It was these elderly frail people who would end up occupying beds for many weeks and months because there was nowhere for them to go. The loss of Accident and Emergency was a change which altered the spectrum of patients. From a professional point of view this was all to the good. The patients who were seen were treatable and it was possible to get them quickly back out into the community. Beds were not blocked, turnover was rapid, there was good educational material, and a good professional sense of doing something that was worthwhile. It may well be that general medicine will continue in that line. Yet there will still be many patients who cannot be so clearly categorised. They will be followed up by a smaller group of doctors who may call themselves general physicians. They may well be, in a large part, geriatricians. There are still physicians with time to do general medicine. When Bill Price retires he will not be replaced with like and he will be the last true general physician to depart the Western. Renal medicine is transferring to the Royal Infirmary, although it may come back in the form of an emergency service. So the near future is likely to involve a group of doctors who are prepared to take on acute medical takes with a fairly rapid turnover and handing over of patients who clearly lie within the remit of one or other of the specialties. Time is needed for audit, management, teaching in a way which will be much more clearly defined than previously. The general medicine sessions will be specifically allocated and there may be less flexibility.

The future of general medicine in a teaching hospital is bleak. It should be considered as internal medicine or emergency medicine in which case its future is not so bleak and may be quite exciting for the relevant person.

Metabolic Unit

In 1952 Dr (later Professor) John Strong invited Dr Reginald Passmore, Reader in Physiology, University of Edinburgh, to collaborate with him in some physiological investigations into possible causes and medical outcome of gross obesity — their mutual interest being 'Why are some people fat?' These initial experiments were conducted, with great difficulty, in the 30-bed general medical 'C' ward at the Western General. Chemical and biochemical analyses were done mainly at the Department of Physiology at the Medical School at Teviot Place. Despite the practical problems, this collaboration resulted in several scientific papers. However, Dr Passmore made it clear that if any further serious work was envisaged at the Western then special facilities would need to be provided on site so that energy intake (food) and energy expenditure (exercise) could be controlled properly and measured accurately. This was taken on board by Dr Strong and thus, with the help of a generous donation from a grateful patient, the Metabolic Unit was born in 1964.

This Unit was designed specifically to provide an area where the patient and the laboratory could meet to facilitate clinical/laboratory research. The initial accommodation consisted of four single bedrooms (each with an attached special toilet facility), a diet kitchen, a clinical experimental area for energy expenditure measurements, a biochemical laboratory, a nurses office, a secretary's office. Later a treadmill was installed. Soon after the building was completed David Shirling was persuaded to move from the Department of Physiology at Teviot Place to the Metabolic Unit. He had a vast experience in the techniques required for energy balance studies. In collaboration with the renowned physiologists McCance and Widdowson he had previously measured energy balance in the crews of submarines, miners working at the coal face, and in individuals moving from a temperate to a desert climate. He was also an expert in weighing fat women under water for the purpose of assessing their relative proportion of lean body mass and fat.

With the necessary facilities and personnel in place classical energy balance studies were performed, initially mainly on obese patients. As time went on other patients with disturbed energy metabolism were studied, such as those with anorexia nervosa, diabetes mellitus and a range of other endocrine and metabolic disorders. These studies were very labour intensive and, by their nature, necessarily prolonged over several weeks or even months. It says a lot for John Strong's personal magnetism that so many patients were prepared to participate in the work and to keep meticulously detailed diaries of their activity and food intake.

Over the next 15 years the focus of the balance work gradually shifted away from energy to minerals (particularly calcium, magnesium, potassium and sodium) and nitrogen. Increasingly, the facilities originally provided primarily for research purposes came to fulfil both service and research functions, with the distinction between the two becoming ever more blurred. The combination of specialist nursing, laboratory and dietetic staff and purpose-built clinical and laboratory facilities (able to provide a range of on-line biochemical results during dynamic function tests) expedited solutions of difficult diagnostic problems. Rapid and accurate assessment of the relative effectiveness of various treatments were possible on short and long-term outcomes as well as information relating to the pathogenesis of a range of endocrine/metabolic conditions. Particularly disorders of bone metabolism (osteoporosis, osteomalacia, and Paget's disease), pituitary dysfunction, and anorexia nervosa.

In 1971 Dr Joyce Baird came to the Metabolic Unit as a Lecturer in Medicine. She had become interested in the clinical and scientific problems posed by patients with diabetes mellitus while working with Professor Sir Derrick Dunlop at the Royal Infirmary. She had previously been attached to the Metabolic Unit from 1965 to 1968 (she worked in a laboratory in the Teaching and Research Centre, recruiting subjects for study from Dr Alan Smith's diabetic clinic at the Victoria Hospital, Kirkcaldy!) as an MRC Research

Fellow. The investigation was of free fatty acid metabolism and insulin/growth hormone secretion in patients with diabetes and in the non-diabetic off-spring of diabetic parents. One of Dr Baird's duties as Lecturer in Medicine was to run the existing Diabetic Clinic at the Western. This consisted of approximately 90 patients and was held in the Medical Out-Patient Department. After two clinics in this setting Dr Baird decided that this was a very poor way of delivering a diabetes service. The most practical way of effecting reasonably rapid improvement was to build on the nucleus of the existing Metabolic Unit. So began the unremitting process of expansion/fund raising which was to continue without a break until Dr Baird retired 23 years later.

The establishment of a comprehensive diabetes service for North Edinburgh based on the Metabolic Unit was a pioneering venture at the time. It incorporated all the features recommended 20 years later by the Departments of Health and the British Diabetic Association for the delivery of health care for diabetic patients through District Diabetes Centres! These included clinics held outwith normal working hours for special groups of patients such as school children, adolescents/young people, and working adults; on-line biochemical results at clinic sessions; open access to specialist advice by 'hot-line' telephone round the clock; a kitchen and other facilities for patient education; accommodation for day patients; and, most importantly, specialist nurses, dietitians, biochemists, and medical laboratory scientific officers. All these various staff were involved in all aspects of the Unit's work. For both patients with diabetes mellitus and the full spectrum of other endocrine and metabolic disorders, with clinical investigations and treatment, patient education in self-management, and research. It rapidly became clear that 6–12 months for new members of staff to acquire all the skills was required to allow them to function independently without direct supervision. Hence it was critical that the turnover of staff was reduced to an absolute minimum. This was achieved by a policy of job-sharing and actively encouraging applications from experienced personnel (particularly staff nurses) returning to part-time work after bringing up a family. The result of this was the creation of a core of mature, highly-motivated, dedicated people, rarely absent through sickness and who remained in post for long periods of time.

Over the years there was a steady rise in both the clinical workload and the research activity of the Unit. In 1976 Dr Baird was appointed to a Senior Lecturer/Honorary Consultant post with administrative responsibility for the Metabolic Unit as an integrated clinical/laboratory facility. The Unit's main problem, namely lack of space, was created by its success. In all, four extensions were added to the original Unit: the first provided two laboratories for basic research; the second an Out-Patient Clinic Suite with seminar facilities and a clinical laboratory delivering on-line results during clinic sessions; the third offices for Dr Baird, computers and scientific staff, along with an enlarged sitting room/dining area for day patients; and the fourth space for additional secretarial staff and clinical records. The result was an extremely effective Unit providing health care for patients with diabetes mellitus and other endocrine/metabolic disorders and excellent facilities for pursuing both clinical and basic research into these conditions. It is interesting to note in passing that, as with so many parts of the Western, the original building was designed for a 10–15 year life-span but 30 years later is still in full use and coping with a volume of work never dreamt of by the architect. Thus in 1993 11,223 patient visits (in, out or day cases) were dealt with and over 120,000 assays performed in the laboratory, while the total number of staff (including research staff) had risen to 40, compared with 7 in 1965.

There is no doubt that the system of health care developed in the Metabolic Unit has proved to be not only effective and user friendly but also extremely cost efficient. There can be few centres in the world which provide a comprehensive service for both diabetic and endocrine patients with a total specialist bed complement of four. In addition the admission rate to the general medical wards for acute complications of diabetes, such as hypoglycaemia and diabetic ketoacidosis, is unusually low. The basic concept underlying the system is that of focusing on the clinical problem and providing the various components of the service required directly round the patient as the central pivot. Working on this principle the facilities created in the Metabolic Unit allow integration of (1) *patient care:* based largely on day stay rather than hospital admission, patient education in self-management, open access to specialist advice round the clock; (2) *training of specialist staff:* doctors, nurses, scientists and dietitians; (3) *clinical and basic research:* aimed at developing better methods of diagnosis and treatment and ways of preventing the development of these disorders; and involvement of all members of the multi-disciplinary staff team in every aspect of the work. Another strength has been the collaboration of University and NHS funded staff at all levels and the fact that the University has played a major supporting role in the work of the Unit since its inception by funding 50% of the medical and laboratory staff posts and laboratory equipment.

One of Joyce Baird's earliest research papers, published in *The Lancet* in 1962, investigated the insulin-secreting capacity of the newborn infants of normal and diabetic women using a bioassay technique to measure the plasma 'effective insulin-like activity'. It took her 3–4 days hard work in the laboratory to produce a single result. In 1971 Isobel Nairn came to the Metabolic Unit as Senior Biochemist. One of her first tasks was to establish radioimmunoassays (delivering results in 1–2 days) for plasma insulin, C-peptide, glucagon and cyclic-AMP. These assays were heavily used for both clinical and research purposes over the next 20 years. In 1993 further development in technology allowed establishment of a Microparticle Enzyme Immunoassay system generating results in one hour. Isobel Nairn also played a major part in the next scientific milestone in diabetes research. This was the development of glycated haemoglobin to assess the degree of metabolic control being achieved in diabetic patients. Measurement of glycated haemoglobin in all diabetic patients attending the Metabolic Unit started as early as 1978 and again was a pioneering venture which formed the basis of regular audit in the Diabetic Clinic. The first audit held in 1980 resulted in several significant changes in clinical practice policy. Audit has been repeated at five-yearly intervals since then. The comprehensive and highly structured computerised case record designed by Dr Baird in 1971 has resulted in a unique database relating to the 4,500 patients seen over the past 24 years. The arduous task of setting up a computer network for the Unit and transferring all the clinical and laboratory data to computer files finally began five years ago. When complete will allow more extensive and sophisticated analysis than was possible with the laborious manual methods originally used. Sheena Douglas, as Dietitian in the diabetic clinic, and David Shirling have played a major role in this audit process.

Other significant advances in diabetes clinical practice developed in the Unit include a method for measuring glycated haemoglobin on capillary blood samples obtained by the patient at home and posted to the Unit (which has reduced the number of clinic attendances, shortened waiting times in clinics, and made consultations more effective and pleasant. This has now been adopted by all other diabetic clinics in the Lothian Area. There is widespread use of meters for the fast and accurate measurement of capillary blood glucose concentrations by patients of all ages. In the Western diabetic clinic patient self-monitoring by urine testing is ancient history.

A milestone in research into insulin-dependent (Type I) diabetes mellitus (IDDM) in Edinburgh occurred in 1982 when Dr Baird established a colony of diabetic BB rats on the Western site. The BB rat develops spontaneous, auto-immune, insulin-dependent diabetes at the age of three months and has proved itself as a valid and valuable model for human insulin-dependent diabetes. Supported by substantial grants from the Medical Research Council, the Wellcome Trust, the Scottish Hospitals Endowments Research Trust, the British Diabetic Association, Action Research, and the Cunningham, Alton and Savena Trusts, important contributions have been made to diabetes research in several cardinal areas. These include the pathogenesis of IDDM; the development of strategies for its primary prevention through targeted immuno-modulation; improved replacement therapy for IDDM by islet transplantation and the use of sustained release insulin implants; the biochemistry of diabetic microangiopathy; and the pathogenesis of diabetic embryopathy. This work has established an international reputation for the BB/Edinburgh colony. This was the basis of Dr Baird's nomination as Banting Memorial Lecturer (the highest accolade the British Diabetic Association can bestow) in 1992. In 1994 the Association officially recognised the value and importance of the BB/Edinburgh colony by designating it as a UK Research Resource and awarding basic support for the next five years. As a Senior Research Technician on the Metabolic Unit staff Bill Smith has been involved with the BB/Edinburgh colony since its inception. He continues to play a crucial part in the research programme, especially that part involving collaborative projects with colleagues in Cambridge, Oxford, Aberdeen and Brussels.

Professor Strong retired in 1980 and was succeeded by Professor Christopher Edwards from St Bartholomew's Hospital in London. At the same time a new NHS consultant post in Endocrinology was created and filled by Dr Paul Padfield. Their academic interest was salt and water metabolism in hypertension (mainly

Dr Padfield) and in classical endocrine conditions (mainly Professor Edwards). In the early 1980s together they studied the place of the angiotensin coverting enzyme inhibitors in the management of hypertension and also their interaction with the endocrine system. Professor Edwards was interested in the role of amplifiers for aldosterone secretion and Paul Padfield in the role of serotonin in aldosterone production. This proved to be a fruitful field of research.

Paul Padfield became increasingly uneasy about the validity of a single clinic blood pressure reading as a predictor of sustained hypertension which led to cardiovascular damage. He began to record blood pressure by electronic methods, with readings initially being recorded manually. Patients were instructed in the use of a semi-automatic electronic sphygmomanometer. It was found that a significant number of patients with a raised clinic blood pressure had completely normal readings in the home situation. Thus patient self-monitoring was a much more accurate method of identifying those with sustained hypertension in need of treatment — a finding which was published in the *Lancet*. Use of the more sophisticated methods of electronic recording showed that the blood pressure fell through the night in a majority of people. Those who did not have a nocturnal dip in blood pressure were at greater risk of developing cardiovascular damage. Much work has been directed towards trying to identify the mechanisms of fall and lack of fall in blood pressure at night. Glucocorticoids, catecholamines and renal function are apparently not involved. An interesting area of research has developed from the use of wrist actigraphs which give a measure of activity and the relationship of activity to blood pressure. These accurately define the sleep-wake cycle and are helping to explain the variability of the blood pressure.

Professor Edwards's current research originated from one young man with marked hypertension and a low serum potassium. This combination is usually seen in patients with excessive secretion of cortisol. However, this particular young man had a very unusual condition wherein cortisol was secreted in normal amounts but not converted to cortisone in the kidney. The enzyme which converts cortisol to cortisone is 11-ß-hydroxysteroid dehydrogenase. Chris Edwards and Paul Stewart went on to show that this enzyme was inhibited by both liquorice and carbenoxolone. This explained why these two substances induced hypertension. Since then, they have shown that the enzyme is present elsewhere in the body and has a ubiquitous function in keeping cortisol away from mineralocorticoid receptors. Professor Barker of Southampton has suggested that much cardiovascular disease in middle age can be predicted from the individual's weight at birth and at one year. This same enzyme, 11-ß-hydroxysteroid dehydrogenase has been shown to protect the foetus from too much maternal cortisol. If the enzyme is inhibited, placental and foetal weight are affected. Hypertension may be due to too much exposure to cortisol in utero. This work has been supported by grants from the Wellcome Foundation, the Medical Research Council and the Scottish Office.

In the early 1980s Professor Edwards and Dr Padfield developed a meeting which has continued to be known as 'Morning Prayers'. The term being coined by one of the SHO's in the early days. Medical students and junior medical staff were taught at 8.30a.m. to 9.00a.m. each morning of the week. In the past both Professor Edwards and Dr Padfield shared this very popular teaching round for junior staff as an educative vehicle. This was a focus for discussing endocrine problems throughout the hospital and including medical students in that teaching process.

From small beginnings the Metabolic Unit has established an international reputation as a Centre of Excellence for both clinical care and research in diabetes, endocrinology and other metabolic disorders. Although new technology has largely superseded the metabolic balance as a clinical investigative tool it is salutary to remember that one of Professor Edwards' major scientific discoveries of the last decade was critically dependent on a metabolic balance study. This was on a the first adult case described with congenital deficiency for 11-β-hydroxysteroid dehydrogenase who was meticulously investigated for more than six weeks on fixed, controlled intakes of sodium and potassium. These studies gave Paul Stewart a Gold Medal for his MD thesis.

Today the Metabolic Unit continues to evolve. In 1993 Lothian Health agreed to fund a new NHS consultant post in Diabetic Medicine and Dr John McKnight took up this post in October 1994 when Dr Baird retired. Since the university intends to refill Dr Baird's post with a physician whose academic interest is in diabetes the profile of diabetes as a discipline in its own right will be strengthened in a major way. Professor Edwards is currently the Dean of the Faculty of Medicine and Provost of the Medicine and Veterinary Medicine Faculty Group. Dr Padfield is Clinical Director of the Medical Unit. A Centre for Molecular Medicine presently under construction on the Western site will contain a floor housing research laboratories for Endocrinology. The site plan for the New Western General Hospital shows a new and larger Metabolic Unit adjacent to the Medical Unit designed to continue operating as an integrated clinical/laboratory facility delivering a patient-friendly, high quality clinical service and looking to basic research to provide answers which can be translated into clinical practice.

The essence of the Metabolic Unit approach is teamwork and the success of the Unit at all levels has depended on the contribution of many people, too numerous to mention individually. The following people have in different ways and at various times made a major contribution to the work of the Unit:

Nursing Sisters: Patricia Peattie, Sandra Main, Nessie Richardson, Nan Campbell, Eleanor Dick, Pauline Burnett.

Staff Nurses: Heather Barclay, Lesley Barrow, Brenda Bolloten, Sally Gobey, Peggy James, Vera Linklater, Veronica McCourt, Mary Norman, Christine Tait, Margaret Van Puyenbroek.

Dietitians:

Diabetes Anne Simpson, Kate Heskith, Sue Helliwell, Sheena Douglas.

Anne Simpson established the whole diabetic set up and the record system for the diabetic clinic.

Metabolic Anne Gibson, June Grieve

The Dietitians were interchangeable and were all involved in the study of severe anorexia nervosa.

Biochemists: Peter Ashby, Adrian Bone, Barbara Brockie, David Crothers, Mark Lindsay, Isobel Nairn, Christine Thin, Susan Walker.

MLSOs: Jacqui Armstrong, Marvin Black, Nicola Christie, Helen Darling, Myra Gilchrist, Sheila Gilchrist, Anne Logan, Eileen McDonald, Susan McIntyre, Carol-Anne McKechnie, David Shirling, Sue Taylor, Joan Yorke.

Secretaries: Elizabeth Holmes, Catherine McDonald, Kathleen McTeague, Karen Tully

Microbiology at the Western; the Central Microbiological Laboratories

Until 1953 the microbiological services to the hospital were the responsibility of the University under the direction of Professor Thomas J. Mackie. By then the clinical pathology requirements of the Northern Hospital Group had so increased that a laboratory for biochemistry and bacteriology was opened at the Northern General Hospital. Dr Andrew MacCabe was appointed consultant-in-charge of the bacteriology unit providing services to all the hospitals in the Group. He was later joined by Dr Nancy Conn in 1958.

There followed a period of rapid growth in demand for laboratory services in the South-Eastern Regional Hospital Board area. Plans were prepared for a new laboratory to house clinical pathology. However, by the time this plan had been agreed it was clear that the concept was too small to provide for the different laboratory specialties. The decision was made that only microbiology should occupy the new building. Dr Cam Gould was appointed Director to the now named Central Microbiological Laboratories (CML), and work started in December 1961. The staff of the Northern General Laboratory joined the new Department. There was a formal opening by the Chief Medical Officer for Scotland, Sir Kenneth Cowan, in July 1962. This was held on the roof of the new building and the large attendance was of much concern to the architect!

The staff from the laboratories at the Sick Children's, Astley Ainslie and East Fortune Hospitals soon joined, and a microbiological service to some 6,000 hospital beds, 150 general practitioners and the Public Health needs of the south-east of Scotland was begun. In addition to the microbiology service a comprehensive service in both microbial, non-microbial and tissue immunology was extensively developed by Dr Kenneth C. Watson who came in 1968. This service was widely used by all the hospitals and general practitioners in the Edinburgh area. The immunological interests of the laboratory highlighted the increased prevalence of 'Farmers lung' and pulmonary fungal infection in patients in certain areas of Scotland. As a consequence, with the support of dermatology and respiratory physicians, including Sir John Crofton and Dr Ian Grant, funding was made available for a Mycology laboratory through the

Scottish Home and Health Department. Dr Leslie Milne was appointed Mycologist (1971) and continues to expand this sub-specialty, which is much sought after by local clinicians and as a reference laboratory by those further afield. The extensive service given by the Central Microbiology Laboratory to users over a wide area required a sizable medical staff to provide clinical advice and a large technical staff led by Mr Douglas Annat to provide round-the-clock examination of specimens. Reports were rapidly prepared by clerical staff under the direction of Mrs Elizabeth Boyle. As the users were widely scattered the efficient collection of specimens and distribution of reports was a major problem. A problem shared by many of the clinical laboratories in the area. Consequently with the help of the Health Board a laboratory van service was developed and by 1972 six vans were operating simultaneously across the city, as far as Belhaven Hospital to the east and Bangour Hospital to the west. These vans had intercalated routes so that their circulation times were short and met at advantageous points to exchange specimens for different destinations. The aim was to have specimens delivered to a laboratory within two hours of sending. This was achieved for a high proportion of specimens. More than 1.5 million items were handled each year (1974) at a delivery cost of a mere 1.5p each, a tiny fraction of the laboratory costs.

Specimens from the Western comprised about one-fifth of the work of the CML. The medical and scientific staff of the laboratories paid frequent visits to the various units and wards, often on a daily basis. There was close clinical contact and consultation available on the significance of results, and the control of infection and treatment. In addition, the laboratories were continuously engaged in a wide range of investigative and research projects, many at the Western. These included extensive surveys of infection and the evaluation of prophylactic and therapeutic antibiotic policies (Drs Selwyn, Samuel, Winton, Bain and Bone), and the value of the Differential Mantoux test in the diagnosis of Mycobacterial disease (Dr Edmond). Dr K. Buchan cooperated with Dr Wilfrid Card and colleagues in the Gastrointestinal Unit in an investigation of intestinal tract microbiology, and programmes to reduce post-operative infection by control of the lower bowel flora were established with Mr A. Gunn. A long term study of prostatitis with Mr Selby Tulloch and Mr M. Henderson produced information on the diagnosis and treatment of this refractory infection.

The Laboratories were involved with Professor Sir Michael Woodruff and Dr John H. Bowie in planning microbiological control in the new Nuffield Transplant Unit. The standards set were proved to be too high in practice, nevertheless valuable information on the aerobiology of this new field was obtained. Much investigative work was carried out with the cardiologists. Dr Michael Matthews, as a cardiologist, recognised the value of the visiting Microbiologist in his lectures to highlight the value of clinical laboratory cooperation. When Dr Richard W. Turner was planning to visit Bhutan in 1965 on a scientific expedition associated with the International High Altitude year it was suggested that microbiologists from the CML accompany the party. Unfortunately this part of the plan did not materialise but a large number of specimens was returned by very special delivery, though somewhat outwith the normal two hours! The results of examination of these specimens were most interesting, particularly in relation to streptococcal disease.

In the field of Public Health, close relations were kept with medical officers of health and environmental health officers. Dr Ronnie Macrae was in charge of this section for a number of years which provided effective bacteriological monitoring of food and water supplies. Several outbreaks of food and water borne infection, both in the general community and hospital, were investigated. These included an outbreak in a hospital near the city and established the source of the causative organism, suggesting it had originated in Roman Pannonian Legions serving in Spain. Another outbreak was related to the Water of Leith and traced back to the Far East before the First World War (Drs Nancy Conn, Sandy Jamieson and Mr Scott).

General practitioners made extensive use of the CML, regularly visiting with specimens, discussing results and receiving advice about treatment. 'Self help' bacteriology was encouraged and reported by Dr James Knox and his general practitioner colleagues at the Muirhouse General Practice. More recently an extensive laboratory and clinical evaluation of a new antibiotic, pseudomonic acid (*Mupirocin*), was carried out in general practice with Dr James Smith.

The Laboratories had an 'in house' Animal House and therefore were able to provide *in vivo* diagnostic and research facilities to other departments. Later a large extension was built with University and other funds and the administration of this facility was transferred to another building. The CML also organised a number of important Symposia, several directly in association with the Hospital, including one on the occasion of the Centenary celebrations (1968). This was particularly notable in using a then novel two-way television link with the Royal Infirmary. The speakers and Western General Hospital audience occupied the lecture theatre in the Teaching Unit. The Royal Infirmary audience sat in the RIE Surgical Lecture Theatre viewing the proceedings and participating in the discussions.

The Central Microbiological Laboratories, despite having other heavy commitments, are an integral part of the Western and have close links with the clinical, administrative and other staff. During the past thirty years many staff have passed through the laboratory. Apart from those already mentioned, consultants have included Dr Brian Watt (1976–82), Dr Keith Cartwright (1977–81), Dr Anne Bushell (1982–85), Dr Archie Scott (1987–92) and Dr Mary Hanson (1982–). Dr Gould retired in 1988 and was succeeded by Dr Watson who retired in 1990 to be succeeded by Dr Scott until 1992. Dr Robert Masterton (1990–) is now in charge, with the support of Dr Mary Hanson and Dr John Coia (1992–). Dr Frank Bone was promoted to be consultant at Dumfries, Dr Roger Farrand as consultant to Bolton, the late Dr Fred Winton as lecturer at the University and thence to Vale of Leven as consultant. The late Dr Betty Edmond also translated to the University, taking over as consultant in charge of the Regional Virus Laboratory. Many Registrars, Senior House Officers and Research Assistants participated in the work of the laboratory and some have continued in microbiology. Mr Douglas Annat the Chief MSLO died in 1981 and was succeeded by Mr Eric Kerr. He remained in post until 1990 when Mr Peter Kale was appointed.

Neurology

Neurology was first practised by General Physicians at the Royal Infirmary. Sir Byrom Bramwell (1847–1931) was an outstanding clinician and published many papers. His son, Professor Edwin Bramwell (1873–1952) was trained at the National Hospital, Queen Square, London before taking up the Moncrieff-Arnott Chair of Clinical Medicine. Dr James K. Slater (1900–65) and Dr W. Ritchie Russell (1903–1980), who later became Professor of Neurology at Oxford, continued the teaching and practice of Neurology. In 1937 Professor Dott had established a Surgical Neurology Unit and appointed two medical assistants Dr Kate Hermann and Dr Ernst Levin. Later, they were joined by Dr W. Sneddon Watson (1916–1989).

After the Second World War Professor Sir Stanley Davidson established a series of specialised medical Units in the old Municipal Hospitals. The Neurology Unit was placed at the Northern General Hospital alongside Respiratory Medicine and Rheumatology in 1953. Dr John Marshall, a Manchester graduate was appointed Physician in charge and remained until 1956 when he moved to a Readership at the National Hospital and subsequently became a Professor there. In 1954 he was joined by Dr J. B. Stanton, a Cambridge graduate, who had worked in Newcastle and had trained in London with Sir Russell (later Lord) Brain. Later, Dr Stanton took over the administrative charge of the Unit until his untimely death in 1970. In 1956 Dr Marshall was succeeded in the academic post by Dr John A. Simpson, a Glasgow graduate, who had trained at Queen Square and developed a particular interest in electromyography and myasthenia. He also carried out experimental work and after promotion to Reader he returned to Glasgow in 1964 to the newly established chair of Medical Neurology.

In 1966 Dr Clifford Mawdsley, a Manchester graduate, was appointed Senior Lecturer in a post that combined clinical duties at the Northern General Hospital and the Royal Infirmary. He was a very dynamic physician. His busy clinical practice was combined at one stage with the task of Secretary to the Royal College of Physicians of Edinburgh. In the same year, 1966, a third post at the Northern General Hospital was created and Dr Ernest H. Jellinek, an Oxford graduate working at Maida Vale was appointed and continued until his retirement in 1987.

Until 1968 neurology was a unit in the Department of Medicine but in that year a separate University Department of Medical Neurology was created. Dr Bryan Ashworth, a St Andrews graduate replaced Dr Stanton in 1971. Bryan Ashworth was also Honorary Librarian to the Royal College of Physicians. His research contributions contained papers on visual function in multiple sclerosis. His interest in Medical History included a biography of the Bramwells. Dr

Roger E. Cull an Edinburgh graduate was appointed in 1981 to a post based at the Royal infirmary when Dr Sneddon Watson retired. His research interest included papers on epilepsy, EEG monitoring and the investigation and management of migraine.

Dr Mawdsley died suddenly in 1983. The University decided that a Chair of Medical Neurology would be created in a joint Department of Clinical Neurosciences based at the Western General Hospital. Professor Charles Warlow, a Cambridge graduate, came in 1987. A few months later, when Dr Jellinek retired, Dr Roger Will a Cambridge graduate was appointed.

Later in the same year the Unit moved to the Western General Hospital. At that time, in order to allow the Professorial Department to be concentrated in one hospital, Dr Ashworth divided his time between the Royal Infirmary and Western General Hospital until he took early retirement in 1992. He was replaced by Dr Robert Grant.

Medical neurology was transferred to the Western General Hospital in 1988 to form the combined Department of Clinical Neurology with Surgical Neurology. This Centre has been a tremendous success. All clinical in-patient services are concentrated in one site. This allows modern neurology to be practised as a combined approach from medical neurologists and neurosurgeons, working with radiologists, pathologists, physiologists and psychologists trained in neurology, all within the environment of a large General Teaching Hospital. The number of consultant neurologists has increased and allows for an acute clinical in-patient and out-patient service. This complements the longstanding acute outpatient service provided by the neurosurgeons. The undergraduate teaching provision has increased in parallel with the overall increase in the size of the department.

In 1993 Dr Roger Cull's inpatient beds were closed in the Royal Infirmary and his in-patient service came to the Western. Professor Warlow has an Medical Research Council Programme Grant. As part of this study Dr Peter Sandercock, a graduate of Oxford University was appointed in 1987 to develop the stroke research programme. This includes international trials in the care of acute ischaemic strokes. Dr Martin Dennis, a University of London graduate, came in 1990 to run the acute clinical stroke service. This has proved to be an important advance in the care of this disabling condition. Initially the post was funded by the Stroke Association, but since 1994 the funding has been undertaken by the Western General Hospitals Trust and the University of Edinburgh. The stroke service is important in its careful research into the development of stroke and the assessment of outcome.

The services to the local Hospitals in the South East of Scotland have been extended by bringing neurology services to the patient's locality. This service, started by Dr Stanton and continued by Brian Ashworth in Fife on a fortnightly basis, was extended by Dr Christian Lueck as a weekly clinic. Dr Lueck is a Cambridge and London graduate appointed in 1994 who has an interest in neuro-ophthalmology. He works closely with Dr G. McIlwaine who replaced Dr Cullen as Consultant Neuro-ophthalmologist to the Department. Neurology clinics are now held in St Johns Hospital Livingstone, (Dr Will), Falkirk (Dr Sandercock), Border's General Hospital (Professor Warlow) and the Edinburgh City Hospital by Dr Grant.

Another important grant came from the MRC Clinical Research Initiative in 1993 as a combined medical and surgical award. This covered the appointment in 1994 of Dr Joanna Wardlaw a senior lecturer in neuroradiology whose remit is research into the imaging of strokes and head injury.

A neuro-oncology service is provided by Mr Ian Whittle, Dr Anna Gregor and Dr Grant. Dr Will is the leader of the Creutzfeldt–Jakob disease (known colloquially as Mad Cow disease) surveillance project for Britain and its relationship to bovine spongiform encephalopathy which is funded by the Department of Health.

The academic and research staff of the Department have grown considerably, so that in 1995 there are more than 70 people on the academic staff of DCN.

Clinical Neurophysiology was established at the Western General Hospital when Dr Horace R. A. Townsend was appointed in 1966 and he continued until 1980 when he obtained a similar post at the National Hospital, Queen Square. He was succeeded in 1982 by Dr Angus D. McInnes who was tragically killed in a climbing accident early in 1993. His successor is Dr Christopher Fisher.

Other important departments within the neurological unit are

Neuroradiology:	Anthony Donaldson, George T Vaughan, Robert J Sellar.
Neuropsychology:	James AL Naughton, Robert Taylor
Neuropathology:	Anthony FJ Maloney, Alexander Gordon, Jeanne Bell, James Ironside

Neuroradiology

Neuroradiology came to the Western General with the opening of the Department of Neurosurgery at the Western General in 1960. This modern Department was the culmination of the efforts of Norman Dott, a pioneer of neurosurgery. Dott ranks with Cushing as the creator of the specialty of neurosurgery. Dott gathered around him a team of surgeons, neuropathologists, neurologists, neuroradiotherapists and neuroradiologists. Dr Donaldson was appointed as Consultant Neuroradiologist. The management of head trauma continued at the Royal Infirmary of Edinburgh, and investigation and surgical management of neurological complaints was carried out at the Department of Clinical Neurosurgery. To meet their needs, Dr Donaldson set up the Neuroradiological Investigatory Unit with angiography, plain films and pneumoencephalography which were then the principal modes of investigation. Dr Donaldson introduced ultrasound to help the detection of shifts in brain structures in 1962, and radioisotopes were introduced in 1966. Neuroradiology was becoming an increasingly powerful specialty with new developments in investigatory practice. Dr George Vaughan was appointed in 1971. Donaldson and Vaughan introduced CAT, (Computerised Axial Tomography) with one of the earliest scanners to be introduced in the UK in 1975. Angiography and CAT scanning became the lynch pin of investigation with CAT scanning permitting a large increase in non-invasive investigations. The Department expanded until 1986, the year that Dr Donaldson retired and Dr Sellar was appointed. These events corresponded with the move to integrate the Departments of Neurology at the Northern General with the Department of Clinical Neurosurgery at the Western General. The new technology of Nuclear Magnetic Resonance was introduced in 1992. Co-incident with this most recent advance in imaging, Dr Roderick Gibson was appointed as a Merck funded scholar. The academic activity in the new Clinical Neurosciences combined Unit has thrived under the combined Professorial Units of Surgery and Neurology. Doppler ultrasound digital subtraction angiography, combination of CAT and MRI have provided an impetus to a high grade academic Unit. In 1990, Dr Joanne Wardlaw, a radiologist, was appointed as an MRC scholar with an interest in stroke. In 1992 she took up her appointment as a neuroradiologist in Glasgow but returned to Edinburgh in 1994 as an academic neuroradiologist with a special interest in vascular disease. Intervention neuroradiology was introduced in the early 1980s by Dr Vaughan and Dr Donaldson with balloon and embolisation techniques. These advancements have been pursued by Dr Sellar with the radiological interventional management of aneurysms and vascular malformations and angioplasty technique.

Surgical Neurology

Neurosurgery, or surgical neurology as Wilfred Trotter and Norman Dott liked to call it, was started as a separate surgical specialty in Britain in the mid 1920s by three pioneers, Geoffrey Jefferson and Hugh Cairns in England and by Norman Dott in Scotland. Dott returned to Edinburgh in 1925 after spending two years in Boston as a Junior Associate with Harvey Cushing. When he first returned to Edinburgh, Dott had to work in general and paediatric surgery, performing neurosurgical operations at a nursing home in Great King Street. Professor Wilkie recognised Dott's needs and skills and lent him beds in his wards at the Royal Infirmary. In 1937 a substantial contribution from Sir Alexander Grant allowed the development of Ward 20 in the Royal Infirmary as a self-contained Department of Surgical Neurology. Dott's work expanded with the development in the field. By the outbreak of the Second World War further neurosurgical beds were allocated at Bangour Hospital for the care of patients with traumatic brain injury.

In the 1950s the Western General Hospital was developing rapidly as the second University Hospital in Edinburgh and had already accommodated the Department of Radiotherapy. It was decided to build a new Department of Surgical Neurology on the western side of the hospital. This was completed in

1960. Ward 20 at the Royal Infirmary took on a new role as a Head and Spinal Injuries Unit. The 60 neurosurgical beds at the Western General were allocated to elective neurosurgery.

There was resident staff accommodation on the top floor of the five storey building, an area for rehabilitation, including hydrotherapy, on the lower ground floor and radiology and twin operating theatres of singular design on the floor above.

The Department in Edinburgh, though now split between accident and emergency and elective, was in essence a Neurological Institute. The staff embraced all areas of neurology, medical as well as surgical, medical psychology and rehabilitation (physiotherapy, occupational and speech therapy), anaesthesiology, radiology and the applied basic sciences such as neurophysiology. Apart from expertise in the fields of trauma, intracranial tumours and aneurysmal malformations, the relatively new specialties of stereotactic and microsurgery were rapidly evolving. Indeed, the new operating theatres were partly designed around the needs of neurophysiological studies for the control of target-siting during operations for involuntary movements, intractable pain and epilepsy. Gradually spinal surgery, apart from trauma, and then paediatric neurosurgery were added. Finally neuro-pathology entered accommodation on the ground floor opposite the operating suite for frozen section work.

When Dott was appointed to the newly-endowed Chair of Surgical Neurology at the University of Edinburgh in 1947 at the Royal Infirmary, he was assisted by Mr George Alexander in surgical neurology and Dr Kate Herman in medical neurology.

Mr Alexander left soon after to head the department in Bristol. Unfortunately Professor Dott required prolonged hospital care and convalescence following a hip operation. Norman Dott was dogged by problems with his skeleton. His original attraction to medicine and then surgery came when he was recovering from a motor cycle accident. He was then an engineer. When he was a young surgeon it is said that he asked the ward sister for a surgical pack. When the Sister came into the doctors' room, Norman Dott was amputating a toe, regarding it as superfluous to effective requirements. His surgical and managerial intelligence were outstanding.

An American neurosurgeon, Dr Berger Thomas, replaced Mr Alexander for two years until the appointment of Mr John Gillingham from St Bartholomew's Hospital as Senior Lecturer and Consultant. Professor Dott returned to full duty in 1952. In 1955 Dr Herman became consultant medical neurologist and three years later Dr Sneddon Watson joined her as a consultant. Surgical neurology was strengthened by the promotion of Mr Phillip Harris from senior registrar. Together with the staff at Eden Hall hospital, he assumed the development of spinal cord surgery and care of the paraplegic in addition to his commitment to general neurosurgery. Professor Dott retired in 1963 and was succeeded in the chair by Mr John Gillingham. In 1965, Mr Edward Hitchcock came from Manchester as Senior Lecturer and consultant. Mr John Shaw was promoted from senior registrar in surgical neurology to consultant in 1965 and began the development of paediatric neurosurgery. Dr A. Maloney also joined the staff at that time as consultant neuro pathologist. Dr James Naughton became a consultant in medical psychology in 1968 and neuro-ophthalmology was added for one session a week by the inclusion of Dr James F. Cullen, consultant in ophthalmology. Dr Horace Townsend took over as consultant in clinical neurophysiology from Dr John Laidlaw in 1970.

In 1978 Mr E. R. Hitchcock, by now a Reader at Edinburgh University, was appointed to the Chair of Neurosurgery in the University of Birmingham (sadly, Professor Hitchcock died suddenly in December 1993). He was succeeded as Senior Lecturer by Mr James Steers. Professor Gillingham retired in 1980 to be succeeded in 1981 by Professor J. Douglas Miller, originally from the Institute of Neurological Sciences in Glasgow but coming to Edinburgh after five years as Professor of Neurological Surgery at the Medical College of Virginia in Richmond, USA.

From the beginning, Dott attracted young aspiring neurosurgeons for further training, from Britain and across the world. He was an exacting task master. Operations took many hours and required concentration and patience, not given to every one. Especially young residents. Nevertheless they all recognised a master of his craft at work. The new developments and modern facilities enhanced the reputation of the department as a post-graduate school for training and this continued over the years. By 1980, 103 of its trainees had become established world-wide, many of them heading departments and ten had taken up university chairs.

During the years of Professor Gillingham's Chairmanship, the Department of Surgical Neurology built up an international reputation in the management of subarachnoid haemorrhage and intracranial aneurysms, and in the practice of stereotactic and functional neurosurgery for movement disorders, most notably Parkinsonism. Professor Gillingham was a kind surgeon but with the same precise approach as Dott.

It can be seen that the department evolved progressively as demands of advancing knowledge were met. Post-graduate training in the clinical fields and research and undergraduate teaching were all increasing the demands on staff. The work was expanded by collaboration with medical neurology at the Northern General Hospital, the newly established MRC Brain Metabolism Unit and the basic sciences. To support research, research fellows and clinical trainees were appointed and supported by grants from the Medical Research Council, British Council, British and Commonwealth Foundation, McRobert Trust, Department of Health and Thistle Foundation as well as a number of major donations. The main fields of research were cerebral vascular disease and malformations, involuntary movements and Parkinsonism, epilepsy, intractable pain and chemotherapy of intracranial tumours.

New procedures were initiated and others developed during the 1960s and 1970s in stereotactic surgery (depth micro-electrode and neuro-transmitter studies), spinal and microsurgery. These were dependent on the revolutionary design of the operating theatres with finely filtered air, controlled temperature and humidity. For example, the operative infection rate was only 1.34%, which was amongst the lowest recorded, essential to the successful outcome of prolonged operative procedures. The theatres were also screened with copper mesh at the time of construction. This was necessary for accurate neurophysiological studies leading to precise therapy.

Television for diagnosis and advice during emergency surgical procedures in Ward 20 was set up in 1968 with a communication cable between the departments of the Royal Infirmary and the Western General Hospital. This was sponsored by the University/Grampian TV Teaching Scheme and was the first of its kind in the British Isles.

Clinical neurophysiology was an early strength in Edinburgh. The EEG service was started by Dr John Laidlaw, then Horace Townsend, and John Gillingham collaborated with Geoffrey Walsh of the Physiology Department in the treatment of movement disorders. Dr Angus McInnes came from Glasgow in 1985 to head this section; he died tragically in a climbing accident in 1993. By this time the department, under the technical leadership of Mrs Marjorie Clarke, was recognised as the premier EEG technician-training centre in the UK. Dr Chris Fisher took over the service in April 1994. Clinical Psychology has always been an important arm of the Department, starting with the contributions of Dr O. Zangwill in Bangour Hospital. He has been succeeded by Jim Naughton, Bill McKinlay and, now, Robert Taylor. Specialist neurological and neurosurgical nursing have also been major strengths in Edinburgh. The first post-basic neurology/neurosurgery nursing course in the UK was and still is in Edinburgh. The Department of Clinical Neurosciences has played a major role in the British Society of Neurological and Neurosurgical Nursing, contributing two Presidents and the Secretary to its organisation. A neurosciences nurse-led initiative in patient focussed care has won a major National Health Service Award and is currently attracting international attention.

In 1986, after several years of planning, the former Departments of Medical and Surgical Neurology were merged to form a new Department of Clinical Neurosciences. By this time, Professor Miller had established a research programme in head injury, in the measurement of intracranial pressure and blood flow and in brain oedema. Professor Warlow brought to Edinburgh an established, Medical Research Council-funded, programme in stroke research where the emphasis was on epidemiology and clinical trials. Dr Peter Sandercock arrived soon after, as an MRC funded Senior Lecturer, now promoted to Reader. These two complementary themes continue in the Department today, boosted by a major Clinical Research Initiative Award from the MRC.

The physical union of the NHS Departments of Medical and Surgical Neurology followed in 1987 with the closure of the Neurology Unit at the Northern General. The addition of twelve beds to the former DSN and the allocation of one of the three ward floors to Medical Neurology produced a 72-bedded Department of Clinical Neurosciences hereafter referred to as DCN. The University provided an academic building adjacent to the main DCN building. At the Astley Ainslie Hospital there was full recognition of the separate subspecialty of neurorehabilitation with the appointment of Dr Brian Pentland, a neurologist, as the Consultant in Neurorehabilitation, holding a joint academic appointment with the Rehabilitation Studies Unit and DCN.

In 1991, Ward 20 was closed and all inpatient and outpatient neurosurgical activity, including the management of moderately and severely head injured patients was transferred to DCN. In 1987, Mr Harris and Mr Shaw retired to be replaced by Mr James Steers who vacated the Senior Lectureship to take over the responsibilities of general and paediatric neurosurgery and Mr Tom Russell who replaced Mr Harris as the surgeon with a special interest in spinal neurosurgery. The Senior Lectureship in Neurosurgery was filled by Mr Ian Whittle who had come to Edinburgh from Sydney, Australia as a New Blood Lecturer a year previously and has now been promoted to Reader. Dr Paul Kelly, a cardiovascular physiologist with a strong interest in pharmacology succeeded Mr Whittle as Lecturer in 1988, and has since been promoted to a Senior Lectureship in Clinical Neurosciences. He heads a laboratory-based programme of study of the cerebrovascular system. The DCN building was expanded by the addition of a four-bed recovery room adjacent to the Operating Theatre, an outpatient clinic, and the Magnetic Resonance Imaging and Spectroscopy Suite, which now has two MR scanning units. A further extension to double the size of the Outpatient Clinic to 12 consulting rooms, and to provide 12 more offices and a seminar room is under construction in 1995.

The Consultant staff in Surgical Neurology have been increased by the appointments of Mr Patrick Statham as Consultant Neurosurgeon. There are also substantial research programmes in the effects of AIDS on the brain, motor neurone disease in Scotland, an interdisciplinary research programme in brain tumours.

Administratively, the NHS Department of Clinical Neurosciences is a Clinical Directorate headed by Mr James Steers. Academically it has one of the strongest research profiles in the Clinical School of Edinburgh University, attracting over £1.5m per annum in research grants currently and producing more than 200 publications per year. Over the years, two of the Professors of Surgical Neurology have served as Presidents of the Society of British Neurological Surgeons. Prof Gillingham has served as President of the Royal College of Surgeons of Edinburgh.

In August 1995 Douglas Miller died suddenly of a heart attack.

Nuclear Medicine

The first isotope tests and the first equipment were installed in Neurology by Tony Donaldson in approximately 1968 for isotope brain scans and isotope encephalograms. This was long before CT was invented. They also used Picker equipment and were able to measure cerebral blood flow using a xenon washout method. These techniques were used mainly for research. Tony Redpath (now in Radiotherapy Physics) and Elizabeth Campbell were the physicists who were involved in the early days.

There was no nuclear medicine in main X-ray until the 'new' Outpatient Department was opened in 1970. A Nuclear Enterprises Mark III Gamma Camera and a Siemens Dual Headed Rectilinear Scanner were bought as part of the original equipment. The radiologist who initiated and ran the service was Danny Sinclair, subsequently a radiologist at Dundee. At the same time Medical Physics acquired a whole body shadow shield counter and equipment for probe renography using 3 detectors, one positioned over each kidney and one over the heart.

Malcolm Merrick was appointed in 1974 on the initiative of John Strong. The reaction of one of the Senior Physicians at the Royal was to enquire whether Malcolm Merrick was to specialise in atomic piles. He came from the Hammersmith where he had been an MRC funded Research Fellow and before that Oxford where he had trained in Radiology. Between Oxford and Hammersmith he was briefly at Northwick Park. There he developed an interest in Nuclear Medicine through a series of coincidences, being in the right place at the right time. The work at the Hammersmith was looking at tumour localising agents using Nuclear Medicine. When he arrived in Edinburgh the equipment used for whole body bone scans and the Gamma Camera were obsolete and of poor performance. The system had some analogue electronics that allowed time activity curves to be obtained and an analogue tape recorder to tape record an examination. These could be played back to examine regions of interest. There was no computer. There was also a 3 probe renography system. The first clinical examinations were bone scans, a few lung scans, many liver scans and a very large number of brain scans. There was good contact with Sick Kids Hospital where Danny Sinclair had started isotope scans in children. These were a novelty for those times and for which Malcolm Merrick had no previous experience.

Dr Merrick's first innovation was to purchase an Ohio Nuclear Model 100 Small Field Scanning Gamma Camera in 1974. This gave a vast improvement in performance over anything available at that time but had a limited field of vision of only 10″ diameter. It was suitable for scanning heads but required several pictures to visualise the whole of the liver or the lungs. The Mark III NE Camera was still used because it had the analogue system for time activity curves and there was no data processing on the Ohio. The first computer was obtained in 1976. This was a Varian V66 and was regarded as being very large having 32k of memory and a 1 megabyte removable disk. This made a substantial difference, to the renal work in particular, making quantitation possible. There was one large X-ray Room which was originally designated the 'Academic X-ray Room'. In order to accommodate the second Gamma Camera it was necessary to discard the Rectilinear Scanner. The new Ohio Camera was a scanning camera, able to scan the whole body for bone images, but took 45 minutes. Nevertheless, the images were much better than those obtained on the old Rectilinear Scanner.

These various improvements lead to a progressive development of a range of investigations. The range included bone scans for the oncologists and orthopaedic surgeons; renal scans for the urologists and the paediatricians, some work for the Medical Renal Unit and lungs and livers for oncology and general medicine. During the early years most of the research was on renal applications. The unit was the first to demonstrate renal scarring in children using isotope imaging. This has since become one of the most commonly used procedures in paediatric nuclear medicine. Dr Merrick has recently published a longterm follow-up of children examined from between 1974 and 1991. This has, for the first time, identified criteria for high and low risk of progressive renal deterioration due to reflux nephropathy. It also enables the avoidance of catheterisation of these children. This study was made possible through a simple system of indexing reports so that all the children's records were returned. This has enabled an almost complete follow-up of children from the Western, the Sick Childrens, Fife and the Borders. Through this follow up system, these children were also followed after referral to the adult urologists resulting in an unusually complete follow-up series.

It was about this time i.e. the mid 1970s, that Malcolm Merrick met Professor George Boyd in Biochemistry in the University. Dr Bierwaltes in Michigan USA had developed an isotope labelled compound for imaging the adrenal cortex. Some time after Dr Merrick came to Edinburgh, he was approached by Amersham (the radiopharmaceutical manufacturer) to test one of two new selenium labelled compounds which they had synthesised as an alternative to the iodocholesterol made by Bierwaltes and his colleagues. Amersham had a very good chemist, Reg Monks, who thought it was possible to label cholesterol with selenium, which he thought ought to be more stable than the iodinated compound. He produced two compounds — one labelled in the Carbon-6 and one in the Carbon-19 position. A group in Germany were given the Carbon-6-labelled compound to evaluate and the Western General Hospital was asked to evaluate the Carbon-19 compound. Dr Merrick went to see George Boyd to ask for biochemical studies on the chemical's metabolism. George Boyd predicted that the compound was likely to be converted into a bile acid. Martin Eastwood, who had worked in Biochemistry with George Boyd on bile acids became involved very early on. The compound was indeed rapidly converted into a bile acid, which was purified and shown to enter the enterohepatic circulation. The compound itself proved to be quite useless in imaging the adrenals. The Carbon-6 compound proved to be the successful agent for imaging the adrenal cortex. However, the group had by this time appreciated the fact that small bowel disease is rather commoner than Cushing's syndrome. Amersham were prepared to produce a bile acid analogue. A number of compounds were tested and a 23-selena compound was selected for clinical trials. This was studied by Dr Martin Eastwood and Henry Nyhlin, who was visiting the GI unit for a sabbatical from Sweden. The compound has proved very effective in identifying problems with bile salt absorption in the distal small intestine.

The Department was the first in the UK, and one of the relatively few hospitals, to provide a seven day, 24 hour on call service for urgent investigations. This is a very cost effective service to provide. Graham Crompton the respiratory physician showed that the mean stay in this hospital with a suspected diagnosis of pulmonary embolism was substantially reduced as a result of this service.

The other major historical development was to take the first new camera made by a small company who rose out of the ashes of Nuclear Enterprises in 1980. The company was at that time called Scintronix and had developed a new large field camera. The department took the prototype for evaluation. Largely because Dr Merrick felt he wanted to support a local company but without expectations, knowing Nuclear Enterprises history. The Department was absolutely astonished to find that this camera was a world beater and far ahead of anything else available. In fact, some 15 years later, most other manufacturers have only just caught up. Unfortunately, the company were better engineers than business men and the company went into liquidation some years ago. There were, however, a number of spin offs. They did succeed in selling about 150 cameras and in order to sell into Europe they had to have various components made by contractors. Because of the requirements in Germany, the steel casting for the gantry had to meet the German DIN quality standard. In order to meet this a foundry in Falkirk became the first UK company to meet the DIN standard in engineering. Also, to build this camera a company who specialised in manufacturing printed circuit boards had to radically revise their techniques. This was necessary to produce what was, at that time, the largest printed circuit board ever made. The surface area was twice that of any one preceding.

The Department has been concerned more in evolution than revolution. There were various building alterations to make better use of the available space. With the progressive development of ultrasound, body Computerised Tomography and Magnetic Resonance Imaging the workload has changed enormously. The unit now does hardly any brain or liver studies but the number of lung, bone and renal studies is increasing steadily. The pattern is that functional investigations are undertaken and anatomical investigations are left to those radiologists who can provide this information with greater precision. The original 32K computer has evolved to one less than a quarter of the size but with 32M of memory and the I Megabyte disc has grown to I Gigabyte whilst the speed of operation has probably increased more than ten thousandfold. Tomographic studies which would have taken weeks to process now take seconds. It is possible to store and retrieve within minutes the raw data of every study performed during the past five years. The wall of filing cabinets has shrunk to a 6 inch cube. Superimposition of nuclear medicine (functional) and radiological (anatomical) data is just around the corner.

The Department is a very active and developing contributor to diagnostics in the Hospital.

Department of Clinical Oncology

The origins of X-ray work in Edinburgh were under the aegis of Dr W. Dawson Turner. In 1897, within two years of the discovery of X-rays, he had installed a primitive X-ray machine in his house in George Square. In subsequent years he had the first supply of radium salts, which were then lent to the Royal Infirmary. Dr Dawson Turner's first appointment was as Assistant Electrician to the Royal Infirmary and he was also appointed to the Royal College of Surgeons. In early days patients from the Royal Infirmary, and other hospitals, were taken to his home, in George Square, for X-ray examination and treatment.

The Radiological Department of the Royal Infirmary of Edinburgh was completed and functioning in 1926. A year earlier the University of Edinburgh appointed a Medical Lectureship in Electrical Therapeutics and Radiology and the first lecturer was Dr J. M. Woodburn. The RIE had an X-ray therapy machine for some years, and a supply of Radium salts which had been purchased by private monies. In March 1930 a loan of radium sources was made by the Radium Commission to the RIE. A special follow-up clinic for patients treated with radium began in the following year. In 1923 the surgeon, Mr J. J. M. Shaw was appointed as the Co-ordinating Clinician. The commitment, enthusiasm and expertise of Mr Shaw ensured that radiotherapy was established in Edinburgh.

Subsequently a Radium Registrar, Dr A. M. Ross, was appointed as assistant to Mr Shaw to help establish Beechmount House as a special nursing home for patients having radium treatment. Dr Margaret Tod also joined the first team of radiation oncologists in Edinburgh. She left in 1937 to join Ralston Paterson in Manchester as Deputy Director of the Christie Hospital and Holt Radium Institute.

In 1935 Dr Morrison was succeeded by Dr A. E. Barclay who agreed to the appointment only if Dr Robert McWhirter was appointed as his assistant. The following year Dr Charles Muirson was appointed as the full-time physicist to the Radiology Department. Dr Barclay decided to return to Cambridge after only a few years in Edinburgh and tragically Mr Shaw was killed on active service in 1940. On the advice of the surgical staff, the Board of Management offered the charge of the department to Dr Robert McWhirter. He introduced the practice of keeping detailed records of patients treated with ionising radiation. These have been retained in Edinburgh since 1930 and from 1937, records of all patients with cancer seen at RIE were included.

Dr Robert McWhirter was recognised to be full of challenging ideas in cancer therapy, particularly in the management of breast cancer. He was the promoter in the 1940s of a management of breast cancer by the combination of surgery and radiotherapy. He was attempting to be more radical. He argued that the radiotherapist was able to irradiate the internal mammary lymph nodes and the lymph nodes of the supraclavicular fossa. This meant that, combined with a simple mastectomy, the patients were being offered the equivalent of the

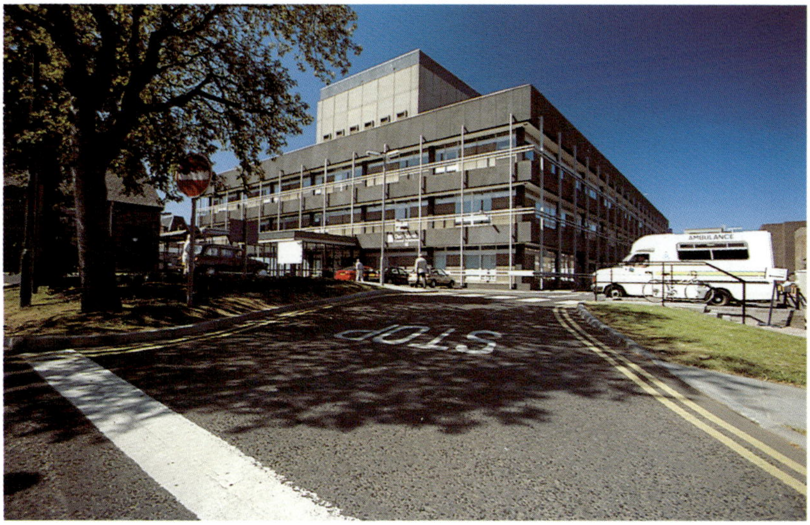

Out-patient Department.

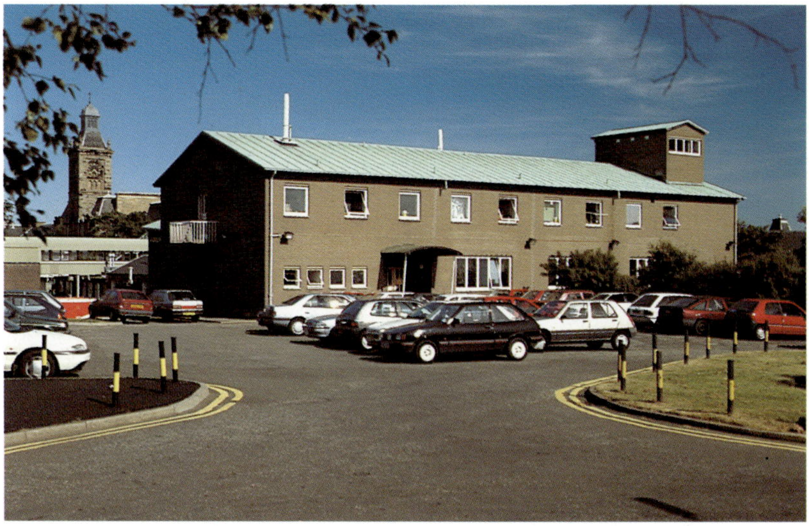

Teaching and Research Centre with clock tower to the left.

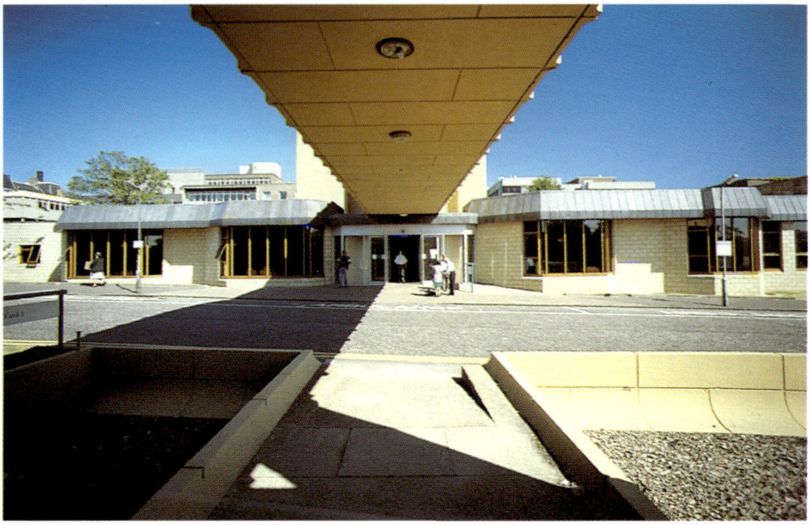

Oncology Unit.

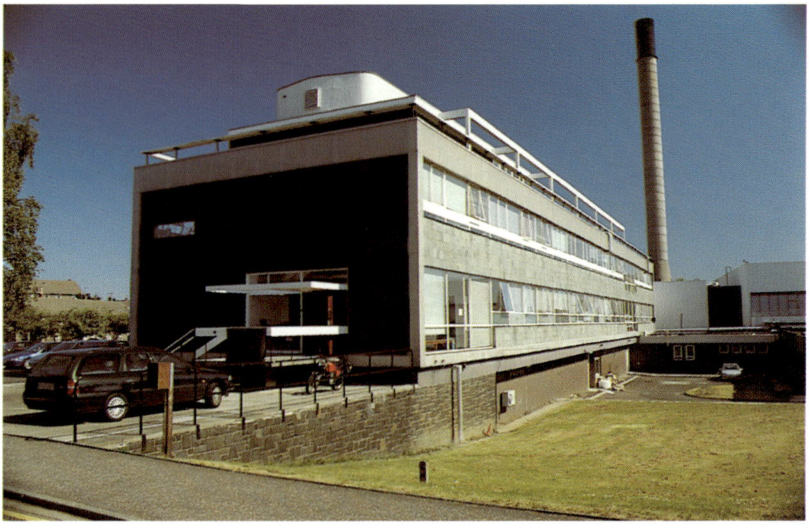

Microbiology Laboratory.

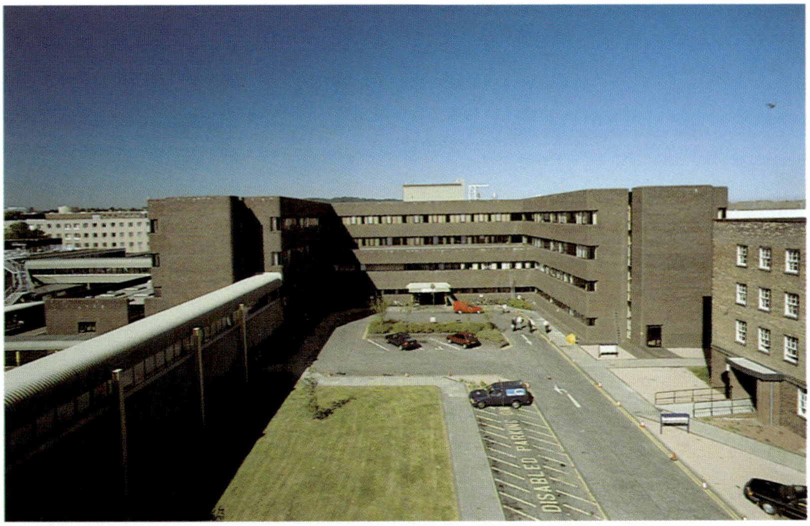

Alexander Donald Building.

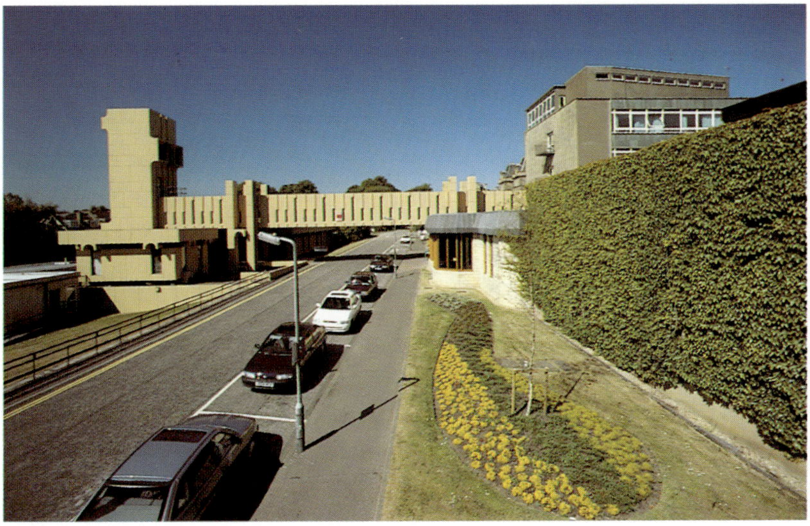

Entrance to main drive; the Transplant Unit
and the new Oncology Unit.

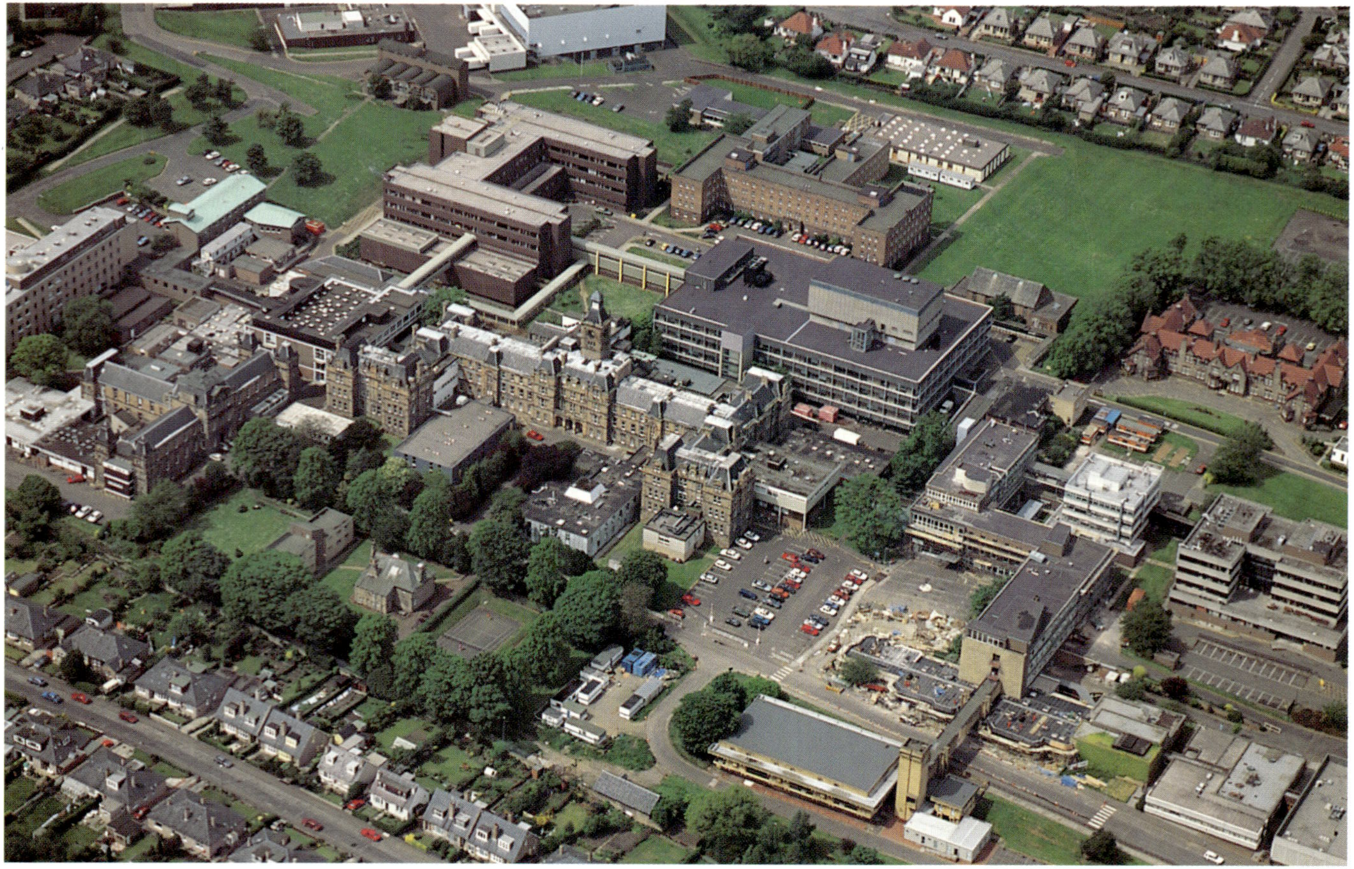

Aerial photograph of the Hospital.

extended radical or super radical operation. The result was less traumatic and disfiguring to women so afflicted with cancer. A crucial scientific meeting was held in the Royal Society of Medicine in 1948 from which his contribution was published in the Proceedings of the Society in 1948, 'The Treatment of Cancer of the Breast'.

An early and important staff appointment was made when Dr William M. Court Brown joined the radiotherapy department in 1947. It was the work of Dr William Court Brown on the hazards of radiotherapy for those patients which contributed to the MRC establishing the Clinical Population and Cytogenetics Unit at the Western General Hospital. This was joined by a link corridor to the Department of Radiotherapy. Court Brown established the Clinical Effects of the Radiation Research Unit which opened in conjunction with the new Department of Radiotherapy at the Western General Hospital. His initial laboratory was designed for biochemistry. He had the remarkable foresight to appreciate the significance of the ability described in 1956 to demonstrate the human genome. He employed three biologists to study the effect of various agents including radiation on the genome. One of these biologists was Karin Buckton. It was the extension of the study of the human karyotype into population studies, such as new born babies, which led eventually to the change to the Clinical and Population Cytogenetics Research Unit.

In 1946 the University of Edinburgh appointed Robert McWhirter to the newly-endowed Forbes Chair of Medical Radiology, a position which he held with great distinction until his retirement in 1970. Soon afterwards, in a characteristically far-sighted way, Professor McWhirter decided that radio-diagnosis, as it was known then, should be a separate department. Professor McWhirter thereafter devoted all his time to radiotherapy.

The Department of Radiotherapy first moved to the Western General Hospital in 1954. At that time a new building was opened to accommodate not only the new X-ray therapy equipment but a Radium Room, special operating theatre and wards providing accommodation for 120 patients. The architect, Mr William Wellwood, and design team were awarded the Architectural Medal of the Royal Institute of British Architects in 1956. On the ground floor a professorial suite of rooms was provided for Professor Robert McWhirter and his staff. The equipment available at that time included a 2Mv Van de Graff generator. There were five Resomax 300 KV X-ray generators installed in the upper ground floor, used mainly for treatment of large numbers, of patients with breast cancer, and a Müller 100 KV unit for treating skin cancers.

When the department first opened at the Western General Hospital, Professor Robert McWhirter was Director of the South East Scotland Regional Radiotherapy Service. The Deputy Director was Dr Kenneth A. MacKenzie, who subsequently moved to Inverness to establish a Radiotherapy Department at Raigmore Hospital to serve the North of Scotland and the Western Isles. The other consultants at that time were Dr Mary Douglas, Dr James F. G. Pearson, Dr Joseph Newall and Dr James McLelland. Mary Douglas succeeded

MacKenzie as deputy director. She was a specialist in cancers of the gynaecological type. In her mature years she married and bought a motor bike, moved for a period to New Zealand and returned to retirement in Edinburgh. James Pearson developed studies on the treatment of cancer of the oesophagus. James McLelland trained originally with Norman Dott and came to Radiotherapy to treat brain tumours and carried out a weekly general radiotherapy clinic in Bangour Hospital for many years. Dr Gordon Ritchie was a kind gentle unpretentious man but a very expert and hard working doctor. He trained with McWhirter and had a special interest in lymphoma. He worked with Dr Norman Allan in combined clinics. They were founders with others of the Scottish and Newcastle Lymphoma Group. Dr John (Archie) Orr was a man of wide interests outside medicine — a polymath. He made major contributions to the neutron trials with a particular emphasis on head and neck cancer and carried out a weekly clinic in Dumfries.

Dr Allan Langlands was another protege of Professor McWhirter. He was involved in research with Court Brown and was particularly interested in the treatment of cancer of the breast in collaboration with surgeons. He took the chair of Radiotherapy in West Mead Hospital, Sydney, which proved to be a great success.

When the Department of Radiotherapy opened in 1954 the number of new patients referred each year was about 2,300, of whom about 1,300 were given radiotherapy. Interestingly, at that time, about 200 patients treated were given radiotherapy for non-malignant diseases — a large proportion of whom had ankylosing spondylitis refractory to other forms of management. A rapid rise in the treatment of patients followed the acquisition of megavoltage therapy in 1955. Before this purchase the number of malignant cases treated was about 1,000 per year and rose to over 1,500 per year within five years. Quite rapidly benign disease was no longer treated by radiotherapy.

A feature of Edinburgh Radiotherapy was the early development of specialist interest in particular tumour sites. There was establishment of joint clinics in which a radiotherapy consultant would care for a patient with the specialist in that field. Careful follow up with tissue identification of results was the basis of progress.

Today the department treats almost 3,000 new patients each year. Few patients are referred for radiotherapy of benign conditions.

Following Professor McWhirter's retiral, Professor William Duncan was appointment to the new Chair of Radiotherapy. Bill Duncan was an Aberdeen graduate who trained in radiotherapy in Manchester. He and his Senior Lecturer, Dr Sidney Arnott, over the following years, built up Edinburgh's reputation as a major cancer treatment centre. Another appointment of great importance was of Miss Gill Kerr as a medical statistician. Notable at this period was the building of the Cyclotron for the assessment of neutrons in treatment of cancer. Neutron therapy was in contrast to the photon irradiation or the more usual radiotherapy. Claims had been made for better effects from the use of the neutron system. Edinburgh embarked on a series of meticulous trials under the leadership of Professor Duncan, working with Dr Sid Arnott. A wide range of tumours were irradiated in a series of trials including cancer of the bowel, bladder, cervix, sarcomas, oesophagus and head and neck. The follow up of patients was close and characterised by biopsy as well as clinical assessment.

The claim for the neutron therapy was not sustained. Neutron therapy was not better than photon and the destruction of normal tissue was considerable. Professor Duncan was awarded the Rontgen Prize by the British Institute of Radiology in 1987. Bill Duncan was interested in urological cancer, including bladder cancer. With Selby Tulloch and Jack Newsam, and later Geoff Chisholm, joint assessment based on cystoscopy in the day bed area was set up as a routine basis followed by meetings to review the pathology.

Bill Duncan was an effective and sympathetic organiser. He inspired young doctors who were genuinely fond of him. Many radiotherapy consultants originally began their training as surgeons, later some were physicians. This surgical background gave an insight into how surgeons think. An insight not given to all. Professor Duncan was heavily involved in the Western General Hospital as a whole, not merely in radiotherapy. He was Chairman of the Clinical Staff. His work there was prodigious yet his style was sympathetic, expert and always acting with the Hospital rather than a facet or faction in mind.

Professor Duncan was appointed subsequently as the head of the Radiotherapy Department in Princess Margaret Hospital, Toronto, where he stayed for five years, designing and establishing a new department. In the interim Professor W. McKillop was appointed for a short period and when he gave up office Professor Duncan was reappointed to his Chair, which he held until 1995. On his return he briefly took up the role of Chairman of the Clinical Staff but had to resign following a myocardial infarct. He regained his habitual vigour following this.

He was also very positive in his welcome to Professor Smyth in Medical Oncology. He made beds available and did everything possible to ensure that Medical Oncology was a success. This approach was not universal in all institutions.

Sid Arnott was promoted from Senior Registrar to Senior Lecturer and was primarily involved in the cyclotron project. His special interest was cancer of the gastrointestinal tract. In particular rectal tumours, an area poorly dealt with previously. He moved subsequently to St Bartholomew's Hospital in London.

When the managerial system of Clinical Director came into the Trust, Dr Hugh MacDougall was the first appointment After training in Edinburgh, he had moved for several years to Ninewells in Dundee. On his return he had promoted the upgrading of the department as a patient care facility. The department, as with many parts of the Western General Hospital were derelict and very poorly provided for. Dr MacDougall obtained a £1 million grant from the Cancer Relief MacMillan Fund, along with further funding from the Lothian Health Board. The facilities to treat patients were transformed and contemporary environment created which removed, in part, the sense of forbearing that a diagnosis of cancer and radiotherapy treatment must arouse. A further enterprise is the further funding from the Cancer Relief MacMaillan Fund to convert the former Renal Transplant Unit into a day Chemotherapy Unit.

Alan Rodgers followed the traditional path of surgery, before coming to radiotherapy. A sabbatical was spent in the MD Anderson Hospital in Houston, Texas. Alan Rodgers took over the breast work. He also had an interest in the Medical Advisory Structure. In the fullness of time he moved to the Alfred Hospital in Melbourne to head Radiotherapy. Another Edinburgh Radiotherapist who migrated to Australia was Dr Sue Ludgate. Dr Howard came from Cambridge after Bill Duncan left for the first time. Grahame Howard looked after the patients with urological cancer. On the same day as he was appointed Valerie Cowie was also successful. Her remit has been gynaecological cancers. Dr Anna Gregor came following Professor Smyth from the Royal Marsden as a radiotherapy research fellow on lung cancer. She was briefly a consultant in Glasgow before returning as an ICRF senior lecturer. Her speciality was neurological, lung and paediatric cancers. Dr Gabber Newaishy came originally from Cairo. His interest has been the irradiation of oesophageal and lung cancers. Sadly his career has been dogged by ill-health. Dr Ian Kunkler came through the Unit's training scheme and moved to a Consultant post in Sheffield. He returned to Edinburgh to replace Alan Rodgers for the cae of Breast Cancer.

The training in the department was superb. An indication of the training provided by Robert McWhirter in the Department was the number of people who travelled overseas to develop and head up Departments there. The present head of the Queensland Radium Institute, Dr Robert Allison, trained at Edinburgh as did Professor Allan Langlands in Sydney. Tom Sandeman, who was an Edinburgh trainee, was the acting head of the Peter MacCallum Unit in Melbourne. Similarly, in Canada, Dr Caskie headed the unit in the Princess Margaret Hospital in Nova Scotia and would only recruit Scottish-trained radiotherapists! It is believed that at one stage there were five Edinburgh trained radiotherapists working there. Jim Pearson headed a new unit, the Cross Cancer Centre, in Edmonton. Others have gone to the United States, perhaps the best known being Joe Newell who became Professor at New York University in the late 1960s or early '70s.

The Superintendent Radiographers have been central to the progress of the department. Miss Diana Foreman was superintendent for many years. A formidable lady at first sight. Her inherent kindness was obvious when she could be seen pushing an ancient pram to collect the children who were coming for radiotherapy from the paediatric ward. She became a Deaconess in the Episcopal Church following retirement. Her successor was Joan Berry who taught radiation oncology to the trainees in radiotherapy. She retired to be succeeded by Martine Jackson from the Cromwell Hospital in London.

Consultant Staff	*Year Appointed*
Professor Robert McWhirter	1935
Dr K. A. MacKenzie	
Dr Mary Douglas	
Dr J. G. Pearson	
Dr J. Newall	
Dr J. McLelland	
Professor Court Brown	
Dr G. L. Ritchie	December 1964
Dr J. A. Orr	
Dr G. A. Newaishy	1964
Dr A. Langlands	1965
Professor W. Duncan	1971
Dr S. J. Arnott	1977
Dr S. M. Ludgate	1981
Dr A. Rodger	1983
Dr R. H. MacDougall	1985
Dr G. C. W. Howard	1986
Dr V. Cowie	1986
Dr I. H. Kunkler	1990
Dr D. Jodrell	1994
Professor W. M. McKillop (from Kingston, Ontario, Canada)	1987–90
Professor J. F. Smyth	1980
Dr R. C. F. Leonard	1981
Dr M. A. Cornbleet	1985
Dr A. Gregor	1986

Orthopaedics

Prior to 1960 the only orthopaedic specialist input into the Western General Hospital were occasional Consultant referral Outpatient Clinics run by the late Robert I. Stirling who was based at the Princess Margaret Rose Orthopaedic Hospital.

With the appointment of Professor John I. P. James to the Chair of Orthopaedics in 1958 elective orthopaedic surgery was established at the Princess Margaret Rose Hospital, major orthopaedic trauma at the Royal Infirmary. The Western General Hospital became a combined elective and orthopaedic trauma service for North Edinburgh.

In 1960 James H. S. Scott returned from Oxford as Senior Lecturer in Orthopaedics to establish the Accident Service in the Western General Hospital. In addition to his considerable experience in orthopaedic trauma he also introduced great interest and expertise in spinal problems which led to the development of a flourishing Orthopaedic Spinal Service within the hospital. At that time W. Veitch Anderson, an Orthopaedic Surgeon based at Princess Margaret Rose Orthopaedic Hospital had developed a leg lengthening technique of international repute. On his retirement this work was handed over to Jimmy Scott and the outpatient component of which was transferred to the Western General Hospital.

Jimmy Scott was soon joined by Douglas Lamb who had just returned from Los Angeles where he had been working with Joseph Boyes, the doyen of hand surgery at that time. In 1967 they were joined by George E. Fulford from the Royal National Orthopaedic Hospital, London who was appointed to the Princess Margaret Rose Orthopaedic Hospital to develop the Lothian Cerebral Palsy Service. His knowledge and expertise in the field of general paediatric orthopaedics resulted in fruitful liaison with the Paediatric Departments within the Western General Hospital. At this time Douglas Lamb gave up his general orthopaedic practice to concentrate entirely on hand surgery in which he developed an international reputation and later became President of the British Society for Surgery of the Hand.

The original orthopaedic wards were situated alongside gynaecology on the top floor of the old building. Geographically this situation could not have been more inappropriate. The wards were not only remote from Casualty, X-ray and the main theatre suite, but the lifts were so small that it was impossible to transport patients without first disconnecting the traction apparatus. A walk-in cupboard between the wards housed the various pieces of traction equipment which were used much more frequently in those days than at present when so many fractures are surgically fixed. The bandages, strings and weights were neatly stored in Huntley & Palmers biscuit boxes awaiting the arrival of new patients!

In those early years Helen Griffin was Sister on the gynaecology and orthopaedic wards, the combination of which defied all medical and nursing logic! She was one of a group of Western General Sisters at that time who had trained at St Thomas' in London. Helen was an outstandingly popular Sister with her nursing and medical colleagues. After she gave up the combined responsibility for orthopaedics and gynaecology she remained in the Western for many years as a Nursing Administrator.

There were two resident student rooms immediately above the gynaecology wards at that time. This gave a unique opportunity for medical students to live in during their senior years and work as locum house staff. At the same time allowing them to join the nursing staff for coffee in the duty room of G12–16 at all times of the day and night. In addition to her efficient running of the ward Helen was always tremendously friendly to the medical students whilst also keeping a watchful eye on 'her girls'.

The medical house staff spent two months in orthopaedics, two in general surgery and two in Casualty which at that time was administered by the Orthopaedic Surgeons. The Casualty Department was located in the Paderewski Building which had housed the Polish Medical School during World War II.

The Casualty houseman covered the Department alone day and night. The off duty was one evening a week and every third weekend. They saw on average about 90 patients a day and did not have the assistance of a plaster technician. As a result, some of the hurriedly applied plasters had the appearance of rather voluminous meringues rather than plaster of paris. The Department itself was remote from the facilities in the main hospital building including X-ray. Ill patients were transferred to the main building for investigation and treatment on a trolley covered by tarpaulin as protection against the elements with a lamp swinging from a drip stand to light their path. The same building housed the main Physiotherapy Department on the first floor but there were no lifts to convey the disabled patients. Presumably some of the most useful physiotherapy was achieved in actually getting the patient up to the Department itself. Most of the orthopaedic physiotherapy was carried out on the wards with great skill by Isobel Bowman, Sheila Cameron, Anne Robertson and more recently Sheila Michael. The Outpatient Department was also housed in the Paderewski Building where Fracture Clinics usually ended with the orthopaedic staff donning waterproof aprons, rolling up their sleeves and applying plasters to the many patients in attendance.

Great support was always given by the secretarial staff of the Department during the G12–16 years. Jean Macleod worked under difficult conditions in the attics above the ward coping with all the in and outpatient secretarial load. From its inception all the inpatient and outpatient orthopaedic casenotes were typewritten which proved a brilliantly simple and effective arrangement. Jimmy Scott dictated during his Orthopaedic Clinics, as he was seeing patients, and was then presented with the letters to sign at the end of the Clinic.

In 1968 the Casualty and Orthopaedic Outpatients moved in to the new Outpatient Building. The newly named Accident & Emergency Department had access to X-rays, plaster room and overnight care area with adjacent operating theatres, one of which was dedicated to orthopaedic procedures between 9.00 a.m. and 5.00 p.m.

The secretaries and medical staff were all housed in what had been originally planned as a children's play area for the Department. As a result the toilet facilities were rather on the low side. They proved to be a very useful parking place for Betty Williamson's old and trusted bicycle which brought her into the Department just after 8 o'clock most mornings. She spent the day frantically typing the huge workload from the inpatients and from burgeoning Outpatient Clinics. If she fell behind she would turn up on Saturday mornings to keep abreast of the workload. The motive for such industry was not monetary but a true dedication to the hospital and the NHS. Indeed Betty had a notice on her desk which stated 'my take-home pay won't take me home'. The NHS has a history of failing to recognise and reward some of its most dedicated and productive staff. After his return from Boston, Peter Abernethy joined the service in 1974 as a Consultant having been House Surgeon, SHO, Registrar and Senior Registrar between 1960 and 1973. He had a special interest in the surgery of arthritis and had a close liaison with the Rheumatology Service which was then in the Northern General Hospital. He also ran the Accident & Emergency Department for the next 14 years until Colin Robertson was appointed Consultant in Accident & Emergency Medicine.

1986 saw great changes in the Department. George Fulford was unfortunately forced to retire on the grounds of ill health at the peak of a highly successful career and an international reputation in paediatric neurological disorders. Jimmy Scott and Douglas Lamb retired, Geoffrey Hooper taking over from Douglas Lamb to continue the successful Hand Surgery Service often dealing with Outpatient Clinics of over 100 patients. Having completed his training in Newcastle and the Mayo Clinic, Richard Nutton replaced Jimmy Scott in 1987. He was responsible for developing the Knee Arthroscopy Service and introducing an interest in shoulder pathology. Later that year James Robb from Leeds and Grenoble took up his post as successor to George Fulford and continued a paediatric interest in the Department. He also had a special interest in Oncology and provided excellent support to the Oncology Department in the Western.

With the opening of the Alexander Donald Building in 1987 the luxury of six single rooms and six four-bedded rooms became available to meet the unpredictable demand of orthopaedic trauma. However in order to meet the pressing need for orthopaedic beds post-fracture patients were transferred after 3–4 days to second line beds in the Northern General Hospital. These patients remained under the care of the orthopaedic surgeons who attended weekly ward rounds on that Unit. In 1992 the Accident & Emergency Department was closed and orthopaedic trauma was transferred to the Royal Infirmary and elective orthopaedics to the Princess Margaret Rose Hospital.

Over the 32 year history of orthopaedics in the Western there were many allied health professionals who contributed to the care of the patients. The care of patients in traction represented a great nursing challenge whilst the rehabilitation of the elderly fracture patient called for skill and patience on behalf of the physiotherapists and occupational therapists. Without the social workers it would not have been possible to discharge patients back to their home or other environment allowing beds to be vacated to cope with the constant influx of new fracture patients. The old plaster meringues from the early days were replaced by lightweight designer plasters, as applied by Archie and Tam the plaster technicians. Recognition is also due to the records staff, who ran the Outpatient Clinics and whose difficult task it was to retrieve the many dozens of casenotes and X-rays required for the nine weekly outpatient sessions.

It is also a pleasure to acknowledge the great contribution by many Orthopaedic Registrars from all over the world. They came to Edinburgh to work on the Orthopaedic Service and spent time in the Western as part of their surgical rotation. Not only did they contribute greatly to the service requirements of the Unit but they also stimulated an exchange of ideas which greatly enhanced the Unit.

Medical Paediatric Unit

Staffing

Until 1948, the Paediatric Unit at the Western General Hospital (WGH) was staffed primarily by the Maternity and Child Welfare Department of Edinburgh Town Council with Dr 'Tiff' Findlay, Senior Maternity and Child Welfare

Medical Officer, and Dr Haldane P. Tait, his deputy, in day-to-day charge. Professor Charles McNeil (University Department of Child Life and Health) was the visiting consultant. Professor R. W. B. Ellis succeeded Professor McNeil in 1946 and assumed the latter's responsibilities at the Western General Hospital. He devolved most of these duties to his Senior Lecturer, Dr J. L. Henderson (later Professor of Child Health in Dundee) and to Dr Douglas M. Douglas who occupied a Senior Registrar/pre NHS Consultant-type post at the Royal Hospital for Sick Children (RHSC).

Admissions to the paediatric wards at the WGH. were predominantly referrals from Clinical Medical Officers and Senior Clinical Medical Officers working in the Maternity and Child Welfare Service and the School Health Service. There was no formal outpatient service. The newborn were under the care of the obstetricians including Dr Ian Morris, later Professor of Obstetrics in Manchester.

With the inception of the NHS in 1948, Dr Douglas carried most of the clinical responsibilities until 1950. Dr Tait was also involved in neonatal follow-up clinics. In 1950 the South-Eastern Regional Hospital Board, as part of the policy of upgrading the WGH and providing a full paediatric service, established a consultant paediatric post designated as 'Senior Paediatric Physician, Edinburgh Northern Hospitals Group'. This post embraced sole consultant paediatrician responsibility for the medical paediatric unit at the WGH (25 beds and the neonatal nurseries), the medical paediatric unit at Leith Hospital (approximately 22 beds), the neonatal nurseries at the Eastern General Hospital and on-call responsibilities to Musselburgh Maternity Hospital and the Vert Maternity Hospital, Haddington. Dr J. O. Forfar, Senior Lecturer in Child Health in the University of St Andrews (Dundee Royal Infirmary and Maryfield Hospital, Dundee) was appointed and took up duty on 15 July 1950. The sff of the RHSC and the University Department of Child Life and Health thereafter ceased to have any responsibility for the medical paediatric unit at the WGH. The appointment meant that a full range of paediatric services was instituted at the WGH including an inpatient service, outpatient clinics and a paediatrician staffed neonatal service. The latter was developed in close collaboration with Professor A. S. Duncan who later became Professor of Obstetrics and Gynaecology in the University of Wales.

Coincidentally with the appointment of a consultant medical paediatrician in 1950 a Senior Registrar in Paediatric Surgery (Mr Ian S. Kirkland) was appointed to the Edinburgh Northern Hospitals Group. The consultant responsibilities in paediatric surgery at the WGH were still with Mr Mason Brown, senior consultant surgeon to the RHSC (and a President of the Royal College of Surgeons of Edinburgh). Later, Mr Kirkland was appointed consultant and undertook most of the paediatric surgery in the WGH until a second consultant paediatric surgeon was appointed.

The responsibilities of the sole consultant paediatrician to the Edinburgh Northern Group of Hospitals (Dr Forfar) were extended in 1956 to include monthly outpatient clinics at both Victoria Hospital, Kirkcaldy and

Dunfermline General Hospital. In addition there was on-call consultant responsibility for the newborn in Forth Park Maternity Hospital, Kirkcaldy and Dunfermline Maternity Hospital (as well as routine monthly visits). As there was no Forth Road Bridge at that time, visits to these hospitals or a call-out by day meant the use of the Forth ferry, with the long waits which that involved. Later, when the ferrymen got to know the 'Fife children's doctor' they would call him to the front of the ferry queue, no matter its length. A procedure which not infrequently evoked sullen scowls from those who had counted the number of cars in front of them and had calculated that they would catch the next ferry. A crisis at night when there was no ferry, usually in one of the neonatal units, meant round trips of 108 miles to Kirkcaldy or 78 miles to Dunfermline via the Kincardine Bridge. In one severe winter a spade and sacking had to be included in the medical equipment. This very large clinical load carried by one consultant continued for four years until a second consultant was appointed.

Dr J. O. Forfar continued as senior paediatric physician until his appointment to the Chair of Child Life and Health of the University of Edinburgh in 1964. His place was taken by Dr Alex J. Keay who had previously been Senior Paediatric Registrar at the WGH and had been appointed as the second consultant to the unit in 1960. Dr James Syme joined the unit as consultant in 1964 and became senior consultant when Dr Keay retired in 1984. For a short period in 1964 Dr David G. D. Barr was a third consultant before moving to the RHSC. Dr Patricia A. Russel was appointed as part-time consultant in 1977 and retired in 1987. In 1984 Dr Alan J. Burt joined the staff as consultant paediatrician.

Dr Keay was to be, at separate times, Secretary and Treasurer of the Royal College of Physicians of Edinburgh. Dr James Syme was also Secretary and then Vice-President of the Royal College of Physicians of Edinburgh.

Because of its pre 1948 association with the Public Health Department of Maternity and Child Welfare, it seemed natural that the paediatric department at the Western should develop a close relationship with Clinical Medical Officers from that Department. Dr Ruth Graham-Youll was therefore given an appointment in the Unit. There was also a close relationship with local general practitioners, many of whom were regular visitors to the unit and its weekly meetings. It was usual for social workers, physiotherapists, dietitians and others to attend ward rounds and demonstrations. Teachers and occupational therapists were involved in the school and playroom associated with the medical and surgical paediatric wards. Unrestricted visiting was introduced long before it was generally accepted in other childrens' units. The common practice in 1950, as seen in the WGH, was for the parents of hospitalised children to be banned from visiting for a week on the assumption that the child would settle down more quickly if he or she was temporarily separated from parents. Thereafter only two visits per week at fixed hours were allowed. Psychological research was indicating, however, that such separation from parents could result in long-lasting post-hospitalisation behaviour disturbance. Early in this period free visiting at all times was introduced into the medical paediatric ward at the WGH. The concept developed that parents were a valuable part of the team looking after their child. This practice was very successful and is now widely accepted. Later, when cubicles were established, it was possible in some instances to admit a mother with her child when she so wished. In all these developments, the medical staff were strongly supported and at times led by senior members of the nursing staff who had trained both in children's and general nursing.

With the increasing development of intensive care for premature and sick newborn babies, more of the effort and resources of the unit were applied to the newborn nurseries. Close cooperation with the obstetric and midwifery staff resulted in paediatricians taking an active part in ante-natal preparation classes and in counselling expectant mothers concerned about their offspring.

Of the postgraduate students attached to the unit, at least three are Professors in Paediatrics. Junior members of the paediatric staff who served in the WGH paediatric unit between 1950 and 1964 include Dr George Maxwell, who was later appointed Professor of Paediatrics in Adelaide, Australia, and Dr Maurice Kibel, who became Professor of Child Health in the University of Capetown. Among those who served in the associated paediatric units in Leith and the Eastern General Hospital were Dr James Knox was later appointed as Professor of General Practice in Dundee and Dr Hamish Simpson, Professor of Paediatrics in Leicester. At least 14 of those who were paediatric SHO's, Registrars or Senior Registrars in the WGH during this period became consultant paediatricians.

Paediatric Teaching

On the appointment of Dr Forfar in 1950, one of the undergraduate paediatric teaching 'cliniques' was allocated to the WGH, and a quarter of the undergraduate paediatric clinical teaching took place there. Dr Forfar was appointed Honorary Senior Lecturer in the Department of Child Life and Health in 1954.

The unit played a full part in teaching within the programme of the Edinburgh Postgraduate Board for Medicine and regularly participated in examination for Membership of the Royal College of Physicians.

From 1950 onwards a scheme of postgraduate attachments to the paediatric unit at the WGH was established. Mostly it was overseas students who took advantage of these attachments, together with the occasional local general practitioners. Among those attached from overseas were Dr Wong Hock Boon, who became Professor of Paediatrics in Singapore, Dr Abd El Khalik Khattab who became Professor of Paediatrics in Ein Shams University, Cairo and Dr So Singh Manchands who became Professor of Paediatrics in Amritsar, India.

The paediatric staff have not confined their activities to the Western General Hospital alone but have been involved in medical education in many parts of the world including, Saudi Arabia, Dubai, India, Malaysia, Singapore, Hong Kong etc. Some of these activities were arranged through the University, others through the Western General Hospital and the Colleges.

Research

During this period a number of active research programmes were pursued in the paediatric unit at the WGH. These involved neonatal staphylococcal infection — so prevalent at that time — congenital abnormalities, urinary tract infection and metabolic problems such as neonatal hypoglycaemia, neonatal hyperbilirubinaemia and idiopathic hypercalcaemia. Arising from the research work carried out in the paediatric unit during this period, over 50 papers were published, two postgraduate students obtained PhDs and at least three members of staff obtained MDs.

Later research by the unit was primarily related to children beyond infancy and concerned subjects such as hypercalcaemia and urinary tract infection. With increasing attention being paid to the newborn, research was carried out on such subjects as neonatal staphylococcal infection, congenital abnormalities, hypoglycaemia and neonatal hyperbilirubinaemia. With the cooperation of Dr Neil McLean of the Pathology Department, pioneer studies were carried out on the incidence of sex chromosome abnormalities in a newborn population using the buccal smear technique. With the development of facilities for chromosome studies in the Medical Research Council Cytogenetic Unit, a long term study of all chromosome abnormalities in a large newborn population was instituted. Dr Shirley Ratcliffe was appointed, first as senior registrar then as consultant paediatrician, to coordinate the large amount of research work and follow-up involved. This work continues and has received international acclaim.

Paediatric Ward Accommodation

In 1950 the accommodation available in the WGH for paediatric patients was most unsatisfactory. The unit was often overcrowded. There were no proper bathing facilities for babies and younger children. A galvanised bath was filled by carrying it over to a tap and when filled was supported on unsteady collapsible legs. There were no cubicles in which infected infants or infants particularly susceptible to infection could be isolated. In 1950 an Edinburgh doctor declared to the newly appointed Western General Hospital paediatrician that he wouldn't have his dog admitted to that hospital. It is satisfactory to record that some years later he was admitting his child patients to the hospital.

The facilities for the newborn were particularly inadequate with no suitable resuscitative equipment, no isolation facilities, no incubators, no proper arrangements for the preparation of milk feeds and no designated paediatric staff. Most of these deficiencies were remedied, albeit slowly. Four cubicles were created and other appropriate structural adaptations made, proper baths installed, a milk kitchen established, and equipment progressively improved.

To extend the accommodation, the upper half of a staircase, a back entrance to the paediatric unit, was closed at the first floor level. The space was used for a sister's room, which extended across the stairway. This had an unexpected consequence. A registrar was appointed who had been a resident in the WGH some five years before but had been in the United States in the interval. A little late for the first morning of his new duties he dashed up the familiar back stair.

Consultation in the sister's room between resident, consultant and ward sister was suddenly disturbed by an ominous bump from below and a perceptible heave of the floor. A few moments later a stunned new registrar holding the crown of his head appeared for duty at the head of the normal stair!

Premature babies needed adequate incubators and higher environmental temperature and humidity. A somewhat singular 'hot room' was created by installing extra heating in a small room and at the same time leading steam into the room. This was very effective in creating a monitored, warm, humid environment but one which was unpleasant to work in. Nurses, on starting in this environment, found it very trying although they became acclimatised to it. On one occasion, a black postgraduate doctor from the Congo, participating in a teaching session in the 'hot room', complained that he would have to leave because he could not stand the heat! Despite so many inadequacies, the fact that the unit consisted of several small wards rather than a single large one was an advantage from a paediatric point of view because it was possible to provide wards for different age groups.

The narrow, ramifying, maze-like corridors of the WGH also proved an advantage on at least one occasion when the hospital received a formal visit from the Scottish Under-Secretary of State for Health. The complaint that the amount of paediatric accommodation was inadequate was in danger of being discounted because, quite unusually, one of the wards was empty. After propelling the Secretary of State through the occupied wards, round the corridors and through some of the ancillary accommodation he was led out of the unit, not through the empty ward, but through one of the occupied wards already visited. His comments about this ward and the unit's occupancy indicated that he did not realise that he had been through the same ward twice.

Paediatric Practice

The 1950s and early 1960s saw many changes in paediatric practice. The advent of antibiotics allowed the treatment of infection in a more effective manner hence reducing the erstwhile major cause of death in childhood. Tuberculosis was still common but was increasingly coming under control as a result of mass miniature radiography and effective anti-tuberculosis drugs. Other striking therapeutic advances included the use of a gluten-free diet in coeliac disease and the diagnosis of phenylketonuria at birth with effective dietetic prevention. Rheumatic fever was still a problem but a diminishing one. In 1950 the average survival time for a child with acute lymphatic leukaemia was six weeks but the first hints were appearing that effective treatment might become possible in the future. Congenital abnormalities remained a major problem, although screening procedures, such as that for congenital dislocation of the hips, were becoming available. Better surgical techniques, for example with congenital pyloric stenosis and cleft lip began to improve the outlook for some children. New diseases, such as idiopathic hypercalcaemia, were appearing and old ones such as pink disease were disappearing.

Perhaps the major charge in this period was the development of a virtually new branch of paediatrics, neonatal paediatrics. The previous arrangement whereby only seriously ill infants were transferred from obstetric care to paediatric care gave way to total care of all newborn infants by paediatricians. The paediatrician now had an important place in the delivery room and the maternity nursery. The practice of screening medical examinations for all newborn infants was established and new therapeutic procedures, such as exchange transfusion for infants suffering from icterus gravis neonatorum, were introduced. More careful long-term appraisals of neonatal management procedures were now being conducted. These showed how vulnerable the fetus and newborn infant were and how dangerous in the long-term were some treatments which in the short-term appeared advantageous. The increasing and mostly beneficial use of oxygen in the treatment of neonatal asphyxia was shown to cause retrolental fibroplasia with permanent blindness in the low birthweight infant. Thalidomide, an apparently safe drug, was widely prescribed to pregnant mothers. The drug turned out to be highly harmful to the fetus — recognised as such only after an inevitable latent period. During this many fetuses became affected. Thus the significant advances in neonatal paediatrics in this period were not, unfortunately, without some attendant tragedies. The neonatal unit at the WGH played its part in advancing neonatal paediatrics but inevitably did not escape some of the tragedies.

The municipal hospital status which the WGH held before the inception of the NHS remained a continuing advantage with a specially close relationship between the WGH paediatric unit and the municipal Maternity and Child Welfare and the School Health Service. Liaison health visitors attached to the paediatric unit played an important part in maintaining this relationship.

Unlike the trainee nursing staff at the RHSC who were training specifically for the Sick Children's Nurse Certificate, the nurses at the WGH were trained in general nursing. To offset this the senior nursing staff recruited to the medical paediatric ward at the WGH after 1950 were holders of certificates both in sick children's nursing and general nursing.

The structure of the wards at the Western General Hospital allowed separation of children by age groups so that it was possible to accommodate teenagers. Because of the close relation with adult wards it was easier to arrange for the long-term management and transfer of children with continuing problems. For some such as those with diabetes, joint outpatient clinics were established. Special outpatient clinics for those with cardiac or growth problems included appropriate specialist consultant cover. Dr Forfar's interest in medical aspects of adoption was taken up by Dr Keay who established a special adoption clinic believed to be the first of its kind.

1950 was in many ways not only the mid-point of the century but also a dividing point between the period when so much of the hospital care of children was in the hands of those whose primary interest was in adults. Their successors were doctors who devoted their professional lives to children. The concept that children could be treated as little adults was abandoned. It was recognised that as infants and children grow, both in body and mind, that they have specific physiological and disease characteristics and a different psychological make-up. Different investigative and therapeutic procedures are required and necessitate specific training, experience and research. With the coming of the NHS, the paediatric unit at the WGH was established to take account of these new developments and played a significant part in implementing them in Edinburgh.

With reorganisation of obstetric and paediatric services in 1991, both the maternity and paediatric services at the WGH were closed, bringing to an end a service which had served a wide geographic area, including Fife and which was held in high regard both locally and internationally.

Although the unit is no longer active there are many former patients, some now themselves grandparents, who can testify to the benefit they received from the paediatric departments at the WGH. Equally significant are the numbers of paediatricians and general practitioners who remember with gratitude the training which they received in this unit. Above all people remember G 7–10 as a happy unit.

Paediatric Surgery

In the fifties and sixties Paediatric surgery was confined to Children's Hospital where the first pure paediatric surgeon was James Mason Brown. Children in the Western General were seen by adult surgeons with an interest in children and included such surgeons as Ian Aird. Mason Brown, although primarily associated with the Children's Hospital would see patients at the Western. The other paediatric surgeons later to be associated with Mason Brown were Frederick Robarts and Rosamund Mackay who also had patients in Leith Hospital.

Ian Kirkland was the first surgeon appointed to the Western with a prime interest in paediatrics. Ian was very much on his own at the Western with Rosie Mackay and Fred Robarts being mainly in the Children's Hospital. Willie Bisset followed Rosie Mackay and worked in both Leith and the Children's Hospital.

Mr William Scobie's appointment in 1971 resulted in four pure paediatric surgeons in Edinburgh. Two, namely Mr Robarts and Mr Bisset, being based in the Childrens Hospital, and Mr Bill Scobie and Mr Ian Kirkland being based in the Western and Leith.

The paediatric surgical unit at the Western was in wards G3–6 and consisted of 25 cots, with beds in two wards and three separate cubicles for babies. The unit was closely associated with the medical paediatric unit on the same floor in G 7–10 and the nursery along in the Obstetric department.

In the early seventies the unit at the Western dealt with all aspects of children's surgery including neonates. All trauma including orthopaedics was dealt with by the paediatric staff. There was a very close relationship between the medical and surgical paediatric staff with outpatient clinics being held at the same time. Medical students spent 10 weeks between the two units.

The surgical staff at the Western also looked after the children in Leith Hospital where traditionally children from West Fife were admitted. There were

20 surgical beds in Leith with a medical unit of similar size. Emergencies were admitted to the Western, Leith, and the Children's Hospital on a rotational arrangement. Both Bill Scobie and Ian Kirkland in the seventies undertook elective plastic surgery including cleft lip and palate, elective orthopaedics including talipes and Congenital Dislocated Hip. Spina bifida was relatively common and was a cause of frequent admissions to the surgical unit. There was no medical oncology in those days so solid tumours were treated by the paediatric surgeons who also managed the chemotherapy.

Ian Kirkland was primarily interested in urology. He was an early pioneer of urodynamics and the study and investigation of the neurogenic bladder often seen in the spina bifida patient. Bill Scobie was interested in gastroenterology, especially Hirschsprung's disease.

In the last 20 years the structure of paediatric surgery in the Western has changed considerably.

In 1976 it was agreed to centralise the surgery of the newborn in the Children's Hospital. This reflected the fall in the number of babies presenting with surgical conditions and the need to concentrate expertise in one centre. The antenatal diagnosis of spina bifida saw this problem gradually disappear. The consequence was that the need for spina bifida clinics disappeared. By 1979 the management of the few babies appearing with spina bifida and hydrocephalus was given over entirely to the neurosurgeons. The trend in recent years has been to refer children with orthopaedic problems to orthopaedic surgeons and the few cleft lips and palates to plastic surgeons. Children with tumours now go to oncologists rather than paediatric surgeons.

The main change in paediatric surgical practice in the last ten to 15 years is a move towards more and more day case surgery. In 1975, 5% of operations were day cases whereas now almost 60% are treated in this manner. This has had a marked effect on bed occupancy and the need for inpatient beds. Coincidental with a fall in the need for inpatient medical paediatric beds, the unit in Leith was no longer required and closed in 1986. The result was a centralisation of all paediatrics on the north side of the city in the Western.

In spite of the loss of beds in Leith, the number of patients attending the Western remained constant mainly due to the expansion of outreach clinics in Dunfermline, West Lothian and East Lothian.

Ian Kirkland retired in 1984 to be succeeded by John Orr. Ian Kirkland had been Chairman of the clinical staff at the Western, during which time he was responsible for a new residency being built for house officers.

In 1990, under the Lothian Health Board's options for change it was proposed to move all inpatient paediatrics to the Children's Hospital. Medical paediatrics moved first followed by surgical paediatrics in 1991. The Children's Hospital did not have enough accommodation to deal with all surgical patients so a purpose-built Day Case Unit was established in the Western incorporated in G3–6. This had ten beds in one ward with the other ward being mainly a large playroom. There were a few additional beds to cater for children coming to the Western for such procedures as radiotherapy, CAT scans, MRI etc. The

Day Case Unit was opened in August 1991 to provide a service for children from the whole of Edinburgh, Fife, West and East Lothian. The result was a very successful unit. With the establishment of Trust status, plans were drawn up to centralise all paediatric surgery in the Childrens Hospital. By the end of 1994 the Day Case Unit at the Western had closed and all paediatric surgery was transferred to the Children's Hospital. The only paediatric service that remains in the Western is an outpatient service.

Pathology Department

The department was founded in 1954 and housed in the two-storey red-brick building on Porterfield Road. Dr J. Murray Drennan (son of Prof Murray Drennan) was appointed consultant-in-charge. Mr Stanley Hay, formerly of the Royal College of Physicians' Edinburgh Laboratories was appointed chief technician. In 1958 Dr Neil MacLean joined the department, initially as Senior Hospital Medical Officer, later Consultant. Formerly there had been a registrar post (including Dr John Webb, 1963–65). In 1969 Dr John Webb was appointed as the third consultant. Dr Anthony Busuttil was appointed consultant when Dr Neil MacLean retired in 1976. When Dr Drennan retired in 1979 Dr Webb became Head of Department and Dr Margaret McIntyre was appointed Consultant.

Dr McIntyre's arrival resulted in a great expansion in the cytology service and she was instrumental in pioneering the introduction of the Fine Needle Aspirate technique at the hospital. Dr Alastair M. Lessells was appointed consultant in 1984 when Dr Anne Le Roux (assistant pathologist) left to become a Consultant in Banbury, Oxon. Dr Jeremy St J. Thomas was appointed Consultant in 1988 when Dr Anthony Busuttil was appointed Regius Professor of Forensic Medicine.

Major building programme in the old building was completed in 1981 to accommodate additional laboratories to cope with the rapidly expanding workload.

In 1988 the department moved to new laboratory accommodation in the Alexander Donald Building. In 1993 there was an amalgamation of Pathology and Neuropathology into a 'new' Department of Pathology with Dr John N. Webb, Head of Department and Mr Robert J. L. Green as Senior Chief MLSO. The presence of Neuropathology at the WGH dates from the late 1970s. Formerly located in the RIE, (Consultants Drs Anthony F. J. Maloney and Alexander Gordon) it moved to accommodation in DSN and then to the Alexander Donald Building in 1988. Currently consultants in Neuropathology are Drs Jeanne E. Bell, James W. Ironside and George A. Lammie.

The Pathology Department has always maintained close links with the clinical Services (Medicine, Surgery, GI Gynaecology, Oncology etc). This is reflected in the large numbers of regular meetings held with clinical colleagues and the numerous published papers on clinically related research. These meetings and close clinical contact had their origins in the regular fortnightly pathology meetings with the combined Medical:Surgical Gastrointestinal Department. The original meetings were held in the lecture theatre of the Teaching and Research Unit. The pathologist discussed a series of slides based on the previous fortnight's work. They would come from surgery and increasingly endoscopic biopsies. The pathologist used a carbon light system to project the microscopic slide through the microscope onto a screen. This was the only uncertainty of the meetings. A combination of hope and inspiration would suddenly be rewarded with the expansion of a cellular structure onto a screen. The present meeting takes place in the comfort of the pathology department seminar room. The microscopic picture is transmitted electronically onto two television screens with breathtaking clarity. A feature of all of these clinical/pathological meetings is the friendship and good-natured exchanges resulting from years of discussing complex and demanding diagnostic problems. The reward has always been the achievement of the highest possible standard of diagnostic service.

There are now plans for yet another move to a proposed new laboratory block on the site. This is part of an integration of the many changes anticipated at the Western General Hospital as part of the Lothian Acute Services Strategy.

Psychiatry

(Liaison Psychiatry)
The fundamental fact of liaison psychiatry, on which all other elements depend, is that the patient is not primarily the psychiatrist's. The patient is referred by another hospital physician, or surgeon or gynaecologist, who retains primary clinical responsibility. The psychiatrist is therefore, although invited, a clinical intruder. Sometimes presented to a patient on sufferance which carries complex professional implications.

The conditions and technical responsibilities to be established, if a psychiatry liaison service is to succeed, must ensure that the psychiatrist can be viewed as helpful. Even when his contribution may turn out to be in respects contrary to the position taken by the primary clinician. He must be positively regarded as a colleague, which occurs only when he has convincingly demonstrated the validity of his subject. Psychiatry, for reasons which may emerge; is still viewed by some as a suspect branch of medicine.

Psychiatrists, therefore, to be clinically effective have to establish themselves as equal among peers. It is therefore hopelessly inadequate for the psychiatrist to view his contribution in the hospital to be only clinical. He has to take part in the administrative structure of the hospital, and indeed in the health services for the total district which the hospital serves. He has to be a partner with his colleagues in planning and conducting medical education. As late as the 1990s, there was much pride that some teaching areas have been equipped in the Edinburgh Faculty of Medicine with feedback lecture rooms. In fact, they were already in use in the teaching unit at the Western in the 1970s. The psychiatrist has also to be socially acceptable, and hence requires to meet the associations and the friendly relations customary among consultants. It is thus evident that the liaison psychiatrist has to be 'on campus' in the most total sense. It does not do in the least for him to edge in unobtrusively from another sector (the psychiatric hospital, say), to materialise episodically, and then disappear. Liaisòn psychiatry depends on continuing, sophisticated, subtle, ongoing, professional interaction and clinical dialogue. The liaison psychiatrist cannot resort to the jargon of psychiatry, but must confer in the language of the other physicians (that is where general medical competence is pertinent). Once his technical reports obfuscate the clinical realities, as the other physicians see them, the purported liaison evaporates.

Psychiatry at the Western in the 1960s

A single psychiatrist operated at the Western prior to, and just into the '60s: Dr William McConnachie Harrows. He was manifestly knowledgeable: he had written a book *Human Person* in 1948, but he had to operate at the negative end of all the elements of liaison psychiatry just specified. He had other work, and would visit the Western only at night, unseen by any clinical colleagues other than night nurses. Referral notes would be left for him in a particular tray. The only sign that he had responded by visiting a ward or seeing an inpatient was evident only from a note left in the same tray when he departed. It was said that he 'padded about' in carpet slippers as a wraith or a spectre. Yet he was a good psychiatrist, coping in a difficult situation.

Feeders

The initiative to develop psychiatry at the Western was taken by Dr Wilfrid Card and his colleagues in the Department of Medicine, John Strong, John Macleod, Michael Matthews, and others. After a number of private discussions with these colleagues, Henry Walton was asked to a working lunch at the University Staff Club with Dr Card and his fellow physicians. The proposal was that he should start a Department of Psychiatry at the Western. Walton was then Senior Lecturer in the University Department of Psychiatry; his main assignments at the Royal Edinburgh Hospital were to set up a unit for treatment of alcoholism. No such unit existed in Scotland at the time, and to carry out a large research project into the teaching of psychiatry.

When accepting the Western assignment, he understood it was to be a major commitment, with the mutual undertaking that it would steadily expand and be enduring. He opened an outpatient department in the Paderewski. Approval was given by the University and Health Board to progressively increase the clinical staff by bringing over colleagues working at the Professorial Unit of the Royal Edinburgh Hospital. There was a gradual build-up of consultant psychiatrists, psychiatrists in training, clinical psychologists, psychiatric social workers, and secretaries etc. The concept adopted made the Western the centre for liaison psychiatry in North Edinburgh, for example, the Superintendent of Bangour Hospital came on the staff and conducted outpatient clinics. The surrounding general practices were systematically contacted and given a psychiatric service. Any patients from these practices treated while in-patients at the Western, were followed up from the Psychiatric Department when they were discharged from hospital.

A serious weakness always was (and emphatically still is) that there is no psychiatric inpatient unit at the Western General Hospital. Edinburgh is characterised by there being no inpatient Psychiatric unit in the Royal Infirmary or the Western: students can gain the impression that decanting into a psychiatric hospital is a normal and customary stratagem. That physical and psychiatric illnesses frequently coexist could remain disregarded. Any Western patient requiring inpatient psychiatric care was spirited away to Professor Walton's or another ward in the Royal Edinburgh Hospital Professorial Unit. For all practical purposes (except for a few interested clinicians) these patients thereupon almost ceased to exist. How they progressed, and what caused them to recover or deteriorate remained a mystery.

Method of Work

The main evidence of psychiatry at the Western came from the *Ward Meetings*. It is perhaps not an exaggeration to say these *Ward Meetings* became famous. In time they were attended not only by the Physician (or Surgeon) Consultant and his full team, with the full psychiatric team also present, but by general practitioners and other visitors concerned with the patient in question or simply interested or curious. The meetings were always held in the ward of the Physician or Surgeon. A mighty effort was required to have the ward senior nurses present also. They, as well as occupational therapists, social workers, etc. required convincing that it was not a waste of valuable time. The convention had to become established that the occasion warranted such concentration of staff, and such intellectual commitment. Ward meetings were held with Dr John Macleod in the first place, and then with Dr Michael Matthews, Dr Arthur Kitchin, and others. An unwritten rule on which the psychiatrists operated was that the Consultants would no doubt remain sceptical, but the junior staff could be expected to perceive psychiatric realities and would be influenced. The adage of William James was not forgotten that: 'by the age of 30 years the mind is set as if in concrete, and will never soften again'. These ward meetings were the occasion for the psychiatrist to do his work in public.

Often there was much evasion and even opposition, when he insisted that the patient also join the ward meeting when the clinical findings could to be demonstrated. Psychiatric interviews were conducted publicly, and relatives were also brought in where relevant. The procedure became nationally known through the publication in *The Lancet*: Macleod, J. & Walton, H. J. (1969). 'Liaison between Physicians and Psychiatrists in a Teaching Hospital'.

The paper remains a classic in this field. Many other publications emerged, particularly as the Registrars in Psychiatry attached to the Western increasingly based their M.Phil theses on general hospital subjects.

Particularly exciting and eventful was the liaison with the Gastro-intestinal Unit, initiated by Dr Bill Sircus and Mr Charles Falconer. The meetings were held in the lecture room in the Teaching Unit. Hilarity was usual: a brave campaign was waged to convince these combined surgeon-and-physician meetings that, in psychiatry, a biographical detail ('his father wanted him to be a girl') was as significant clinically, potentially, as a physical sign (e.g. a palpable liver).

Full Recognition

The Psychiatry Department moved from its initial poorhouse accommodation into the new Outpatient Building. When, good fortune for psychiatry, the Venereal Disease Unit was located on another site. It was thought beneficial, by some, that the windows stopped above head level, and what went on would not be evident from the outside.

In addition to proper accommodation, a Second University Chair of Psychiatry was established and, although the designation was feebly contested, was accepted to be based at the Western.

Solid progress was made. A letter to the District Medical Officer, dated 15 August 1974, could refer Dr Ferguson to the following ten points:

1. Northern Division of Psychiatry established, H. J. Walton as Chairman and A. K. Zealley as Secretary.
2. Administrative charge: the Department of Psychiatry was an academic department and provided active outpatient services for all patients from North Edinburgh, with an active ward liaison service.
3. Development was continued of the academic outpatient suite, first floor, Phase 1 building.
4. Social worker posts were established, based on the Psychiatry Department.
5. Clinical psychologist posts administratively with the Department were established.
6. Outpatient facilities for psychiatrists not on the staff of Western General Hospital were provided: e.g. Dr Sam Robinson, attached to the Royal Victoria Hospital, and Dr Lyndon Murray, Consultant appointed in 1975 to the REH required their status at the Western Department to be clarified.
7. Records: psychiatric case notes needed to be filed separately from the Western Case Record Department, and for this purpose the Royal Edinburgh Hospital Records Department liaised with that of the Western.
8. In-patient facility. The very pressing need for psychiatric beds at the Western were to have been provided by a psychiatric in-patient provision in Phase II of the Western building programme, regarded as an urgent necessity since 1962.
9. Specialist Advisory Group in Psychiatry: The University of Edinburgh Department of Psychiatry supervised post graduate training for the Lothian, the Borders, Forth Valley and Fife. Edinburgh University was second only to the Mawdsley Hospital at the University of London in

the size of its psychiatric training programme. Registrars in Psychiatry rotated to work for planned periods at the Western General Hospital.

10. *Royal Victoria Psychiatric Centre* A Day Psychiatric Centre was planned and now operates at the Royal Victoria Hospital.

Aftermath

Professor Henry Walton retired as Professor of Psychiatry at the Western General Hospital on becoming Professor of International Medical Education (and President of the World Federation for Medical Education) in the '80s. By all accounts, the story since then has been one of steady decline, attributable as much to diminishing concern by the physicians and surgeons at the Western General Hospital as to psychiatric withdrawal of commitment. The present position could have been different had the Western Clinical Staff insisted that without Liaison Psychiatry, up to contemporary standards, their clinical service was deficient. There has even been an understanding, bruited abroad, that of late, Western patients showing any psychiatric component are referred to their general practitioners from some clinical firms at the Western.

Radiology

Dr Hunter Cummack was appointed in 1947 as Consultant Radiologist to the Edinburgh Corporation based at the Western General Hospital. He was also Radiologist to the Northern General Hospital, Eastern General Hospital, City Hospital and Gogarburn. Those commitments remained unchanged at the inception of the National Health Service in 1948. Today there are eleven Consultant Radiologists staffing these hospitals. In 1948 the X-ray department was in a room off the main hospital corridor. It consisted of one X-ray room with two tables, one horizontal and the other erect, the patient having to be moved from one to the other if supine and erect films were required. Today there are 24 X-ray rooms. The dark room had no ventilation. The film processor was made by a local joiner. The films were dried by hanging them from a washing line attached to the ceiling. There were two mobile units, one of which was United States army surplus stock.

There was a waiting room for patients, part of which was screened off with a mobile screen and this served as the radiologist's office and reporting room. There were no toilet facilities in the department. Patients who had experienced a barium enema examination had then to go to a toilet down the main hospital corridor. When Dr Cummack requested toilet facilities for these patients, he was advised by Hospital Board officials that patients should use a bucket in the X-ray room.

In 1948 the department was staffed by two radiographers, Mrs Bell, the senior radiographer and Miss Johnstone and two student radiographers. Today there is a complement of 42 radiographers. In 1953 a second X-ray room was added and Miss K. Fegan succeeded Mrs Bell as superintendent radiographer.

In 1955 Dr Norman Thomson took over the radiological service at the

Eastern General and City Hospitals from Dr Cummack. Dr William A. Copland was appointed the following year to cover the radiotherapy diagnostic X-ray work, at the Northern General Hospital and the increasing volume of work at the Western General Hospital. In succeeding years the department continued to grow in size so that by 1968 there were five X-ray rooms, a new dark room with automatic film processing and two radiologists' offices. In 1971 the main department moved into new premises with 16 X-ray rooms in phase I. In 1969 Dr Cummack published his much acclaimed work '*Gastrointestinal X-Ray Diagnosis*'.

Over the next two decades the specialty advanced rapidly. An ultrasound service initiated by Dr Sinclair in 1973 was carried on and expanded by Dr Roger Wild. The nuclear medicine service which was initially based in the DSN X-ray department was taken over by Dr Malcolm Merrick from his appointment in 1974. The Western General was the first centre in the UK to use nuclear medicine techniques in the investigation of children with urinary infections and these techniques are now generally accepted. Another important nuclear medicine innovation was SeHCAT used in the diagnosis of diarrhoea. In 1986 the first mitral balloon valvuloplasty in the UK was performed by Dr T. R. D. Shaw and Dr Turnbull.

Following Dr Cummack's retiral in 1977, the Gastrointestinal Radiological Service was provided by Dr Martin Fraser who made an extensive contribution to the literature on double contrast barium radiology.

Internationally acclaimed radiology has been developed by Dr Douglas Grieve in the main department and this has included renal and splenic embolisation, renal angioplasty and percutaneous biliary drainage. At DCN Dr Robin Sellar has developed interventional radiological techniques treating arterio venous malformations with glue and particles, carotid cavernous fistulas with balloons and aneurysms with coils. ERCP techniques were introduced by Mr John H. Saunders and Dr John Cruickshank and continued by Dr Kelvin Palmer and Dr Douglas Grieve. A general practitioner open access service was introduced in the early 1970s. In the late 1980s film reporting and patient appointments in the department were placed on computerised systems. In 1992 a body CT scanning service was established in the main department and an MRI service was set up in the hospital.

In 1992 there were also major administrative changes, Dr Wild being appointed as clinical director and Mrs Louise Abrahams as Business Manager.

Radiologists

Dr D. H. Cummack	(1947–77)
Dr W. A. Copland	(1956–85)
Dr A. A. Donaldson	(1957–1986)
Dr G. M. Fraser	(1968–91)
Dr D. J. Sinclair	(1970–75)
Dr G. T. Vaughan	(1970–
Dr J. G. Cruickshank	(1973–93)

Dr M. V. Merrick	(1974–
Dr S. R. Wild	(1975–
Dr D. C. Grieve	(1978–
Dr C. M. Turnbull	(1979–
Dr S. Mackenzie	(1985–1989)
Dr A. J. M. Stevenson	(1989–
Dr A. R. Wright	(1992–

Superintendent Radiographers

Mrs Bell	(?–1953)
Miss K. Fegan	(1953–79)
Mrs L. S. Abrahams	(1979–

Renal Transplant Unit

The Renal Transplant Unit owes its origin to the work of Professor Sir Michael Woodruff FRS and Dr James Robson in the Royal Infirmary. Professor Woodruff had been Professor of Surgery at the Medical School of the University of Otago in Dunedin, New Zealand. He was appointed to the Chair of Surgical Science in 1957. He had a distinguished background in transplantation and on arrival in the chair considered the time suitable for the transplantation of a kidney. However the conservatism of the Edinburgh of that day required success. Therefore he waited for identical twins. It happened that a patient with terminal uraemia was used in the membership examination. He was asked by a candidate in that exam, who had heard a lecture on transplantation by Professor Woodruff, if he, the patient, had a twin. This turned out to be the case. The AB blood groups were equivalent; the twins looked alike and finger printing reported in the press to be identical. The chief constable was alarmed by this but was reassured by Sir Michael, that while the finger prints showed areas which were identical, there were other areas that were markedly different. The skin grafts were interchanged between the two men and survived indefinitely. A kidney from one brother was transplanted into the other without immuno suppression. It worked. Curiously enough, both brothers died with carcinoma of the stomach some five years later.

Another curious story of that first operation is that a distinguished urologist scrubbed up for the operation. Whilst Professor Woodruff went through to the other room to pick up the recipient kidney, the colleague felt in the pelvis and felt a mass. He declared that the patient had a carcinoma of the bladder. This turned out to be the inflated balloon of a Foley catheter.

The next transplant at the Royal Infirmary was between a brother and sister who were compatible in many respects. The only way to prevent rejection at that time was whole-body irradiation. The radiation however proved to be too much and the recipient died of infection.

One of the next patients was a young boy of eleven whose father offered his kidney. In many respects they were identical for the blood groups and HLA factors. At the same time the distinguished transplanter, Dr Joseph Murray, came to Edinburgh and was a guest of Professor Woodruff at the Annual Meeting of the Association of Surgeons of Britain and Ireland in Swansea. It was raining during the meeting and Professor Woodruff was wearing his overcoat. When he checked it in, he was given a tag bearing the number 322. Dr Murray looked with amazement because Burroughs Welcome 322 was the name of a new drug they were using for transplantation. This was used with the young man and the kidney has lasted until the present day.

Transplantation took place in rather inadequate surroundings at the Royal Infirmary. At that stage, whilst azathioprine was the treatment of choice, it was felt that it would be better to be closer to the radiotherapy in the Western General Hospital. Professor Woodruff had developed a new method to reduce the lymphocyte originating rejection of the implant. Antilymphocyte serum was made, which was an heterologous serum produced in horses, but this was only used in combination with other agents.

Professor Woodruff approached the Nuffield Foundation, who gave £100,000 to build a unit. He gave this sum to the South East of Scotland Regional Health Board on condition that six nurses were provided and two junior doctors. He approached the Regional Board Architect who felt a building with a curious function should have a curious building, and produced a circular building. This was not acceptable so Mr Womersley was invited to produce a building. This turned out to have a rough finished style, with horizontal surfaces all over the place which collected dust. This was started in 1965 and completed in 1969. By the time it was built, the use of irradiation had been abandoned. However the building provided many other facilities, insofar that there were two theatres always available, sterile rooms and an opportunity for visitors to speak to the patients without coming into contact. The building was opened by Sir Peter Medawar.

In 1960 the physicians were Dr Robson and Ann Lambie of the Royal Infirmary, helped by Dr Anderton and Dr Winnie. The surgeons were Professor Woodruff, Mr Bernard Nolan and later Mr Sandy Jenkins. The first sister was Sister Weatherspoon.

In 1971 Dr John Anderton was appointed physician to the Unit. A series of problems were identified. The first one was that the transplantation programme was in conflict with the dialysis programme at the Royal Infirmary. This programme was based on the concept that dialysis was an assured success and therefore obligatory for individuals between the ages of 15 and 60. Renal transplantation was undertaken in the extremes of age, that is under 15 and over 60. This affected the prognosis. The other group offered for transplantation were the very ill and those who had run out of arterial sites. Another problem was that the waiting list was very small. This meant that when a kidney was made available the choice of immunologically compatible subjects was small. Ideally a transplant programme should have a large waiting list so that there is a choice of compatibility.

In the first year after opening, disaster struck. A patient who was not thought suitable for long-term dialysis because of hepatitis, came to the dialysis unit and was transplanted. The consequence of this was that hepatitis swept through the transplantation team. A visiting locum registrar Dr Nick Asfiz from Greece, a lecturer in surgery, Dr John Clark FRCS, and a receptionist, Pamela Scott, in haematology all died. This was a terrible experience and put the transplantation programme out of business for at least a year. The patient who had been transplanted was probably infected by two viruses, non-A non-B, B. Professor Barry Marmion in the bacteriology department looked at the virology of this curious and deadly outbreak.

Another surgeon who was involved at this time was Mr George Abouna. Many overseas doctors were trained in the unit. Professor Woodruff retired in 1976. Professor Chisholm took over the directorship of the transplant unit and gradually the urologists at the Western General Hospital became involved. Mr David Hamer Hodges was appointed to undertake transplantation and was responsible for a vigorous recruitment of kidneys and successful transplantations.

Now the transplantation is conducted entirely by urological surgeons, Mr Tim Hargreave and Mr Gordon Smith. The procedure has now become a very straightforward process. The rejection phenomenon is contained by Cyclosporin A. Throughout this time Dr Anderton has been in charge of looking after medical aspects of the renal patients. One problem was that the patients before transplantation were dialysed in the Royal Infirmary, or in the corridor of the transplantation unit. This meant that there was very limited availability for transplantation. Then by virtue of John Anderton's vigour and that of Mrs Maida Fairbairn a kidney unit appeal was established and £300,000 raised. This enabled nine dialysis patients to be looked after in an extension of the unit. The unit was opened by the Princess of Wales. It is now possible to have 18 patients on dialysis at any one time.

At the present time the limiting factor in transplantation is the availability of kidneys. The acceptance rate is 75% but the number of people being asked is not sufficient. Nevertheless between the opening of the unit and 1994 some 800 patients have had kidney transplantations.

In 1995 the Transplantation Unit was transferred to the Royal Infirmary.

Respiratory Unit: Northern General Hospital

When Professor (now Sir John) Crofton was appointed to the Chair of Tuberculosis and Respiratory Diseases on 1 January 1952 the 400 or more beds he inherited in three hospitals were occupied by patients suffering from tuberculosis. There were no medical facilities in Edinburgh for the investigation and treatment of non-tuberculous respiratory disease. With the active support of the late Sir Stanley Davidson, a Respiratory Medicine Unit of 30 beds and an out-patient department, staffed by two consultant physicians, Professor John Crofton and Dr Ian Grant, was opened at the Northern General on 1 August 1952. The Unit was planned and organised to fulfil the following functions:

1. To provide a specialist in-patient and outpatient service for the investigation and treatment of non-tuberculous respiratory disease in the South Eastern Region of Scotland.
2. To advise on the management of in-patients with respiratory disease under the care of physicians and surgeons in other hospitals in the Region.
3. To participate in undergraduate and postgraduate teaching in the Edinburgh University Medical School.
4. To undertake clinical research.

The Unit has continued to perform these functions to the present day. Until the early 1970s its staff also provided in-patient and out-patient services at the City Hospital and the Royal Victoria Dispensary, mainly for patients with pulmonary tuberculosis.

The main events in the history of the Unit can be summarised as follows:

1953: In conjunction with Dr John Marshall (then in charge of the Neurological Unit) facilities were established for artificial ventilation, initially for acute poliomyelitis. Later an intensive care area (also used for bronchoscopy) was opened for the treatment of all types of acute respiratory failure, including severe acute asthma and respiratory failure of neurological origin.

1957: The Unit was heavily involved in the influenza outbreak which struck Edinburgh in the autumn of 1957. Extra wards had to be opened, and at one stage the two consultants had charge of 120 acute medical beds in Edinburgh.

1958: The Unit investigated a large proportion of the patients who had been found to have abnormal chest X-rays in the Edinburgh Mass Radiography Campaign.

1960: With the opening of the Professorial Respiratory Unit at the City Hospital Professor Crofton relinquished his post at the Northern General Hospital, leaving Dr Grant as the sole consultant, supported by a senior registrar. The unit, however, continued to be affiliated with the University Department of Respiratory Medicine at the City Hospital, and later also joined the University Department of Medicine at the Western General Hospital.

1968: Dr Edward Harris, from Auckland, New Zealand, was appointed as a second consultant physician, but resigned the following year, to return to a more senior post in Auckland.

1968: An 'epidemic' of deaths from asthma, most of them outside hospital, prompted the inauguration of a self-admission scheme whereby patients attending the Unit who were known to be at risk could be admitted directly to the Intensive Care Area.

1969: Dr Graham Crompton was appointed consultant physician in succession to Dr Harris. Dr Crompton played a large part in formalising and publicising the Edinburgh Emergency Asthma Admission Service (as it is now known) which became a model for similar schemes elsewhere in Britain, Australia and New Zealand.

1973: Facilities for pulmonary function measurements were expanded with the opening of a new Pulmonary Function Laboratory at the Western General Hospital under the direction of Dr Ross McHardy, and local facilities at the Northern General Hospital were upgraded.

1974: The Unit consultants took over responsibility for Respiratory Outpatient Clinics, bronchoscopic examination and in-patient consultations at Peel Hospital and Hawick Cottage Hospital in the Borders Health Board Area, and for an out-patient clinic at Edenhall Hospital, Musselburgh. The commitment in the Borders ended in 1979 when a consultant physician with a special interest in Respiratory Medicine was appointed to Peel Hospital. Clinics at Edenhall Hospital continued to be held.

1978: Dr Grant was seconded to the Chair of Medicine at the National University of Malaysia, Kuala Lumpur, for one year, at the request of the Commonwealth Fund for Technical Cooperation, and Dr Ian Paterson took his place as locum consultant.

1979: In collaboration with Professor John Smyth a Joint Oncology Clinic was established at the Northern General Hospital to supervise the use of chemotherapy in the treatment of lung cancer.

1984: Dr Grant retired and was replaced by Dr Andrew Greening.

1991: The Unit was transferred from the Northern to the Western General Hospital.

1992: An Adult Cystic Fibrosis Service Centre funded by the Scottish Office was set up.

1993: Dr J. Alastair Innes was appointed as additional consultant funded by the National Cystic Fibrosis Service Contract.

Research and publications

Members of the Unit have published extensively in scientific journals and the number now exceeds 250 articles in medical journals since 1952. These report original work on a wide range of subjects including the treatment of bronchial asthma with bronchodilators, oral and inhaled corticosteroids and sodium cromoglycate, the problem of corticosteroid resistance, the prevention of deaths from severe acute asthma, antibiotic therapy in chronic bronchitis and pneumonia, extrinsic allergic alveolitis, fibrosing alveolitis, fungal infections of the lung, pulmonary eosinophilia, bronchopulmonary aspergillosis, treatment of bronchial carcinoma, artificial ventilation for neurological diseases and bronchoscopic examination.

In addition, past and present members of the Respiratory Unit have been authors of 15 chapters in textbooks and one book.

Rheumatology

It is probably true to say that rheumatology, as a subdivision of general internal medicine, remained a rather poorly defined specialty well into the early decades of the present century. Just before the Second World War, however, the Empire

Rheumatism Council was established to encourage education and research into the rheumatic diseases. Edinburgh was perhaps fortunate that the Chairman of its Scientific Committee was Sir Stanley Davidson. In the Western, during the years of the War, patients with rheumatic problems were seen by general physicians. Dr J. G. Sclater, however consulted in the Royal Infirmary and subsequently set aside beds at his Unit in the Eastern General Hospital for the care of patients with rheumatic diseases.

After the Second World War, however, and particularly after the establishment of the National Health Service in 1948, there was considerable change. It has been recorded elsewhere how Sir Stanley Davidson, who then held the Chair of Medicine at Edinburgh University, decided to establish specialised units and physicians as senior lecturers within the Department of Medicine in the hospitals in the north side of the city. Among these was Dr J. J. R. Duthie, who had worked in Sir Stanley's Department in the University of Aberdeen before the War. He established a Rheumatic Diseases Unit in the Northern General Hospital. After a few years, with financial support from the Nuffield Foundation, Dr Duthie was able to establish a new Department. This combined facilities for inpatient and outpatient treatment of patients with rheumatic diseases and also facilities for teaching and laboratories for research. The Unit increased in size over the years with support from benefactors such as the McFarlane brothers who provided funds for the building of a new wing in the 1960s. The Arthritis and Rheumatism Council, as it came to be known after the War, made funds available for the extension of laboratory areas. Thus was established a Unit with consulting rooms, patient waiting and dressing areas, laboratories, a library, teaching facilities, facilities for record storage, secretarial accommodation and even an experimental orthotic workshop. During the 1950s and 1960s Dr Duthie was joined by Dr Robert J. G. Sinclair, Dr W. Rowland, Dr M. Alexander, and Dr Jacobus L. Potter who was a Senior Research Fellow at that time. Dr Potter subsequently became the Executive Dean in the Faculty of Medicine in the University of Edinburgh.

During this period outpatients were also seen at the famous 'Blood and Rheumatic' Clinic above ward 27 in the Royal Infirmary. This was staffed by Drs John J. R. Duthie, Robert J. G. Sinclair, J. G. Sclater and J. G. Macleod. The siting of this Department was unfortunate. Many arthritic patients were so disabled that they were unable to climb the stairs to the eyrie and the Consultants had to come down and examine them in the side room of ward 27!

Thus, between 1948 and 1977, there was a period of expansion in several directions. Major efforts were made to study the natural course of diseases such as rheumatoid arthritis. Large groups of patients were followed for many years to provide data for critical analysis of their progress. Exploratory studies were carried out into the fields of biochemistry, haematology, immunology and microbiology. This was also a period of expansion in the field of therapeutics with the introduction of many new anti-rheumatic drugs. The Department was involved in many exercises testing the efficacy of therapeutic measures by properly designed and conducted controlled clinical trials. During the 1960s there was nurtured the concept of a combined surgical and medical approach to the management of patients with diseases of bone and joint. This led to the setting up of combined clinics with Mr Douglas L. Savill. This development proved so successful that the demand for surgical intervention soon outstripped the facilities available. The inevitable consequence was the creation of long waiting lists. The rheumatologists at that time were also conscious of the need for close liaison with the professions allied to medicine and the necessity for close collaboration with the Departments of Occupational Therapy, Physiotherapy, Social Work and Nursing Services. At this time too the Department was fortunate in Dr Duthie's choice of Miss Margaret Daniel to be OIC Nursing as Departmental Sister until her retirement in 1984.

Mention should also be made of the valuable contributions to our knowledge of the biochemical aspects of the rheumatic diseases by a series of lecturers in biochemistry appointed, by Professor Duthie, to work in the unit's laboratories, namely Linda Roy, Isabel Nairn (nee Bell) and Harry Rylance. Close collaboration between them and members of the clinical and nursing staff yielded fruitful studies later published in the literature.

In the 1960s another important contribution was the setting up of an Industrial Survey Unit under the aegis of the Department to study rheumatic complaint rates in industrial establishments in and around Edinburgh. All these activities provided training for many young physicians who were given the opportunity and encouraged to develop their ideas and talents. Many subsequently achieving Consultant status at home and abroad and thereby doing a great deal to foster the development of rheumatology as a specialty. All these activities attracted many interested visitors from overseas as the pages of the Unit Visitor Book of the day testify.

In 1972 the Unit suffered a tragic loss with the death at a young age of Dr Rowland Alexander — a physician of whom Sir Stanley Davidson wrote '*as portraying at an early stage in his career a remarkable combination of the science and art of medicine*'. He was replaced in the Unit by Dr John N. McCormick who brought with him laboratory expertise acquired in England and the USA. In 1972 Dr R. J. G. Sinclair retired and was replaced by Dr T. M. Chalmers who, like Dr McCormick, had spent several years training in the Edinburgh Unit prior to his appointment in 1967 as a Senior Lecturer to Professor J. H. Kellgren in the University of Manchester. Professor Kellgren occupied the first University Chair in Rheumatology to be established in the United Kingdom.

In 1969 Dr Duthie was given a personal Chair in Rheumatology by the University of Edinburgh. When he retired in 1970 the Arthritis and Rheumatism Council and the University combined to set up an established Chair in Rheumatology in the Faculty of Medicine. The first incumbent was Dr George Nuki who had been senior lecturer in the University of Wales in Cardiff. He had also spent some earlier years in research in the United States. He brought with him an unextinguishable enthusiasm for all things rheumatological and an enviable clinical flair. He also brought an obvious concern for the part that rheumatologists should be playing in the education of undergraduate and postgraduate students. It was shortly after his appointment that the Arthritis and Rheumatism Council funded the extension of the laboratory facilities at the Northern General Hospital. The council also provided funds for the remuneration of a series of lecturers appointed to conduct investigations and projects covering many areas of the whole field of connective tissue disease. These included Dr David M. Reid, who subsequently became a Consultant Physician in Aberdeen and whose main interest lay in the study of metabolic bone disease. Subsequently, Dr Gordon Duff was appointed as Senior Lecturer in the Unit and supervised and initiated much research into the part played by the cytokines in the development of inflammatory joint disease. He subsequently was appointed to the Chair of Molecular Biology in the University of Sheffield. Most recently the Consultant staff has been greatly strengthened by the appointment of Dr Nigel P. Hurst as Consultant Physician. Dr Hurst had worked with Professor Nuki during his days in Cardiff and had spent several years as a Consultant and Senior Lecturer in the Department of Rheumatology in Adelaide in Australia. He brought with him considerable expertise in both the laboratory and the clinical aspects of the practice of rheumatology. Since his arrival he has made great efforts to update the technology of research and communication within the Department.

In 1991 Lothian Health Board, who had been responsible for the maintenance and upkeep of the Department, decided to close the Northern General Hospital and to transfer the specialised Units in Rheumatology, Neurology and Respiratory Medicine to the Western General Hospital. This move was initially very disheartening for the staff of the Department, as it appeared to undo in one fell swoop all that had been achieved by constant enthusiastic effort over a period of over 40 years. It is to be hoped that in time these facilities will be reproduced within the Western General Hospital and allow the teaching activities, clinical and research activities of the Unit to flourish again. It is also to be hoped that provision of these facilities will help to encourage the most recently appointed Consultants in this specialty. Dr Rashid Luqmani and Dr C. Michael Lambert have both demonstrated talent, ability and enthusiasm which are to be fostered as valuable assets in present day medicine.

General Surgery

During this period there were, in effect, two areas of surgical endeavour — the established general surgical unit, and the more recent component of the combined Gastro-intestinal unit.

There was a general surgical unit in the days of the Municipal Hospital, under the successive direction of the University Professor of Surgery, Sir David Wilkie and Sir James Learmonth. While they were responsible they worked mainly by proxy, their lecturers doing what surgery was required. Charles Illingworth was attached to the Western before moving to the Chair of Surgery in Glasgow. In 1948, John Bruce was appointed as an NHS consultant surgeon, the University being represented by Sandy Slessor. This was an uneasy union of NHS and

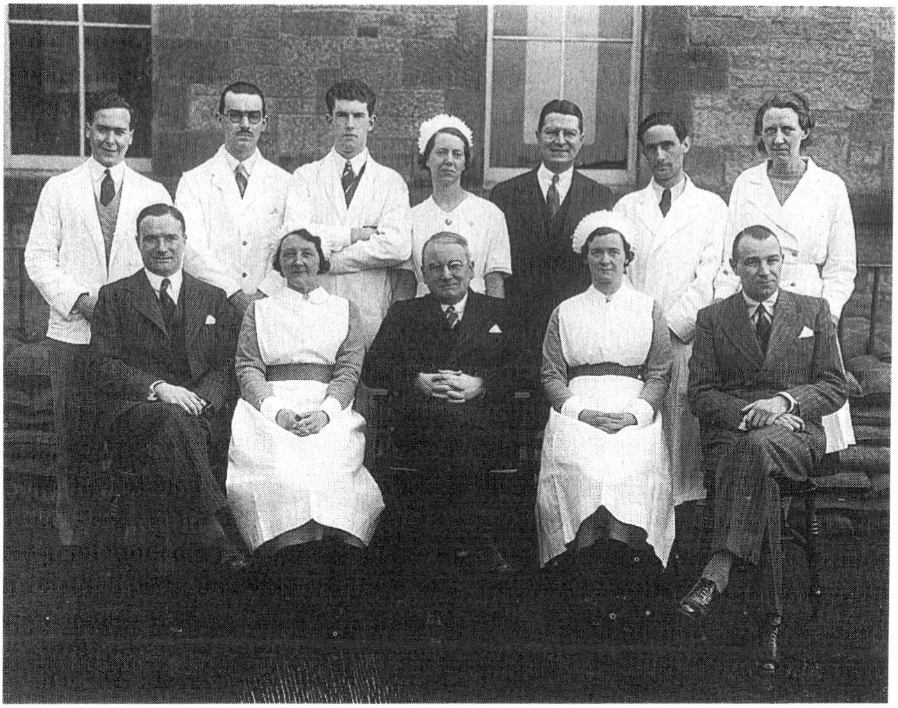

Group which includes, in front row, Mr AB Wallace, Sir JK Learmouth, Mr David Band. Late1930s

University. Much of the restrictions from the old municipal hospital days remained. No outpatient clinic referrals were allowed, direct referral by GP's forbidden, mandatory admission on the order of the Medical Officer of Health etc. This subordination to the Municipality and to the University was broken at a famous meeting between John Bruce, Richard Turner and the Professors of Surgery and Medicine in about 1950. The meeting was precipated by a visit to the Western General Hospital by the Regius Professor of Surgery Sir James Learmonth, a man of great presence who was to operate on the King. He came expecting the surgical practice to be varicose veins and hernia surgery. John Bruce had been a Brigadier in General Slims's army, friend and confidant to this famous commander in the ferocious battles in Burma. John Bruce was a well known member of Edinburgh's surgical and social world. He had established an advanced surgical practice with a team of young surgeons, some of whom were ex-army. The visit was memorable for its vigour. The line of command, with Sir James Learmonth as titular head of surgery WGH, was identified by a plaque in the entrance to D block. The new independence of the WGH surgeons came with the forceful removal of the plaque by the surgeon who was to succeed Sir James and who was to become Professor Sir John Bruce!

Two quite different consultant surgeons of equal quality were appointed in the early years, Charles Falconer in 1950 and Bill Small in 1955. Through their

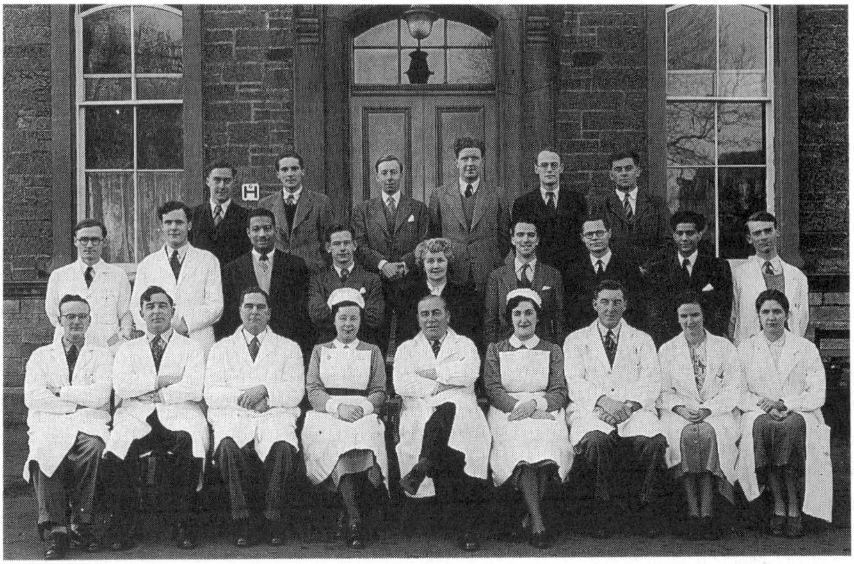

Surgical Clinique, 1951. Sir John Bruce, centre front row; Sister Nimmo, front row, who later became Matron

very astute clinical approach and technical ability they were able to establish a practice of surgery in which all felt confidence. They were comfortable clinicians, aware of changes in practice and able to develop when necessary. Charles Falconer was John Bruce's senior registrar, and became very much the leader of the surgical practice when John Bruce moved to the Royal Infirmary. The standard of training was high with a focus on skill, a healthy respect for the basic premises of surgery, coupled to self examination on the results. Charles Falconer was a good endocrine surgeon as well as having skills as an gastrointestinal surgeon.

Mr W. P. Small came to the WGH as consultant surgeon in general surgery in 1955, to join John Bruce and Charles Falconer, to fill the vacancy caused by the untimely death of Sandy Slessor. In effect this severed the link with the University and General surgery. Yet Bill Small was to develop an academic theme in the unit with the Gastric Follow up clinic. This was a careful follow up of the patients who were operated upon for duodenal ulceration. Bill Small was a skilled surgeon who taught generations of surgeons to do and think about what they were doing and the long-term consequences of what they had done. Later University links came to be re-established on an informal basis with Adam Smith's attachment to the GI Unit.

The general surgical unit rose to a consistent peak in the 1970s which has been sustained since. All-round surgical experience was offered to the junior staff in training in all branches of surgery except Urology, and this gap was filled by a system of secondment. It held the highest rate of application of any unit in Edinburgh for undergraduate student cliniques and for house surgeon appointments. The link with Urology led to the collection, combined treatment and subsequent publication of one of the largest series of vesico-colic fistulae with a re-appraisal of the conventional method of management. Charles Falconer and John Strong together did much to improve the diagnosis and isolation of parathyroid tumours. With Norman Allan, splenectomy for platelet and blood disorders was established on a joint basis and the results subsequently reported.

Day care surgery was another pioneering area. Dr James Ferguson, the then Medical Superintendent, and Mr Vaughan Ruckley establishing this approach to surgical care within North Lothian and subsequently publishing what was to become the basic reference work. Vaughan Ruckley trained as surgical registrar and senior registrar in the Western General Hospital. He was involved in the initiation of Audit in the Edinburgh Hospitals. Bill Small was an influence on him through the Gastric Follow-up Clinic. Vaughan Ruckley held a philosophy that if it was worth while to keep a record of one's work and its outcome then there is merit in pondering on the results from time to time. Surgeons in all units in Edinburgh kept records of their operations and deaths over a period of more than 20 years. This collection of data owed its origins to the Saturday morning Surgical Meeting established by Sir James Learmonth just after the War. One of Vaughan Ruckley's first projects was to look at the post-operative problem of pulmonary embolism. Autopsy studies showed that pulmonary embolism was the commonest acute lung disorder in Hospital patients and a major cause of death after operation. Yet the Edinburgh surgical statistics showed that the incidence of pulmonary embolism post-operatively had fallen over the 20 years prior to 1981. This was due in part to improving techniques; early mobilisation, early discharge, better anaesthetics, more frequent regional and local anaesthesia, better control of fluids and electrolytes, and less post-operative sepsis. This enabled a routine thromboembolism prophylaxis programme to be established on a basis of informed logic. Vaughan Ruckley also looked at the surgical management of varicose veins. Before 1970 there was little or no outpatient varicose vein surgery. Hernia and haemorrhoid surgery and varicose vein surgery were moved to the short stay and outpatient surgical field. This meant that the main acute surgical ward became a combination of intensive care and geriatrics. Vaughan Ruckley, Charles Falconer, Bill Small and Adam Smith promoted a study in which 2,000 consecutive newly-referred surgical patients were followed from their first Clinic visit to the final outcome. This study extended over a two year period. 30% remained minor outpatients, 8% major day care and 34% were managed in a five day ward. Only 28% of all surgical patients needed to be cared for in conventional acute surgical wards. This led to the almost unacceptable, in those days, concept that there was a serious discrepancy between the needs of the population and the surgical facilities provided. Once this revolutionary thought was accepted there was a need for an increase in short stay beds, of which day care beds are the most important. Dr James Ferguson was the Medical Superintendent and he lent his considerable influence to the promotion of this concept. He was a clinically sensitive administrator. These proved to be an economic way of treating patients. Five day care is a variant of conventional care which makes possible a saving in staffing at weekends. The average amount of time spent with patients by GP's post-operatively was only eight minutes longer in the day care group than the ward group and 42% had no direct contact with their GP's in the follow-up period.

The opening of the Day Bed Area in Phase I of the reconstruction of the Hospital was a great innovation for the Western. The principal users of the Day Bed Area were:

Urology:	Endoscopy; Vasectomy.
Gastro-intestinal:	Endoscopy.
General Surgery:	Varicose veins; Hernia; Haemorrhoids; Breast Biopsy.
Haematology:	Venesections; Transfusions; Marrow punctures.
Gynaecology:	D & C; Sterilisation.
Radiology:	Arteriography; Cholangiography.

The Day Bed Area consists of three six-bedded wards and six small cubicles giving a total of 24 beds. It was adjacent to the main hospital outpatient reception area, the endoscopy suites and outpatient theatres. The original nursing staff consisted of a Charge Nurse, two State Registered Nurses and an Auxiliary Nurse. The selection of patients for outpatient surgery was in the Clinic at the first referral. Surgeons decided which would be the most appropriate approach to day or conventional ward admission dependent on the patient's general health and home background. Routine screening tests, urine tests, blood count, electrolytes, chest X-ray and ECG were arranged. The great merit was that patients could be given the date of their operation, and the general practitioner and district nursing staff could be notified of the arrangements by carbon copies of the letter to the patient. Three lists of outpatient general surgery were conducted each week. The patient was transported home by ambulance and often a district nurse was ready to greet them.

Patients who had stripping and ligation of varicose veins, surgery for hernia or operations of equivalent severity had a complication rate of 10%, the main complications being delayed wound healing and chest infections. Of 300 patients, only nine had to be kept in and the discharge delayed and only six had to be readmitted. There were no serious complications of this procedure. In 1975 a five day ward was established with ten beds provided. Among other advantages the system allowed the employment, or re-employment of married, part-time nursing staff. Men and women were admitted on alternate weeks. Operating lists were on Monday and Wednesday afternoon and even included some cholecystectomies, and mastectomies but largely comprised varicose veins, haemorrhoids and recurrence of hernias. This was still in the era of open surgery and before key hole surgery. However, highly selective vagotomy, thyroidectomy, carotid endarterectomy, simple mastectomy and haemorrhoidectomy were performed. An important feature was the back-up of the main ward for those patients who required a longer stay. The system went well and according to plan in 82% of admissions. The community nurse and the general practitioners also enjoyed looking after patients who were discharged early. As a result of these two measures, the increased turn-over eliminated the waiting list to the extent that a direct booking admission policy became possible. However, the basis of all this was an enthusiastic team. This became less the case after Vaughan Ruckley moved to the Royal Infirmary.

The intensive care recovery ward in the main theatre was a direct result of the efforts of the general surgical unit. It is from this beginning that the present specialist unit developed.

The general surgical unit attracted a very high calibre of nursing and medical staff. Staff nurse posts in the wards were sought after just as much as the medical jobs. As a result, with the experience and encouragement gained, the output of ideas and the standard of patient care reached an all-time high, as evidenced by the requests by patients admitted 'elsewhere' for transfer to the Western. Apart from a high standard of care, the friendly, understanding approach of the nursing and auxiliary staff was a major factor in what was a successful and very happy unit.

Mr Charles Falconer retired in 1978 and was replaced by Mr John Saunders who had a joint appointment between Leith Hospital and the Gastro-Intestinal Unit. Mr (now Professor) C. V. Ruckley was appointed to a new Consultant post at the Western. When he transferred to the Royal Infirmary to establish the Vascular Unit there, he was replaced by Mr David Hamer-Hodges who was given the brief of further developing day care surgery at the Western. In 1985 Mr Bill Small retired and was replaced by Mr Iain Macintyre who transferred from Leith Hospital. In 1988 the Leith Hospital Surgical Unit was formally transferred to the Western, bringing Mr John Saunders into the Western as a full time surgeon along with Mr Steve Nixon. These General Surgical Units moved into the new Alexander Donald Building which was physically separate from the Gastro-Intestinal Wards and Laboratories. Thus began the loosening of the ties that was eventually to result in the break-up of the integrated Gastro-Intestinal Medical and Surgical service. Mr Graeme Wilson was appointed Consultant Surgeon in 1994.

In the most recent period, 1985–94, considerable changes have occurred in surgery. The most significant of these have been in gastroenterology. Important contributions have been made by all the surgeons. Adam Smith established the Anorectal Laboratory, developed for pioneering sphincter-saving pouch surgery in Lothian, becoming Wade Professor and subsequently Vice-President of the College. David Hamer-Hodges continued to develop thyroid and parathyroid surgery and surgery of inflammatory bowel disease. John Saunders helped to establish the Endoscopic Retrograde Cannulation of the Pancreas (ERCP) service. When laparoscopic cholecystectomy was described, allowed this hospital to establish what was regarded as the best training course in the United Kingdom. This led to the publishing of the largest British series. Steve Nixon developed information technology and audit techniques within the Surgical Unit and beyond. Such audit techniques and information technology are becoming commonplace throughout Britain but owe a great deal to Steve Nixon's work.

Surgical audit, the critical examination of clinical practice to bring about constant improvement, has been a feature of the surgical units at the Western since the 1950s. Annual reports detailing both outpatient and inpatient workload figures and mortality have been presented at the Lothian Surgical Audit Saturday morning meetings since that time. Considerable improvements in data handling became possible with the introduction of microcomputers in 1983. The WGH was amongst the first to use the BBC micro as a powerful audit tool which was to spread across all Lothian surgical units and beyond. The software was written by the surgeons themselves based on the, now famous, Lothian surgical codes. This work was acknowledged by the National Audit Office and received praise in the Government White Paper 'Working for Patients' published in 1988.

The limitations of the BBC microcomputer storage capacity required an increase in computering capacity. IBM compatible computers allowed a marked increase in the number of data items which could be collected from just 15 per operation to over 150. By 1990, a surgical office package had been developed in the Western which took over the day to day running of the entire surgical unit. With the help of the secretaries, a sophisticated suite of programs was designed. This now serves the dual purpose of offering our secretaries a friendly, computer based, word processing package whilst providing the surgeons with an extensive range of audit data. This was originally planned as a 'stand alone' system for the surgeon and his secretary. There is now a complex information network reaching throughout the hospital with up to 30 users at any one time. Surgeons were the first to use the network-wiring introduced throughout the Western in 1992 and remain the major users to this day. Other specialties within the WGH have adopted the system and it has been introduced in Edinburgh Royal Infirmary, other Scottish hospitals and in an increasing number of English centres.

The surgical system for recording patient details has now been introduced to the Gastro-Intestinal Unit through a system called networking. The word processors for secretaries in the Typing Pool, Day Bed Area, Endoscopy, Surgical Office and Gastro-Intestinal Unit Offices are all networked and can transfer information from one word processor to another. The system established in the Western General Hospital has influenced the Scottish Office and with the development of the Scottish Audit of Surgical Morbidity, of which Steve Nixon is the Chairman. Graham Wilson is auditing minimal access surgery using the same system as Steve Nixon's.

In general, major central investment in information technology has largely failed to deliver on promises. Yet interested and informed surgeons, with a clear practical idea of what is required on a far lower budget have made great strides forward.

The present system in use in the Western General Hospital allows more than 150 items and every typed text to be recorded on the computer and be readily retrievable. Originally the documentation was the operation and whether or not the patient died. Now it is possible to identify morbidity, case mix and the outcome measures of the operation. The system also allows the operation complication rate to be calculated for the whole of Lothian and also for individual surgeons. This is based on a structured form which forms part of the day to day care of the patient. It also enables surgeons in training to identify their work and how they are doing in terms of what happens to their patients after the operation. All of this can be collected prospectively.

Steve Nixon has also further developed minimally invasive surgery from the firm basis established by John Saunders. Mr Nixon has performed the largest series of laparoscopic splenectomies in the United Kingdom to date.

No account of the General Surgery unit would be complete without recognition of the part played by generations of nurses and nursing sisters. The Nurse Manager, Mrs Betty Sutherland, and her Sisters and the Charge Nurses; Linda Tucker D5, Mary Archibald D7, Ruth Swanson D5, Audrey Cowie D5, Mary Alexander D7 and Jane Fraser D5. They have adjusted to totally new surgical techniques and nursing care in a skilful and caring manner which characterises their work.

Urology

For some 18 years after the inauguration of the National Health Service, the urological unit at the WGH served the South Eastern Regional Hospital Board, Scotland, which covered Edinburgh, the Lothians, Fife and the Borders. The two consultants were the only surgeons in the Region who confined their work to urology, although in all hospitals in the region much urological surgery was performed by general surgeons, some of whom had a special interest in the specialty.

The first of the urological surgeons to be appointed in 1948 was Mr David Band. He started as a general surgeon with a special interest in Urology, but then devoted himself to Urology, becoming the first Consultant Urological Surgeon to the South East Regional Hospital Board, Scotland. He was a Reader in Surgery in the University of Edinburgh, a founder member of the British Association of Urological Surgeons and for many years Editor of the British Journal of Urology. His major research interests were renal tuberculosis, and bladder dysfunction which he studied with a cystometer which incorporated a smoked drum. He retired in 1966.

In 1948, Mr William Selby Tulloch, always known as Selby Tulloch, returned to the Western General Hospital, after demobilisation from the RAMC in which he had served with distinction, first as assistant surgeon and became, in 1948, the second Consultant Urological Surgeon. He started the first Edinburgh clinic for the study of male infertility. These clinics were held from 7.30 to 9.30p.m. on two evenings each week, in the expectation that men would be more likely to attend in the evenings than during the day. Apart from his commitments in Edinburgh, Mr Tulloch was also responsible for the urology service in Fife and did one theatre session and one outpatient clinic every Monday at the Victoria Hospital, Kirkcaldy. Mr Tulloch retired in 1978.

Mr Jack F. Newsam, who had been a Senior Registrar in the Unit since 1958, became a Consultant Urological Surgeon on the retiral of Mr Band. He always described himself as a general urological surgeon, a typically modest appraisal. He was the author of a textbook, *Urology and Renal Medicine* with a renal physician Jim Petrie, which ran to three editions. He also wrote the urology section of Cushieri's Modern Surgical Practice. Mr Newsam retired in 1990.

In addition to the two consultants, the unit had a senior registrar and a senior house officer, though it often failed to attract a senior house officer. The unit consisted of two wards, D4 for males and D5 for females, an endoscopic theatre which opened directly off the main hospital corridor opposite what until 1995 was the Chief Executive's office. They shared with the gynaecologists the 1914–18 operating theatre constructed of creosoted timber. This theatre became the CSSD after extensive upgrading. Outpatients were seen in what had been the Paderewski Hospital.

The operations during this period were both endoscopic and open. The endoscopic operations consisted of cystoscopies and retrograde pyelographs and the purpose was mainly diagnostic. Therapeutic endoscopic procedures were confined to urethral dilations, the crushing of bladder stones (litholapaxy), the electrocoagulation of bladder tumours and the attempted removal of ureteric stones using Dormia stone dislodgers, blindly or under X-ray control. The open operations were prostatectomies, usually by the transvesical route, pyelo and uretero lithotomies, nephrectomies for tumour, stone or infection, and uretero colic anastomosis, with or without cystectomy. Most invasive bladder tumours were treated primarily by irradiation given externally or interstitially using radium needles or radon seeds.

In 1964, the new Renal Transplant Unit at the Western General Hospital opened under the direction of Michael F. A. Woodruff, Professor of Surgical Science, who had previously carried out renal transplants in his Wards 13 and 14 in the Royal Infirmary. He and his surgical colleagues in Wards 13 and 14, Mr Bernard Nolan and Mr Sandy Jenkins, continued to be responsible for all renal transplantation in the South Eastern Region and Tayside. The Urological Surgeons had only a minimal involvement.

Professor M. F. A. Woodruff retired in 1976 and after much thought and not a little intrigue it was decided that his successor should be based at the Western and should, among his other duties, be Director of the Renal Transplant Unit. Professor Woodruff's Wards in the Royal Infirmary would become a Vascular Unit.

Professor Geoffrey Chisholm was appointed Professor of Surgery at the Western General Hospital. Geoffrey Chisholm was born in Hawera, New Zealand of Scottish ancestry. He was an expert in renal transplantation at the Hammersmith Hospital in London. He came to the chair of surgery at the

Western General in 1977 and he developed the department of urology into one of the foremost in Europe. He collaborated with immunologists, especially Professor Keith James, and was an international contributor to the understanding of prostatic cancer. In this field he worked with the biochemist, Fouad Habib on the hormonal control of the prostate. Geoff Chisholm was editor of the British Journal of Urology and a contributor to many books and papers. His greatest honour, of which there were many, was to be the President of the Royal College of Surgeons of Edinburgh, from 1988 to 1991, which was a time when the Colleges began to revise the whole concept of surgical training. He was also chairman of the Joint Committee on Higher Surgical Training for the United Kingdom and Ireland. Most of all he was a kind and caring man, who was responsible for so much progress in Edinburgh surgery and in surgery internationally. He died, in post, in 1994 aged 63.

Mr Timothy B. Hargreave joined the Department in 1978, some months before Mr Tulloch retired in September 1978, Mr Hargreave was appointed Senior Lecturer and Honorary Consultant Urological Surgeon. He became a National Health Service Consultant when Mr Newsam retired in 1990. Amongst his other work, he took over the male subfertility clinic. He has become a world authority on this problem and with members of the MRC Cytogenetic Unit has carried out fundamental research some of which has been recently published in '*Cell*'.

In 1954, Hopkins and Kedansky demonstrated that images as well as light could be transmitted along a bundle of glass fibres. This principle was soon utilised by gastro-enterologists and respiratory physicians. It was not until 1968 that good images be obtained with fibreoptic instruments small enough to pass safely down the urethra and into the bladder.

In the 1970s endoscopic procedures were revolutionised by the introduction of fibre optic lighting and the rod lens telescope. By the early 1970s, more than 90% of prostatectomies and all bladder tumour resections were carried out endoscopically. Urethral strictures were treated with an optical urethrotome instead of blind dilatation. Nowadays many check cystoscopies use fibreoptic cystoscopes under local surface anaesthesia.

Radiological imaging of the urinary tract also advanced. Ultrasound, in particular, became as valuable in the visualisation of the kidney and bladder as it had been for many years in the visualisation of the foetus in the gravid uterus. Improvements included intravenous urography and the introduction of CAT scanning. Further developments were the ureteroscopes introduced in the 1980s. They enabled urologists to view the interior of the ureter. By the 1980s the vastly improved imaging of the kidneys enabled radiologists and urologists to insert accurately needles through the skin into the pelvic-cortical system of the kidney. A silicone stent could be inserted through the lumen of the needle and left to drain an obstructed kidney. This technique soon led to percutaneous renal surgery in which the needle track was dilated until a 30 F tube could be passed into the pelvic cortical system. An endoscope and other instruments could then be passed through the tube and used to crush and remove stones, biopsy and electro coagulate tumours of the pelvis and cortex and incise obstructed pelvi-ureteric junctions.

Other advances of the 1980s include the development of urodynamics for the investigation of bladder and urethral function, of artificial sphincters for the treatment of urinary incontinence, of complex reconstructive operations on the bladder for serious bladder dysfunction and of continent urinary diversion operations. The 1980s also witnessed the rise and fall of transfemoral embolisation of the renal artery in patients with renal cell carcinoma.

The establishment of the Scottish Lithotriptor Centre at the Deaconess Hospital in the second half of the 1980s brought Extra Corporeal Shock Wave Lithotripsy (ESWL) to all in Scotland. This rendered obsolete most operations, even percutaneous ones, for stone, except for staghorn calculi in non-functioning kidneys. The Lithotriptor Centre along with the urological unit at the Deaconess Hospital moved to the WGH in 1991. In 1993 a mobile lithotriptor mounted in an articulated van was obtained. This travels to the major medical centres in Scotland, taking the service to the patient, whereas previously patients had to come to Edinburgh for treatment on the lithotriptor.

In the transfer of services from the Deaconess in 1991, the two established surgeons Mr James Fowler and Mr David Tolley, and the senior lecturer and honorary consultant, Mr Gordon Smith, together with their staff came to the Western General Hospital and occupied the wards vacated by the general surgeons when they moved to the Alexander Donald Building.

Laparoscopy has been an essential diagnostic and therapeutic tool of gynaecologists for many years, but used by few surgeons until recent years. It has now become the main instrument in the new branch of surgery called Minimal Invasive Surgery (MIS). Urologists have been slow to use it for operations, including nephrectomy. Training courses have been established to teach MIS to surgeons brought up in the days of the large incision. As Ambroise Paré said in the 16th Century, 'We now know so much about surgery, its inconceivable that there are still major advances to be made.'

Senior Registrars

Mr Dermott O'Flynn 48/52	became a Urologist in Dublin and recently was President of the Royal College of Surgeons in Ireland
Mr A. Robb 52/55	became a Surgeon in Inverness
Sir James Fraser 55/58	became a Professor of Surgery in Southampton
Mr J. E. Newsam 58/66	Surgeon, Western General Hospital
Mr G. F. Murnagham 59/62	worked as an Honorary Senior Registrar and became Professor of Surgery in Sydney, NSW

M. Henderson 66/68	became a Surgeon in Dumfries
Mr G. Foster 68/71	became a Urologist in Ayr
Mr J. O'Brien 71/74	became a Urologist in Birmingham
Mr G. Carswell 74/78	became a Urologist in Monklands
Mr J. Hindmarsh 78/81	became a Urologist in Middlesburgh
Mr L. Beynon 81/84	became a Urologist in Wolverhampton and, sadly, died in 1987
Mr A. Ritchie 84/88	became a Senior Lecturer in Edinburgh, now a Urologist in Gloucester
Mr M. Lucas 88/91	became a Urologist in Newport, South Wales
Mr S. Prescott 91/93	became a Senior Lecturer in Urology, Edinburgh, and in 1995 a Urologist in Leeds.

Department of Clinical Psychology

The post held by Dr Tris Buckley evolved from the original post instituted by Professor Henry Walton when he first established the University Department in Psychiatry in the Western General Hospital. At that time, about 30 years ago, the multi-disciplinary model was in vogue. In addition to sessions provided by Professor Walton, his senior lecturer and junior medical staff, there were also two psychiatric social workers and a clinical psychologist.

For the last 14 years or so, in the first instance Dr Ann Cull and Dr Buckley shared the post, following which Dr Buckley took the post in a full time capacity. There have been many developments in liaison services in general, but in psychology in particular. Health Psychology is a well recognised specialty in its own right. Previously, the clinical psychologist tended only to have an input to patients who had a psychiatric status or diagnosis. Now the discipline has a much broader base of application where a contribution is made to all aspects of health; in the promotion of good health practices; the prevention, therapy and management of illness; and to health care in general. This is a highly regarded service to the clinicians. A history of the hospital would be incomplete without reference to a famous psychologist — a neuropsychologist, Oliver Zangwill — who worked for a time in the Department of Surgical Neurology as it was then called. He was followed by Jim Naughton who had studied medicine as his first degree before proceeding to psychology. Dr Robert Taylor is the current incumbent.

Dietetic Department

When Miss Constance Cameron came to the Western in 1961, the establishment was two full-time and one part-time Dietitian. There was a large Diet Kitchen, separate from the main kitchen, providing all special diets, mainly gastric, diabetic, low fat and low salt diets. The number of special diets varied, but could reach 100 in a 500-bed hospital. This reflected sadly on the quality of the general food supplied to patients at that time.

The Dietitians' office-cum-cloakroom was a space approximately 8ft by 6ft partitioned off the Diet Kitchen. It contained a wardrobe, two shelves, a desk and three chairs. As the partition was only head-high, it was not the quietest place in which to work. In fact the working conditions were horrible. The Dietitians' work consisted mainly in visiting ward patients, arranging their meals for the day, and instructing them in their diets to be continued at home. A considerable time was spent in serving and checking the meals leaving the Diet Kitchen, seven days per week. The Dietitians were involved in the supervision, cooking and serving of meals. This was particularly the case when the Diet Kitchen at the Western was three times the size of the present one. A complete Unit separate from the kitchens was used. The kitchen was provided with its own supplies and the meals were cooked under careful supervision.

One session each week was spent in the Outpatient Department at the Diabetic Clinic. If any other outpatient required advice, the receptionist in Outpatients would ring for a Dietitian to attend.

At this time, plans were already in hand for the Metabolic Unit, indeed the first two balance studies were carried out, with some difficulty, from the Diet Kitchen. When the Metabolic Unit was opened, the establishment was increased to three full-time Dietitians, one being employed there. Later, the Diabetic Clinic was transferred to the Metabolic Unit, requiring a part-time Dietitian. The opening of the new Outpatient Department made the dietitians work easier. They were given a suite of rooms, two offices for interviewing patients and a demonstration room where classes were held for some of the many overweight patients. About this time, the Department was approved for the practical training of Dietetic students. They took part in all aspects of dietetic work, including advising patients at the Ante-natal Clinic on their general nutrition.

When the Nuffield Transplant Unit was opened, the Diet Kitchen had to be reconstructed to make room for a small kitchen for the preparation of sterile meals for these patients. At the same time, two offices were made available for the use of Dietitians.

The next major improvement was the introduction of patients' menu cards and a plated meal service for all patients. The Dietitians were involved in the composition of the menus and the organisation of the servery. This needed further alteration of the Diet Kitchen, reducing its size to allow for the larger servery. This considerably changed the Dietitians' work, as much of the food for special diets came from the main menus. Less time was spent supervising the preparation of meals and more in instruction of patients in their choice of menu.

Miss Cameron retired in 1978 and was succeeded by Mrs Christine Johnson. As the hospital became more specialised, the role of the Dietitian changed accordingly. Previously diets were very structured, and the patient had to adapt to the diet rather than the diet fitting in with the patient's lifestyle. Diets are now more complex and dietetics as a profession is becoming more and more scientific. By the late 1980s the majority of the prescribed food was cooked within the main kitchen and the diets integrated into choice menus.

The number of Dietitians at the Western General Hospital has not changed from 1973 but there is now a Dietitian working part-time at the Royal Victoria Hospital and a Scottish Office-funded post devoted to cystic fibrosis.

The office accommodation has improved from two small rooms off the Diet Kitchen to a large open plan office for the Dietitians. Outpatient accommodation has deteriorated from a suite of offices to one very small office on the Outpatient Clinic floor.

Diets have altered considerably as new drug treatments are available. In the past one of the mainstays in the treatment of duodenal ulcers was the gastric diet. This white unappetising diet associated with duodenal ulcers is no longer used. Patients with dysphagia due to carcinoma or other problems are now on food which is of a fine consistency. The Dietitians work very closely with the Speech and Language Therapist to assist safe swallowing. A very central point of dietetic care is the use of nasogastric feeding for patients who are not able to take food orally, because of conscious level, or patients requiring extra nutrition. Other forms of feeding are percutaneous endoscopic gastrostomies (PEG tubes which are inserted in the anterior abdominal wall in the stomach) or total parenteral nutrition (TPN). Such new feeding systems use defined commercially prepared feeds whereas previously the Dietitians made feeds from milk, eggs, Complan etc. The Dietitians are aiming to increase awareness of the role of nutritional status in recovery and now have a programme for the screening of every hospital patient to identify those who may be nutritionally compromised.

These assisted feeding systems require professional input from Dietitian, Nurses, Clinical Chemists, Pharmacists, Physicians and Surgeons. This has resulted in the development of a Nutrition Team in which all these are represented. Dr Martin Eastwood has chaired the group; Betty Sutherland, Fiona Phillips, Juliet MacArthur, Sheila Selkirk, George Lindsay, Gillian Blundell, Liz Clinton and Edith Skutecki have been important members in the group.

The dietetic care of patients with cystic fibrosis is an important new interest under the supervision of Rosalind Yuill. These young patients present great problems with their limited capacity to absorb food. Another group of patients for which specialist care is provided are those who suffer from inflammatory bowel disease and coeliac disease. The Metabolic unit has dietitians (June Grieve and Sheila Douglas) looking after the complex problems of the diabetic patient and also the obese.

The Physics Service to Radiotherapy

The radiotherapy service moved from the Royal Infirmary to the Western General in 1954, Dr Charlie Murison, who had been the sole physicist in that service from his appointment in 1936, also moved to the Western. Here he was joined by an expanded team of physicists and technicians who were recruited for the installation of the linear accelerator in radiotherapy. This gave more penetrating X-ray beams than had previously been available, and it was therefore much more suited to the treatment of deep tumours. This accelerator was of a type which was the first to be commercially available for radiotherapy in Britain. The machine installed at the Western was one of the first half dozen to be used. The maintenance was, as now, 'in house', no equivalent commercial support being available. This work and the associated treatment planning and dosimetry required additional expert staff, and the provision of a comprehensive workshop.

Dr Murison was assisted by a succession of able physicists up to his retirement in 1972, when he was succeeded by Dr John Law. Amongst many physicists who served in the department in these periods, particular mention should be made of Dr Tony Redpath, who joined the department in 1967 after completing a PhD in the Medical Physics Department at the Royal Infirmary. He was in charge of developing computer facilities for detailed patient treatment planning on the original accelerator, and on all subsequent machines of its kind at WGH. He was in the forefront of this development at national and international level. The techniques he developed have been copied widely throughout the world in a form often referred to as 'the Edinburgh software.' More recently Dr David Thwaites has been in charge of patient dose measurements. He has established an international reputation through his original research work, and by membership of national and international committees who are charged with establishing sound protocols for radiotherapy dose measurements. He has been closely associated with the development in the 1980s of electrons for radiotherapy as an additional modality to the more familiar high energy X-ray treatments.

In 1954 the chief technical officer newly appointed to take charge of the workshop was Mr Roy Cowtan. On his departure to join the Scottish Office Equipment Supplies Team in 1959 he was succeeded by Bill Jackes, who was in turn succeeded in 1975 by Lewis Mackie, both of whom had been on the staff since 1954. Mr Mackie retired in 1993 after 38 years continuous service in radiotherapy physics.

The importance of this workshop to the physics service and to the radiotherapy service as a whole cannot be over-emphasised, since without it the cancer treatment equipment would rapidly cease to function reliably, or even at all. The workshop has been staffed throughout this time by a remarkable body of men, who have all shown the highest dedication to the service, despite the fact that their skills have been in considerable demand outside the National Health Service. They could often have improved both salary and career prospects had they chosen to make a move. In more recent times, especially since

1975, this has also been true of the smaller number of electronics technicians, who are just as crucial as those in the workshop. They were recruited against fierce competition from local industry in what was known at the time as 'Silicon Glen'. The hospital as a whole has great cause to be thankful to this team.

Genetics

In 1956 the Medical Research Council established a small group, under the leadership of Dr (later Professor) Michael Court-Brown, which became the 'Clinical Effects of Radiation Research Unit.' The group occupied one floor of one wing of the radiotherapy department. The broad terms of reference were to study the delayed effects of radiation exposure in humans, with particular emphasis on leukaemogenesis. At that time, radiotherapy was used in the treatment of several non-malignant disorders, particularly ankylosing spondylitis. These patients, among others, provided the information for longitudinal studies which continue to the present time. In collaboration with Sir Richard Doll, Michael Court-Brown and his colleagues demonstrated that the incidence of leukaemia in patients exposed to radiation is proportional to dose. They were able to deduce a quantitative relationship that is used internationally as a basis for determining acceptable levels of industrial and medical radiation exposure.

The late 1950s saw major technical advances in human chromosome analysis. Since it was known that in many species chromosome damage provides a measure of exposure to radiation it was natural that the Unit should turn its attention to cytogenetics. This lead to many major discoveries on the population distribution and clinical consequences of constitutional chromosome aberrations in humans. Drs Patricia Jacobs and Karen Buckton were at the forefront of these laboratory developments. Their principal collaborators, Dr Tom MacGregor, Professor John Strong and Dr Neil MacLean (gynaecologist, physician and pathologist respectively) played major roles in establishing the international reputation of the Unit which became a World Reference Centre for human cytogenetics. Somewhat belatedly, in 1967, the Unit's title was changed to 'Clinical and Population Cytogenetics'. By 1964, the Unit had expanded and now occupied a new four-storey building on the Western site, linked to its original premises by a bridge.

The scientific interests of the MRC staff also expanded to include the role of viruses in cancer and as agents causing chromosome damage. Dr (later Professor) David Harnden was head of the 'Experimental Studies' group. Among the clinicians actively engaged in these early studies of the molecular genetics of cancer were Dr Albert Baikie and Dr Allan Langlands. Dr Bill Price was head of the 'clinical section' which took responsibility for the follow-up of patients with chromosome abnormalities. This section also followed a programme of research on the genetics of cardiovascular and connective tissue diseases.

A satellite section had been established in the early 1960s in London under Dr Denis Rulovitz. Its remit was to develop automated facilities for the analysis of visual images, including of course chromosome spreads. Some of the technology was applied to cervical smear screening.

By 1972 the Unit had continued to grow. An additional linked building was added (officially 'opened' — but in fact declared 'more open than before' in November 1974 by the Duke of Edinburgh). The London group was 'brought home' and soon the total complement of MRC and associated staff had grown to over 200, making this one of the largest of all the MRC units. Professor Court-Brown had foreseen the need for the new building and had obtained approval for the necessary developments before his untimely death in December 1968. His successor, as Director, Professor John Evans, has overseen the Unit's growing involvement in the molecular biology revolution as well as its continuous contributions to ever-more sophisticated cytogenetics. Following the departure of Dr Ed Southern from Edinburgh to Oxford in 1985, the MRC Mammalian Genome Unit at Kings Buildings was subsumed into the Western site and by 1987 there was a further related change of name to the 'Human Genetics Unit'. The research activities of the Unit now encompass human gene mapping, developmental biology, fundamental molecular genetics and structural studies on human chromosomes, the molecular biology and genetics of common cancers and of certain specific diseases such as schizophrenia and cystic fibrosis. There are numerous collaborative programmes with clinicians in Edinburgh and far beyond. The Unit attracts research grants for National and International Agencies and is host to many visiting workers from all over the world.

While actively supporting research under the aegis of the MRC, the University also recognised the need for clinical services, teaching and research in Human Genetics. In 1967 a new clinical department was established at the Western with Professor Alan Emery as its first head. The department moved into the top floor of the new MRC building in 1973 and that remained its base until Professor Emery's retirement in 1983. Thereafter it became a sub-department of Medicine at the Western, occupying a 'portacabin' laboratory at the foot of Porterfield Road. Dr David Brock, who took over as head of the sub-department, was awarded a personal chair in 1986. The continuing growth in the importance of clinical genetics, as well as the international reputation of the Edinburgh centre, was recognised with the provision of new purpose-built accommodation for the department in the Molecular Medicine building, work on which started in 1993.

Physiotherapy Department

The development of this Department has been consistent through the years, keeping pace with each and every new Unit and specialty as the hospital has expanded.

Staff over the years have come from many parts of Britain and Ireland, Europe, USA and Canada, bringing new and different thoughts and ideas on patient care. Post-graduate education of the staff has always been a priority in keeping up to date with the ever-changing new techniques of treatment. Regular liaison with the other colleagues, such as GPs, speech therapists, and dietitians is considered vital. Placements are found for students not only from the Edinburgh School but from many others, as some students choose their own elective placements.

It took 40 years for the accommodation of the Department to be improved from a cupboard in a wooden shack behind D3 to a modern architect-designed Department in the Alexander Donald Building.

The inclusion of the Department in the ADB building is very appropriate. It was Dr Alexander Donald who helped to engineer the first move from D Block to the Paderewski building, initially on the ground floor on the west end of the building, but as the Casualty Department expanded, the physiotherapists had to move upstairs to the east end of the building. A retrograde step, really, as the patients had to be able to climb stairs before starting their rehabilitation. In the past all inpatient rehabilitation had to be in the ward areas because there was no covered walkway from the main hospital to the Paderewski building.

In the early days of the Department's existence in 1947, there were only two members of staff. As the scope of the work developed and was recognised, and changes in the hospital occurred, different types of patients were treated and staffing levels rose accordingly. By 1951, six members of staff were involved in the Children's Unit and in ante and post natal care, as well as in the general medical and surgical wards.

The next major development in 1956 was the addition of the Radiation Therapy Unit. This offered a new and very varied challenge for the staff which continues to the present time.

In 1960 the opening of the Department of Surgical Neurology, with its own Physiotherapy Department and small treatment pool, brought staffing levels to 11. Helpers were recruited to assist the professional staff with patient care and the many clerical duties.

In the next few years, more and more demands were being made for outpatient care. New developments in physiotherapy techniques for back and neck pain became available. Orthopaedic techniques became more intricate and more rehabilitation was needed. The care of stroke patients became more time-consuming and continued long after patients left inpatient care.

By 1966 the staff were becoming involved in the early and longer term care of patients in the Nuffield Transplant Unit.

In preparation for the next major development, that of Phase II, the new Out patient building and casualty department, the staff increased to 17 physiotherapists and five helpers, and, for the first time, a receptionist/typist. There was a recognised need for a physiotherapist to attend morning Trauma Clinics and Orthopaedic Clinics, to give on the spot advice and early care. In 1974 the Department was relocated in the old Radiotherapy Department in the main corridor of the hospital, a purpose designed reconstructed Department, with important drawbacks. No natural light and no fresh air. At last there was adequate space available. Another advantage was that the occupational therapists were there too.

Eventually the inpatients came to the gymnasiums and treatment rooms, the children to a special area of their own, and staff could use all the modern techniques especially in the rehabilitation of the early stroke patients. Many more orthopaedic cases could be seen because the gym space had doubled and there were no stairs to negotiate.

In 1982, through a request from the general practitioners in the district, GP open access was agreed. GP's could refer patients directly to the Department without first going through Consultant Clinics. A senior physiotherapist was appointed to assess the patients referred, to treat, or give advice, or to return to the GP, if it was felt that physiotherapy was not appropriate. This was one of the first such projects in Britain, Birmingham and Aberdeen followed. It was an exciting development mainly because patients with back, neck and shoulder problems principally could be seen much sooner after developing symptoms. Consequently the success rate improved.

The Department was soon bursting at the seams and so the prospect of the new Department development in the Alexander Donald Building was welcome. This Department included a hydrotherapy pool, as well as two larger gymnasiums and a much larger treatment room, paediatric room, and staff facilities. All close to the new ward areas and connected to the clinic areas and the old part of the hospital by covered walkways.

The staff moved into the new Department in the Alexander Donald Building in 1987–8 with the Princess Royal performing the official opening in July 1989. At this time the Intensive Care Unit was opened, which again involved physiotherapists treating these acutely ill patients. By this time physiotherapists were working in all areas in the hospital. In 1989–90 the Head injury Unit moved from RIE to DCN.

Option 2 re-organisation altered physiotherapy input at the Western General Hospital, some specialties were lost and others gained. Luckily no staff were lost in the transfers but some changed direction and specialised in new areas.

In 1991 Rheumatology and Medical Respiratory Unit moved from the Northern General Hospital to Western General Hospital.

Orthopaedic inpatients and Outpatient Clinics and Accident and Emergency moved to RIE. Nevertheless all patients attending these RIE departments still have their physiotherapy outpatient treatment at the Western General Hospital if they live locally.

In 1991 Antenatal and Obstetrics moved to the Eastern General Hospital/ Royal Infirmary; Paediatric inpatients transferred to the Royal Hospital for Sick Children and Breast Surgery from Longmore came to the Western General Hospital. ITU beds increased from six to eight.

By 1992 things had settled once again as the new clinical specialties established themselves in the Western General Hospital. The Physiotherapy Service underwent a reprofiling and skill mix exercise which created changes within the management structure. The Unit (RVH and Physiotherapy Service, WGH) was working well. The Superintendents at WGH (Miss Fiona McDonald)/DCN (Miss Beverley Bryan) and RVH (who has also a Unit Superintendent, Miss Wendy K. Ross) co-ordinated the physiotherapy input to all areas within both hospitals as well as providing an outpatient service for patients with musculo-skeletal problems.

1993 saw the development of a Stroke Rehabilitation Team and Regional Adult Cystic Fibrosis Unit. This resulted in two senior physiotherapy appointments. The Department began a Unit-wide programme of risk assessment and training to address the problems associated with manual handling.

By 1995 the Western General Hospital Physiotherapy Department is still situated in the ground floor of the Alexander Donald Building alongside Occupational Therapy. The physiotherapy service is run Trust wide. The current staffing level, including DCN, for the Western General Hospital is now more than 30 whole time equivalents (40 staff). The most recent development was to offer the Minor Injuries Unit a daily weekday Clinic so patients with acute soft tissue problems are seen within 24 hours.

Superintendents of Physiotherapy were:

1. Betty King
2. Sheila Cameron
3. Anne Robertson
4. Fiona McDonald — present superintendent.

Association of Friends

The Association was formed at the initiative of Dr Sandy Donald and Mr Selby Tulloch in 1957. The official inauguration date is December 1962, which is the date on the Incorporation. Although registered as a charity it went a step further than was required. The Association was registered under the Companies Act because it was felt that the annual Financial Statement should be published. The Chairman was Sandy Hodge, the Treasurer was David Alexander, who was the Head of the Royal Bank of Scotland in St Andrews Square, John Shaw was the Accountant and David Illingworth was on the list of Directors as the only medical representative. Sandy Donald and Selby Tulloch were advisers on things medical but not as Director. The finances of the Association were primed by a substantial donation from Ferranti's. This gift being obtained on the recommendation of Dr 'Ekke' Kuenssberg who was the Medical Officer to Ferranti at that time.

The aim of the Friends was to provide amenities and comforts for the patients in the hospital. The objectives specifically stated that the function of the Association was not to provide equipment which was regarded as being a proper call on the resources of the Health Service. Similarly, providing finance to members of the staff of the hospital was specifically excluded so that no-one could be accused of having any vested interest in the monies raised. To start with, the Association confined itself to supplying curtaining round the beds, easy chairs, chairs for visitors, part of the Social Service Department, part of the Patients Library with the provision of talking books and the television sets and trolley telephones. Over the years its funds have increased through donations and this is one of the reasons why a number of the legal representatives were on the original list of Directors so that they could encourage bequests. These, in fact, never amounted to a great deal in any one year. For quite a number of years the biggest single donation made to its funds came from the sponsored cycle run. This was enthusiastically run by Bill and Tordis Small with the unstinting and cheerful support of the staff of the Gastric Follow-Up Clinic. They were succeeded by Martin Eastwood and Anne Jenkinson. Each year cyclists left the Western General Hospital and rode approximately 30 miles. The route passed through Kirkliston, Linlithgow, stopping at the Hawes Inn in South Queensferry and home. There were teams from the gastric follow-up clinic, surgery, gastroenterolgy, physiotherapy, oncology and elsewhere. This was a social event of the year with children and parents having a lovely and exhausting ride into the country. There were also a certain number of fund-raising events and, of course various collecting boxes placed in the wards and corridors throughout the hospital.

When Sandy Hodge retired as Chairman, Sandy Donald took on that role until he in turn retired, when Bill Small became Chairman for the next nine or ten years. The Hospital Chaplain, Melville Schofield, is the present Chairman. The Royal Bank of Scotland has provided the Treasurer ever since the beginning. David Alexander retired, and was followed by John Burke. Now the Treasurer is Kenneth Aitken, the present Senior Manager of the Royal Bank of

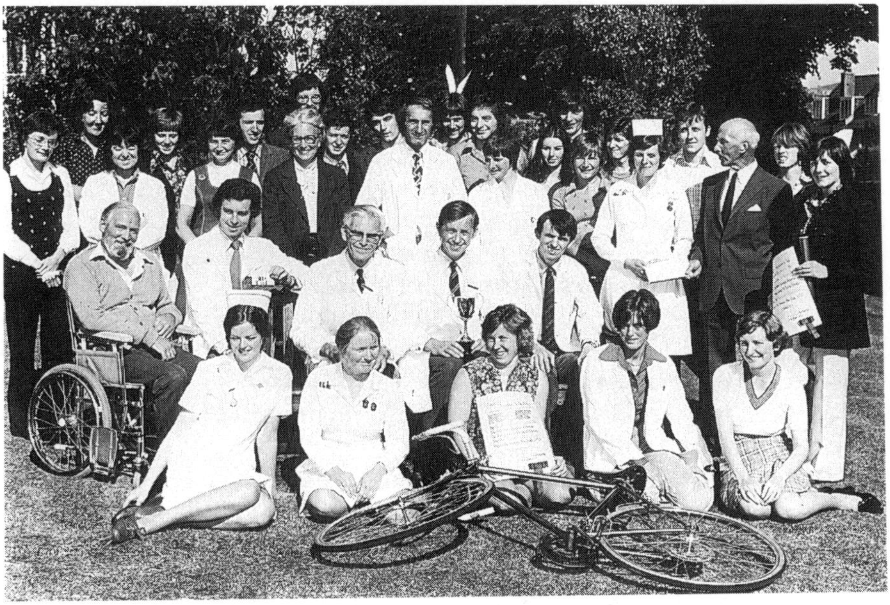

One of the Association of Friends' Cycle Runs. Mr WP Small, third from left front row; Dr Sandy Donald second right second row

Scotland's main office in St Andrews Square. A feature of the Association is that none of the office bearers receive any remuneration. In fact, all money donated is spent in support of the hospital. There have been no overheads. The present address is the Chaplaincy Centre, which provides facilities for the meetings and also a good deal of secretarial help, particularly with Melville Schofield becoming Chairman. Over the years the attitude towards the provision of facilities has broadened quite considerably. The Association provides substantial items of equipment where there is an immediate benefit to the welfare of patients. The computer facilities to the CSSD and some quite expensive urological equipment to Professor Chisholm's Department. The Association also supports further education of nursing staff by an annual grant. This is monitored by a panel, the idea being that nurses requiring or benefiting from further experience will, through their increased expertise, benefit the hospital and patients. The Association continues to provide telephone facilities and has also provided much help with refurbishing, including the landscaping around Raeburn House. There are no longer collecting boxes around the hospital, fearing that they probably did not do the image much good. Instead they have been replaced by 18 purpose designed holders of brochures.

Quarterly meetings of the Directors are held and an Annual General Meeting at which the Accounts are presented, duly audited and then submitted to the Company Office in George Street. There is much support for the work of the Association. There is no evidence that this support by patients or the welcome that it receives is diminished with the coming of Trust status. The Association belongs to the National Association of Leagues of Hospital Friends. On the occasions when Mr Small has attended their Annual Conferences there is a justified feeling of a very happy liaison throughout the hospital and its administration. Unlike some Leagues or Associations, the Friends of the WGH do not run shops. These are the remit of the Womens Royal Voluntary Service with whom there is a cordial association. They have from time to time helped with the sale of articles such as the cook book, post cards and some of the furry toys and items which are donated by well wishers.

Chaplaincy in the Western General Hospital

Between 1948 and 1971, two full-time Chaplains held office in the Edinburgh Northern Group of Hospitals, the first being Mr Walker. He was succeeded in 1959 by Rev. John L. Douglas, who came to the post from being Minister of Newhaven-on-Forth Church.

With the appointment of Rev. David Lyall, formerly Minister of Park Parish Church, Ardrossan, chaplaincy was established on a slightly different basis. In a period of 18 months in 1970–71, the three full-time Hospital chaplaincies in Edinburgh all became vacant. In each case an appointment was made by which the Chaplain had Honorary status within the University's Department of Christian Ethics and Practical Theology. This carried the responsibility for developing the training of divinity students in the care of the sick. In 1970, Murray Leishman was appointed to the Royal Edinburgh Hospital, Stewart McGregor to the Royal Infirmary, and in 1971 David Lyall to the Northern Group.

The major problem confronting the Chaplain was ministry to a Group of hospitals, for included with the Western were the Eastern General, the Northern General and Leith Hospital (and, to begin with, Musselburgh Maternity Hospital). How could a Chaplain, even supported by a full-time assistant and part-time Roman Catholic and Episcopalian Chaplains, possibly minister to over 1,000 patients whose average stay was six days? In truth, priorities had to be set. The Radiotherapy Unit and the Department of Surgical Neurology tended to take up a great deal of time. Not only through pastoral care of patients but through being available to anxious relatives and, not infrequently, being available to staff.

Baptisms, weddings and funerals took up a significant amount of time. The baptisms were usually anxious affairs in the Special Care Baby Unit, where there was a degree of concern for the life of the baby. Interestingly, the number of 'emergency' baptisms has dropped significantly over the years. This was partly a result of a decline in religious interest in the community, and partly because of the decreased number of births. The introduction of new drugs and techniques reduced such conditions as respiratory distress in the new born and fewer babies were terminally ill.

Weddings could be both happy and sad: happy when a member of staff asked the Chaplain to officiate, and sometimes a bit of each. Especially when the wedding had to take place in hospital because of a concern for the health of one of the parties involved.

In a sense, for the Chaplain to conduct a funeral service marked a kind of failure on the part of the Chaplain. This meant that no meaningful link had been made with a local minister. Sometimes because of the intensity of the pastoral bond that can be created with both patients and families in the crisis of hospitalisation, it was entirely appropriate that the Chaplain conducted the Funeral service of someone who died in hospital.

In the early days, accommodation was always a problem for the Chaplaincy. In 1971 the Chaplain worked from a tiny room, next door to the old mortuary (opposite the entrance to the present OPD). Its furnishings consisted of a table, a chest of drawers, an electric kettle and two cups! In the 1970s two moves were made; first of all, to the Paderewski Building (bigger, less smelly, but still inaccessible to patients); then to a new room opposite the Snack Bar. There were, however, a number of staff who were conscious of the need for adequate chaplaincy accommodation, and were prepared to work to make it possible. Over coffee in Mat Flat one morning, Miss Stephen, the Maternity Superintendent, said to David Lyall, 'You may not have a Women's Guild, Mr Lyall, but you do have us.' From that moment, the building of the Chaplaincy Centre was inevitable! A fund-raising committee was set up, chaired by Professor Bill Duncan of the Department of Radiotherapy. Large donations came from the WRVS, Hospital Endowments, the major denominations and individual congregations. Many events were organised and, in 1979, the Chaplaincy

Centre — costing approximately £65,000 — was opened. It was a multi-purpose Centre, with facilities for worship and meetings, and a place where people can come just to be quiet, as well as offices of the Chaplains. The architect was Stewart Tod, an Edinburgh Architect, with much experience of church design. The tapestry in the apse was designed and executed by James J. More, of the Galashiels Textile College, and the Communion Table was gifted by Dr and Mrs Alex Keay, in memory of their son.

Over the years, a succession of assistants and colleagues made outstanding contributions to the work of chaplaincy. Miss Phyllis Bain, a Deaconess of the Church of Scotland, was in post before John Douglas arrived. She retired in 1972. She had a prodigious capacity to visit patients and really did see most of them at least once during their stay. She was succeeded briefly by Miss (now Dr) Barbara Boal, a former Baptist Missionary in India who went on to post graduate studies at Edinburgh University. From 1974–82 Mrs Myra Hutchinson was Chaplain's Assistant, having previously been Matron of Tumu Mission Hospital in Kenya. Mrs Hutchinson exercised a profound pastoral ministry and shared fully in the developing work over these years. This included not only the building of the new Centre, but in responding to an ever-increasing number of invitations to take part in interdisciplinary team meetings. This period was also marked by a deeper involvement in nurse education, contributing, among other topics, to seminars on terminal care, and on issues in medical and nursing ethics. In 1982, the Rev. Gillian Morton joined the team. Her ordination as a Minister marked a high point in the story of chaplaincy in WGH — and with two ordained Ministers in post, it also became possible for each to have genuine time off! Gillian made her own distinguished contribution to all aspects of chaplaincy, not least in the Nuffield Transplant Unit. A dissertation written for her BD Degree subsequently was published, and became recognised far beyond WGH, as a significant contribution to chaplaincy. In 1988, Gillian was appointed first Chaplain of the new Borders General Hospital, and has continued to do pioneering work there.

A feature of chaplaincy at WGH in recent years is that it has been as ecumenical as wider church politics has allowed, with a genuine sense of being a team, helped along of course by working together from the new Centre. The Revds. David Jowitt, Philip Price, Reg. Henning, George Spencer and Diana Forman, for the Scottish Episcopal Church; Fathers Birnie, Kiernan, Gallagher, and Sisters Ita and Felix for the Roman Catholic Church, all exercised a pastoral and sacramental ministry which was appreciated by members of their own denominations and beyond. On many days, those members of the team present ate sandwiches together after hospital prayers held each day around 1 p.m. Frequently, students who were present on placement, said that they learned more about ministry by taking part in these conversations, than from any other source. In 1987, David Lyall left for an academic post, first in St Andrews and then back in Edinburgh. He was succeeded by Rev. Melville Schofield, Minister of the Laigh Kirk, Kilmarnock, who was introduced in March 1988. Melville Schofield introduced a different style to the chaplaincy, not inconsistent with the previous chaplains. His ministry is based on a lifetime in the Parish. He is a well recognised figure throughout the hospital. His ministry extends to the staff as well as the patient population.

The Rev. Alison Barclay was ordained to the post of Chaplain's Assistant on 1 November 1988 and retired in January 1991. Regrettably, because of a financial crisis, the Board could not see its way to appointing someone in her place and the full-time Chaplain once again found himself on his own.

A significant and traumatic period of change in the organisation and thrust of the National Health Service coincided with this new appointment. The introduction of the Purchaser Provider Philosophy and uncertainties regarding the Trust Status meant that the Chaplain was now involved with staff at all levels and of all disciplines. He now takes part in all orientation programmes for new staff, seeking to enhance attitudes in hospital. The Chancel part of the Chaplaincy remains open 24 hours a day. Other departments have been encouraged to use the lounge area for meetings, relaxation sessions for oncology patients, various groups supporting patients and relatives affected by strokes, brain tumours, breast cancer, and grief and loss.

The Association of Friends of the Western General Hospital, under the present Chairmanship of Mr William Small, also use the Chaplaincy Centre as the 'headquarters', from where a great deal of financial assistance is given for various projects throughout the hospital.

Money has been raised through various Guilds and outside organisations. A significant sum was given by the WRVS to provide equipment to broadcast the morning prayers and the Sunday service to those wards capable of receiving them through the hospital broadcasting system.

Someone once described hospital chaplaincy as being a matter of 'loitering with intent'. Certainly, those Chaplains who have been accorded the privilege of 'hanging around' the Western General Hospital have found themselves involved in ministries which have been as fascinating as they have been demanding, seeking to exercise pastoral care in an institution which always tried, and usually succeeded, in affirming what was essentially human, while pushing forward the boundaries of medical science and technology.

Patients' Library

In 1943 Mr Butchard, a librarian of Edinburgh City Libraries, suggested that there should be a hospital library service for six hospitals. By 1944 he had produced proposals. The town council approved the idea in April 1946 and this finally happened in October 1946. A small library was established at the Western General. Twice a week a member of the Public Library staff visited the Hospital to distribute the books. Books were sent to other Edinburgh hospitals but evidently the Western General scheme was established on a more ambitious scale than the others. It was proposed that a small room in each hospital should initially stock one book per patient increasing to at least two. With 2,365 beds in the hospitals to be supplied, approximately 5000 volumes were required. The books had to be 'mostly recreational, cheerful in tone, well printed and easy to handle'. The stock was sometimes supplemented with gifts from members of staff. The initial cost for staffing (one assistant working 4 days in hospital) and fitments was £500 per annum. In 1957/58 the patient library was moved to the then new Radiation Therapy Unit which made it more accessible to mobile patients. Because of the development of the patient library a request was made for more staff. This was rejected on financial grounds and it was agreed to consider voluntary assistants. As a result the Womens Royal Voluntary Service was approached. In 1961 a scheme was put into operation for two WRVS helpers to come twice weekly for ward round duty with the library staff.

Miss Lilias Tait was the librarian who originally set up the library service, not only in the Western General but in other Edinburgh hospitals. When she first started she personally went round bookshops choosing stock. Today the suppliers come to the Central Library, George IV Bridge, where the librarian calls once a week.

In 1964 the Friends of the Western General Hospital funded an investigation into the possibility of using tape recordings in the hospital to include talking books and music. Thanks to their continued help it has been possible to expand this lending capability. At this time large print books were included for partially sighted patients.

When the new Medical Library was built, provision was made for the present Patients' Library which was a big improvement. There are now 2700 books per month distributed throughout the Western. Stock also includes videos, story and music cassettes, reminiscence material and jigsaws.

The Librarian also provides information on a range of subjects, including health.

Librarians:

Ms Lilias Tait	1946–1975
Mrs Jane McDonagh	1975–1982
Ms Gail McKinley	1982–1984
Mrs Christine Craig	1984–present

Medical Library

The Western General Hospital Library was originally kept in a small room in the attics above A Flat where the respiratory medicine offices are now located. The books were not infrequently given by members of the staff. Many members of staff gave their Journals to the Library and a small useful and compact Library was established. A series of professional librarians, appointed by the University of Edinburgh, were in charge. It was clear that the requirements of the Library were not sufficient for the hospital. Thanks to the endeavours of Professor Strong and the members of the Library Committee, Dr Ted French and also

Dr Neil McLean, the Pathologist, and Mrs (later Dr) Rita Neilon who was Chairman of the South East of Scotland Health Board, and Dr Campbell the CAMO, money was made available to build a new Library. This was sited off the main corridor and opened in January 1980. The Library expanded rapidly and a number of Journals relevant to a teaching hospital were introduced. The donated Journals remained an important contribution to the Library's well-being. In the early 1980s there was a strong feeling from the clinical staff that the hours provided by the Library were insufficient — the Library opening from 9.00 a.m. until 5.00 p.m. The then Chairman of the Library Committee, Dr Martin Eastwood, approached all the Departments within the Western General Hospital, asking them to make an annual contribution to the expansion of the Library service. Some made contributions of £150 per year from their various endowment funds. Funds from North Lothian District enabled a further extension to opening hours. The response was uniformly generous and typical of the Hospital, to meet a problem generously and imaginatively. The result was that the Library was able to open from 9.00 a.m. until 9.00 p.m. and on a Saturday morning. The librarian who took the Library from the small attic Library through to its present modern systems was Anne Kennett, 1973–1988. As part of Edinburgh University Library, staff and the Library benefited from the strong connection with other parts of the University Library system.

The Library has further developed this strong connection through the activities of Mrs Dorothy Walker and also Dr John Webb, Chairman of the Library Committee from 1983 onwards. The Library nowadays is fully computerised and has ready access to the Erskine Medical Library in the University and the British Library and to information databases such as Medline. The Medical Library has been a truly combined endeavour between the University of Edinburgh, the Lothian Health Board and the Hospital.

Librarians in Charge:

Mrs E. MacLean	1966
Miss Crowe	1969
Mrs Morrison	1969
Mrs Valentine	1973
Mrs Anne Kennett	1973–1988
Mrs Dorothy Walker	1988–1993
Mrs Alice Langdon	1993–

Chairmen of the Library Committee:

Dr E. B. French	1966
Mr C. V. Ruckley	1976
Dr M. A. Eastwood	1978
Dr J. N. Webb	1983

Number of books held:	3,500
Current journal titles:	240

Medical Records and Secretarial Services

At the inception of the National Health Service in 1948, all previous records of the hospital were removed to the city's archives. The military records associated with the Paderewski Hospital which was situated in the grounds of the Western during the war, were subsequently removed by the military authorities.

The Medical Records Department started from humble beginnings in an Enquiry Office at the main entrance to the hospital (under the clock tower) in 1948–49. Two members of staff, Margaret Ferguson and Helen Fox were original members of the newly-formed department. They were responsible for the documentation of all admissions to the hospital and the compilation of routine activity statistics. An Appointments Office was established in the basement of the Surgical Block, this was maintained by the surgical and urology secretaries.

Very few departments at that time had their own personal secretaries and a small typing pool was situated in the main corridor of the Medical Block. As the workload grew more secretaries were appointed and attached to individual units.

Outpatient clinics were held in a hut off the main drive of the hospital.

As was customary in all hospitals around this time, each clinical department maintained and stored their own patients' medical records. In 1959, a new innovation from America, the 'unit medical record system', was introduced, i.e. all medical records relating to a patient were contained within the one case-folder, and for the first time, they were stored in a central records library. This practice was gradually extended to the whole hospital. As the number of outpatient clinics expanded and the need for more space for the Medical Records Department grew, both departments were moved to the Paderewski Block, which also housed the Accident and Emergency Department, and a small typing pool. The typing pool, under the supervision of Clare Wardlaw, provided a secretarial service to the various outpatient clinics and back-up to the unit secretaries.

In January 1960, the first Group Medical Records Officer (Ray Hopkins) was appointed to develop the medical records functions of the Edinburgh Northern Group of Hospitals, based at the Western General Hospital. Professional advice and supervision was provided to the Medical Records Departments of the Northern General, Leith and Eastern General Hospitals.

Plans for building the new Outpatient Department (Phase 1) were being developed during the early sixties. In 1965, trials of several 'remote control dictation systems' were conducted with a view to installing one of them in the new building. Unit records were allocated to the typing pool on a rota basis to test these new systems. Remote dictation failed to find favour with the secretaries and consultant staff and the project was abandoned. Individual dictating machines were installed and quickly replaced shorthand dictation for clinical correspondence. The clinical Units retained their personal secretaries.

Two other new developments were introduced about this time:

Mechanical Documentation — embossed metal plates containing the patient's identification details, which enabled the Records Office to produce adhesive labels for the first time.
Microfilming of medical records — as clinical science advanced, the amount of paper accumulated for each patient grew in scale. When the National Health Service started it was possible to store between 100–120 records per linear foot of shelving. By the mid-seventies this figure had been reduced to around 70 records per foot. Today the figure is nearer 26–30. By the mid-sixties the pressure on available storage space increased and micro-filming offered an easy solution. However, microfilm was not very popular with the clinical staff, recall rates were very low, and this facility was eventually replaced by a destruction policy.

In 1971 the Department moved to the basement of the Phase 1 building into new and much extended accommodation. In the mid-sixties, medical records and secretarial staff numbered 49. In the years following the move to the new building the number of staff quickly increased to over 100 as improved clinical and paramedical facilities were brought into use.

Few technological advances were made between 1971 and the early eighties. A massive revolution followed. This saw the introduction of computers, replacing outdated mechanical documentation equipment, and manual patient indexes. The word processor and inter-ward process networking system make for a ready interchange of information. This was followed in 1987 by the introduction of the HOMER Patient Administration System which revolutionised medical records procedures.

An important sub-division in medical records is Coding, which enables a summary of the Hospital's work to be made available to local and national authorities. Mr Alan Hinton has led this unit through many complex changes.

The introduction of the 'internal market' in 1991 has placed major demands on the medical records and information staff with the requirement to 'track' patients from areas outwith Lothian, or who belong to GP Fundholding Practices. This will allow the 'purchasers' responsible for the patients' health care to be invoiced accordingly.

In 1948 the administration saw the benefits of centralising as many of the medical records functions as possible in order to obtain economies of scale and the standardisation of procedures. Today, with the development of Clinical Directorates, medical records resources and functions are being devolved, leaving only medical records library and appointment functions under the control of the medical records office.

Medical Records Officers have included in succession Ian Laing, Jim Knowles, Douglas MacKensie.

Portering

Charlie Wood started work as a general porter in the Western General Hospital in October 1960 when the Portering Department consisted of approximately 26 porters and one Head Porter. There were 19 day-shift, three back-shift, three night-shift and one permanent mortuary porter. Duties comprised the collection of refuse, to burn and clean out the incinerator, to deliver all types of stores, the collection and delivery of pharmacy baskets, as well as patient movement, and the movement of furniture and other items.

The Radiotherapy Unit had three porters for patient movement only. DCN had four porters, two for general duties within DCN and two for theatres and X Ray department only. Laundry had two porters, Mail one porter, and Accident and Emergency three porters for patient movement only. Four shift porters in the main building covered almost everything else.

This was the situation until the Bacteriology Department opened, when the employment of an additional porter brought the staff level to 27.

From 1960 to 1970 the NTU unit, Haematology Laboratory and Clinical Chemistry Laboratories were completed. This required more portering service and one porter was employed for the laboratories, and three for the NTU — one day-shift, one back-shift and one night-shift. By 1972 the number of porters totalled 31. Phase one was opened and this meant the closing of the Paderewski building where physio, A&E, records and clinics were located. A further eight porters were employed — one for A&E, one lift attendant, one back-shift, one night-shift, one deputy Head Porter, three day-shift Phase One. Also four porters were made up to charge-hands, bringing the total to 39. This increased to 40 when X Ray moved from main corridor to Phase One.

In the 1980s Phase Two was opened thus creating more portering duties. Pharmacy, Physio, Occupational Therapy, Domestic Dept, changing accommodation, mortuary, neurology, pathology, and wards, were all transferred to Phase Two. Five more porters were employed raising the total to 44.

Charlie Wood was head porter from 1969 to 1990. After he retired he was succeeded by John Diamond who during the introduction of new managerial systems in the hospital, became manager in charge of portering services.

The Portering service has always included great characters. Some of whom coped with disabilities, which in no way prevented them from giving commitment to the Hospital. Many patients have gained support and cheer whilst being transported about the Hospital to unknown and sometimes anxiety producing experiences. Often on trolleys and chairs that had a will of their own.

Central Sterile Stores Department

In 1960 a working party of Dr Donald, the Medical Superintendent; Miss Estelle Adamson the Matron; Mr James Bee the Theatre Charge Nurse and Mr Alex Campbell the Supervisor established a Central Sterilising Room (CSR) at the Western General Hospital. This was originally in the temporary wooden surgical theatre which was built during the 1914–18 War. Until that time, all instruments and sterilisable equipment in theatre and in the wards had to be cleaned and sterilised by the nursing staff. This was an exacting and time consuming task. The Western General Hospital piloted this comprehensive service. At this time the Royal Infirmary only had a Syringe Service Centre. The service provided sterile dressing materials, instruments and glass syringes to all theatres, wards and Departments within the Group. An additional service of cleaning, drying and powdering rubber macs and gloves was also provided to all theatres.

Items for sterilisation were packed into drums, and sterilised in an Arnold Downward Displacement Steriliser. The CSR had three sterilisers, one for selected rubber goods, one for metal/glass items and one for dressing materials. The sterilising cycle was slow by modern standards and included a cooling cycle between 2¼ and 3½ hours. This is very different from the approximate 30-minute cycle of today.

High risk items, where hepatitis was suspected, were autoclaved three times to ensure sterility! In addition to this, the Department had two genito-urinary manual sterilisers for processing catheters and bougies from Mr Tulloch's GU Sessions, and Radiotherapy Theatre lists and clinics.

Another innovation came in 1960 when the Department of Surgical Neurology opened — CSR staff had the use of a High Speed High Vacuum Autoclave which was placed beside the Neurosurgical Theatres. However, in 1964 and 1965, the Manlove Alliot Autoclave was transferred from DSN to CSR and an additional machine was purchased for the CSR.

When the Department of Surgical Neurology opened, an Electric Razor Cleaning Maintenance Service was introduced. This was for the shaving of patients' scalps before neurosurgical operations.

The name of the unit was changed a year later, in 1966, and became the Central Sterilising Supply Department (CSSD).

A further development, which was quite revolutionary in its time, came about when Colonel John Mackie and Miss Sheila Scott from the South Eastern Regional Hospital Board introduced a project to provide a Ward Procedure Pack System, to be supplied from a Commercial Source. The two companies chosen were Johnson & Johnson and Smith & Nephew.

The Procedure Pack System was available by 1969 for all the hospitals in the South East Regional Hospital Board. Both training demonstrations and film shows were organised to promote correct use of these new packs. The result of this was that CSSD stopped the production of all packs available communally, but continued the in-house production of 'specialised' packs only. Shortly after the Procedure Pack System was introduced, as part of a Sterile Service Reorganisation, the Royal Hospital for Sick Children CSSD Edinburgh and the Victoria Hospital, Kirkcaldy CSSD provided a service of 'soft' goods CRHSCD and intravenous cut down, stitch and aspiration trays (VHK) to all Lothian Health Board users. This service was phased in over a period of months.

In 1970 a Manlove Alliot Autoclave MKII was purchased to replace existing old machinery. This acquisition provided the means to attain a higher, more monitorable standard of autoclaving. A further autoclave was purchased two years later because of the increased workload.

During this period, the CSSD service consisted of the purchase and distribution of commercially produced Ward Procedure Packs and supplementary items. There was inhouse production of 'Composite' packs, individual instruments, 'soft' goods, and minor instrument trays, including a tray service to the Family Planning Centre at Dean Terrace, thereby supplying Lothian Health Board Family Planning requirements. Even so, there were insufficient stocks of theatre instruments within the Western. This meant that theatre staff (nurses) were still having to sterilise baskets of theatre instruments within the main theatre suite. In 1976 the Royal Infirmary established a Theatre Service Centre (TSC). After further developments this service provided the Western General Hospital Main Theatre Suite with instrument trays and some supplementary instruments.

A further development in Sterile Service Centralisation came when a new 'Area' Sterilising Centre at the City Hospital site was built in 1981–83. The plan was that all three centres, the Royal Infirmary Theatre Services Centre, the Royal Hospital for Sick Children CSSD and the Western General Hospital CSSD would all be provided from a central complex in the new centre.

In the meantime the Western General Hospital had increased its service to include all the hospitals within the Northern Group i.e. the Northern General Hospital, the Royal Victoria Hospital, the Eastern General Hospital, as well as Edenhall Hospital, GP surgeries, and the Community needs of the North West Community.

However, in 1985 the requirements of the Royal Hospital for Sick Children CSSD were transferred to the new centre at the City Hospital. Despite the fact there were minor problems and upheavals, the service was maintained.

In 1986 when the Royal Infirmary was transferred to the new theatre supply system, there was a catastrophic upset to the service previously supplied by the Royal Infirmary. Problems included the 'Red Alert' situation, the failure of the service to provide what they were identified to do for at least two weeks. This required theatre sisters from within the Lothian Health Board Area volunteering their services to pack theatre instrument trays. This was not helped by strike action by ancillary staff within the new centre. This was a time of considerable disruption within the service. It took approximately one year for the problems to be resolved and a satisfactory service to be provided from the new centre.

In 1988 it was suggested that the Western General Hospital CSSD would transfer to the Area Sterilising Centre. Nevertheless, within that year the Western General Hospital CSSD supplied sterile packs to the newly opened ITU at the Western General Hospital. By 1989 the prospect of the Western General Hospital CSSD transferring to the new centre became increasingly unlikely.

It was recognised in 1990 that the accommodation for the CSSD was in a poor state of repair and was never intended to be a CSSD building. The building had been designed to be a surgical theatre in the 1914–18 War, and did not meet the guidelines of the Good Manufacturing Practice Guide for NHS Sterile Service Department (1989).

In 1990 the Western General Hospital Unit General Management Team decided to close the CSSD because of the unsurmountable problems of the building. It suggested that the Neurosurgical Mini Theatre Services Complex, soon to be refurbished, could be considered as part of a contingency plan. Throughout the year there were suggestions that CSSD should close and a costing exercise was made by the Theatre Clinical Nurse Manager. This included the removal from the site of the services provided by CSSD. The problem then arose about where would 'sterile' and 'dirty' instruments be stored in the event of the closure of CSSD?

The increased work capacity of the Area Sterilising Centre went a stage further when they took over the services provided by the Victoria Hospital, Kirkcaldy.

In 1991 the CSSD had to tender for the work which it had hitherto provided. By 1992 the discussions were still continuing about the future of CSSD. Yet, in late 1992, CSSD Assistants began training to become proficient in packing Neurosurgical Theatre Instrument Trays to provide a much-needed service for the Neurosurgical Theatre Service Centre (this work was being carried out by theatre nursing personnel). After much discussion in 1993 it was agreed that the Western General Hospital CSSD would remain open to provide an in-house medical equipment service, neurosurgical TSC service, cleaning and packing service of all items requiring gas EO2 sterilisation at the Area Sterilising Centre. Also the purchase and distribution of commercially produced disposable items (sterile), and collection and distribution of all manner of items produced by the Area Sterilising Centre.

Throughout this period the Centre was led by Mr David and Mrs Sheena Henderson. However in 1993 as a result of the competitive tendering and rationalisation it was decided that the post of Deputy CSSD Manager would be lost in order to produce savings against a competitive tender exercise. David Henderson transferred to a post in Human Resources. Later that year the CSSD Chargehand was upgraded to Supervisor Grade to deputise for the Sterile Services Manager, Mrs Henderson. In February 1993, as a result of liaison between the Area Sterile Centre and the Western General Hospital Managers, there began the transfer of agreed workload from the Western General Hospital CSSD to the Area Sterile Centre. The services of the Western General Hospital CSSD continue under Mrs Henderson's supervision.

Womens Royal Voluntary Service

When volunteers first came to the Hospital in 1953 they belonged to the Womens Voluntary Service (WVS). The WVS began their work in the hospital in approximately 1953 providing a tray of tea and biscuits in the

Waiting Room at the Outpatient Department. The Outpatient Department in those days was in the Paderewski which was a cold, vast building. Patients had to wait a long time, and they were seen collectively in a large room, an entirely unsatisfactory system. Volunteers collected stores from a remote Steward's Office and carried trays up and down stairs. They served tea to Maternity Outpatient Clinics from a small table. Then a trolley service for Outpatients was requested. Later on the WVS agreed to take complete charge of hospitality to patients. Over the years the volunteers have developed fully-stocked trolleys covering all sections of the hospital. The takings were varied. Initially the takings were as little as 9d a day (4–5p). The service was much appreciated by patients who, in those days, often had a long wait. In 1959 Dr Donald, the Medical Superintendent, asked the WVS to start a shop which would be open every day. This entailed recruiting many members who then had to learn the mysteries of buying and accounting on a larger scale than most had been accustomed to.

The old Dining Room was converted into an attractive Sandwich Bar to cater for medical staff unable to use the Staff Canteen because of the way that their day was progressing. This bridged the period between the availability of the old and new canteen. Further help was given in the Teaching Unit by serving snack lunches outside the room when there were lectures in the Teaching Unit Theatre.

In 1966 the WVS became the Womens Royal Voluntary Service, a tribute to the work that is a national endeavour.

The initial rota of six members has extended to over 350 volunteers involved in WGH projects at the present time. All the profits earned by the WRVS are used for the benefit of the hospital. This means that there is a very warm and caring relationship between the WRVS and the hospital as a whole. The profits were spent after consultation with the Medical Superintendent and the Matron in the past, and now with Management, in the buying of amenities for the staff and patients. To begin with these were in the flower glass type of purchase. The expenditure and scale of purchase has risen as profits have increased. These range from television sets to chintzs for the Nurses Home, ward cubicle curtains, upgrading of china etc. They have even financed extensions to buildings, such as the veranda for ward D1. During 1993/94, the WRVS projects within the Hospital funded items were valued at £55,000, including medical equipment, specialised beds, mattresses and screens, carpets, curtains, lockers, flowers and televisions.

An important development was the Hospital Library Service which developed to include talking books and other aids for partially sighted patients. Many partially sighted patients have been introduced to the Ulverscroft large print books as well as to the British Library of tape recordings for hospital patients. There are over 50 such specialist books. Many books have been loaned throughout the hospital and the Nuffield Talking Book Library for the blind has loaned books.

With the opening of the Alexander Donald Building a further shop was started here in 1987. An outpatient tea trolley was developed in November 1990. Ward flower arrangements by the WRVS began in 1991. A further extension of their work was the Guides to help in Oncology and the Outpatient Department and this started in November 1992. Now there is a Tea Bar in the Oncology Department which was started in 1993. From 1993 the WRVS has also assisted with stroke patients on the ward, reading to them and taking them to the Canteen for a cup of tea.

Each project has its own rota keeper. Many of the ladies who work in the WRVS have worked for 10 or more years. There are also a number of men working in a voluntary capacity.

The Future

From its humble beginnings (127 years ago) the Western General Hospital has gone from strength to strength caring for its local community and, since the end of the war, has become a major teaching hospital in its own right. Its full potential has yet to be realised but the next decade will be critical in this development.

By the end of 1995 the Molecular Medicine Centre adjacent to the MRC Human Genetics building will be commissioned and will add a complete new dimension to medical research, not only in Edinburgh but in the United Kingdom. Funded by the Wolfson Foundation, Cancer Research Campaign, Lothian Health, ROW-FOGO and Robertson Trusts, University of Edinburgh and SHERT this enterprise again emphasises the need for collaboration between all those involved in health care to support research.

Also in 1995, the original Medical Superintendent's House — subsequently part of the Medical Residency — is being radically upgraded to allow patients, referred from a distance, to stay on the campus following invasive cardiology procedures. The house will be renamed Turner House, in memory of Dr Turner and his major contribution to cardiological investigation while a consultant here.

1995 will also see the completion of a Clinical Research Initiative to allow an expansion of the Out-patient Facility and office/research accommodation for Neurosciences.

In 1996 the current Nuffield Transplant Unit will also be rejuvenated to become a Day Chemotherapy Centre, closely integrating the skills of the individual specialties, such as, Haematology with those of Oncology, and Pharmacy. The Macmillan Fund has agreed to be a major benefactor in this major step forward for such patients.

Work started in 1995 by clearing the site previously occupied by the Bank of Scotland, and the Linen Store, to allow the building of a new four storey block to house the Breast Unit Out-Patient Department, an extension to the Breast Imaging Department and also an in-patient and academic Haematology Department.

In 1996 clinical haematology in Edinburgh will be amalgamated at the

Western allowing maximum utilisation of the skills, experience and research facilities presently split between the Royal Infirmary and the Western. All haematology in-patients will be the natural focus for academic Haematology, and a new Chair of Haematology will be created. The Leukaemia Research Fund have agreed to be a major contributor to this development, and the Research area is likely to be called the John Hughes Bennett Laboratory, in memory of Dr Bennett who first described leukaemia following his observations in Edinburgh in 1845. There will also be an expanded Blood Transfusion Service on site.

The University has also agreed that two further Chairs be created at the Western: Diabetic Medicine and Clinical Pharmacology. The former is a tribute to the pioneering work of Dr Joyce Baird who retired as Reader in Medicine in 1994, and who — like so many before her — has to be replaced by at least two consultants to cover the same work load! The appointment of Dr David Webb to the latter will greatly strengthen the Clinical Research Centre and add a new dimension to the Drug Development aspects of the current centre.

The real challenge of the next decade will be the bringing to fruition of the Lothian Acute Services Strategy. The end result will be two major acute hospitals in Edinburgh — an expanded Western General Hospital and the Royal Infirmary transferred to a green field site at Little France. The closure at that time of the Eastern General, the City Hospital and the Princess Margaret Rose Hospitals has implications for the Western — Infectious Disease and HIV will transfer, as will gynaecology. The future of the maternity/obstetric service within the City is still under debate, but hopefully will be sited where patients will gain most advantage rather than directed by any particular pressure group.

In practical terms this will mean that at the Western a new theatre block of around 16 operating theatres will be required to rationalise the current, rather scattered, theatre facilities. A large new ward block will be built on the present site of the nurses's home and will incorporate the principle entrance to the hospital, including a reception area and a shopping facility. It is hoped that a major University Academic block will also be an integral part of this ward block.

Who knows, we may even achieve a realistic multi-storey car park on four levels, in the north east of the site, to accommodate the needs of staff, patients and their visitors. That alone would be a major achievement!

The future of the hospital, the Trust and patient care, lies entirely in the skills, enthusiasm, experience and knowledge of the staff. The advent of Trust status has brought us a most powerful and understanding Chairman in Michael Walker, and a Chief Executive, John Connaghan, whose experience (albeit in the West of Scotland) has already imbued a sense of urgency, clarity of thought and action, with a determination to improve the service, which comes as a breath of fresh air to many of us. Hopefully the next generation of managers will continue to be of such highly motivated calibre.

We now stand on the brink of yet another challenge to improve the health and care to our patients. On the basis of past experience, and the inspiration which has been referred to so often in the chapters of this book, the staff of the Western, both present and in the future, will accept this challenge and again amplify their ability to provide leadership and academic prowess in the years to come.

Dr J. B. Scrimgeour
Medical Director

References

1. Maitland's History of Edinburgh, 1753.

2. University of Edinburgh and Poland. Edited by Tomaszewski, W. Edinburgh 1969.

3. 'A Doctor and two Policemen' A History of Edinburgh Health Department. H. P. Tait, 1974.

4. Nicholas Pevsener. Buildings of Scotland.

5. Dialysis-Associated Hepatitis in Edinburgh; 1969–1978 Marmion B. P., Burrell C. J., Tonkin R. W. and Dickson J Reviews of Infectious Diseases, 1982; **4**, No. 3 619–637.

6. Royal Commission on Poor Laws and Relief of Distress. Report. London 1909

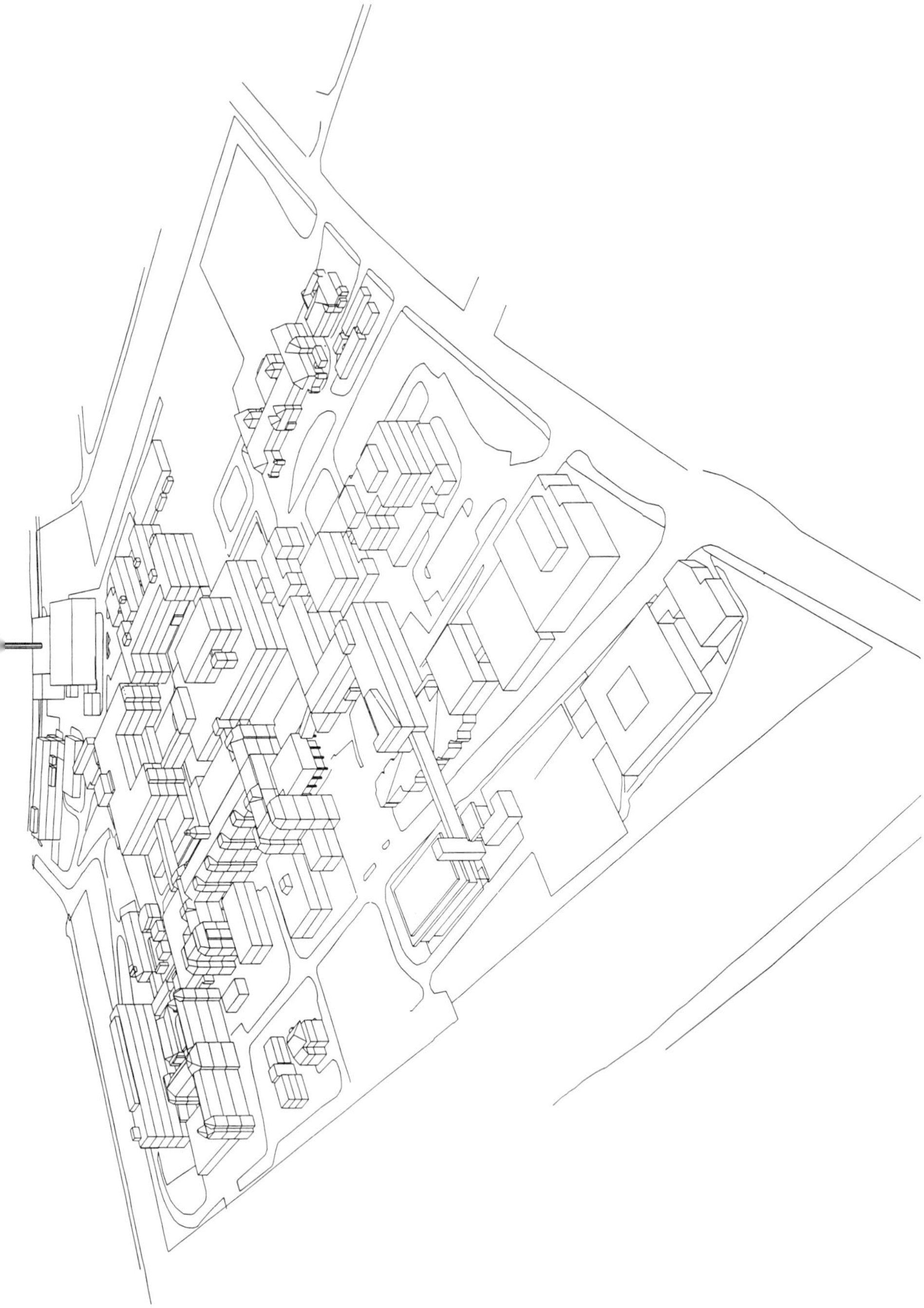

The Future

Western General: Outpatient & Day Cases by Specialty for 1970, 1980 & 1990

Specialty	*Total Attendances*	
	1980	1990
General Surgery	6791	6294
Orthopaedic Surgery	13171	14955
ENT	5532	5804
Ophthalmology	313	179
Urology	4008	4621
Neurosurgery	2347	2617
Dental Surgery	3890	0
General Medicine	13118	7629
Cardiology	0	3339
Metabolic	810	5163
Neurology	0	0
Gastroenterology	3261	4848
Nephrology	752	1846
Chest Medicine	0	0
Radiotherapy	1039	1940
Medical Oncology	0	2200
Surgical Paediatrics	2960	3140
Medical Paediatrics	4418	2723
Pain Control	0	1030
Gynaecology	4266	4425
Obstetrics antenatal	10810	7238
Obstetrics postnatal	812	1186
A & E	30756	50030
Mental Illness	2546	1734
Haematology	2315	3021
Genetics	313	689
Others	811	525
Totals	115039	155306

Western General Hospital — Bed Usage and Inpatient Activity for 1970, 1980 & 1990

Specialty	*Bed Complement*			*Total Number of Inpatients*		
	1970	1980	1990	1970	1980	1990
General Surgery	53	46	84	1532	1356	3130
Orthopaedic Surgery		13	30		637	1454
Urology	28	29	29	887	1434	1518
Neurosurgery	60	60	48	1287	1373	1402
General Medicine	111	98	89	2381	2877	2625
Cardiology		0	0		0	1299
Metabolic		4	4		150	320
Neurology		0	24		0	777
Gastroenterology		32	23		680	866
Nephrology		8	13		193	290
Diagnostic Radiology		0	0		0	2
Radiotherapy		111	111		2257	2333
Medical Oncology		0	12		0	1079
Surgical Paediatrics	25	25	22	958	1058	1026
Medical Paediatrics		25	23		966	929
Anaesthetics		0	0		0	105
Gynaecology	22	23	23	1137	1293	1385
Obstetrics	42	47	47	1601	1629	2150
Special Care Baby Unit		14	14		693	544
Intensive Therapy Unit		0	12		0	1204
Geriatric Assessment	0	0	15	0	0	19
Haematology		0	0		0	261
Staff Ward		5	0		31	0
Others	32	10		541	56	0
Total	373	550	623	10324	16683	24718